MEDICAL LIBRARY, NATHAN CUMMINGS CENTER
MEMORIAL SLOAN-KETTERING CANCER CENTER
1275 YORK AVE., NEW YORK, NY 10021

WITHDRAWN

MEDICAL LIBRARY, NATHAN CUMMINGS CENTER
MEMORIAL SLOAN-KETTERING CANCER CENTER
1275 YORK AVE., NEW YORK, NY 10021

MEDICAL RADIOLOGY

Diagnostic Imaging and Radiation Oncology

Editorial Board

L. W. Brady, Philadelphia · M. W. Donner, Baltimore
H.-P. Heilmann, Hamburg · F. Heuck, Stuttgart

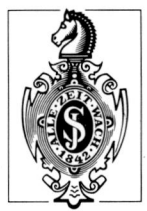

Radiation Therapy of Benign Diseases

A Clinical Guide

Stanley E. Order and Sarah S. Donaldson

Foreword by
Luther W. Brady and Hans-Peter Heilmann

With 103 Tables

Springer-Verlag Berlin Heidelberg New York
London Paris Tokyo Hong Kong

STANLEY E. ORDER, MD, ScD, FACR
Director Radiation Oncology
The Johns Hopkins Hospital
Baltimore, MD 21205, USA

SARAH S. DONALDSON, MD, FACR
Professor of Radiation Oncology
Stanford University
School of Medicine
Stanford, CA 94305, USA

MEDICAL RADIOLOGY · Diagnostic Imaging and Radiation Oncology

Continuation of
Handbuch der medizinischen Radiologie
Encyclopedia of Medical Radiology

ISBN 3-540-50901-1 Springer-Verlag Berlin Heidelberg New York
ISBN 0-387-50901-1 Springer-Verlag New York Berlin Heidelberg

This work is subject to copyright. All rights are reserved, whether the whole or part of the material is concerned, specifically the rights of translation, reprinting, reuse of illustrations, recitation, broadcasting, reproduction on microfilms or in other ways, and storage in data banks. Duplication of this publication or parts thereof is only permitted under the provisions of the German Copyright Law of September 9, 1965, in its version of June 24, 1985, and a copyright fee must always be paid. Violations fall under the prosecution act of the German Copyright Law.

© Springer-Verlag Berlin Heidelberg 1990
Printed in Germany

The use of registered names, trademarks, etc. in this publication does not imply, even in the absence of a specific statement, that such names are exempt from the relevant protective laws and regulations and therefore free for general use.

Product Liability: The publishers can give no guarantee for information about drug dosage and application thereof contained in this book. In every individual case the respective user must check its accuracy by consulting other pharmaceutical literature.

Typesetting, printing and bookbinding: Appl, Wemding
2113/3130-543210 – Printed on acid-free paper

Foreword

The radiation therapist's primary concern is the treatment of patients with malignant disease. However, there are definite indications for radiation treatment for benign diseases that do not respond to conventional methods of treatment. It may be the treatment of choice in the unusual instance of a life-threatening benign disease that cannot be surgically or medically managed.

The present volume by Order and Donaldson represents a major statement on the utilization of radiation techniques in the management of benign disease.

The initial report of the Committee on Radiation Treatment of Benign Disease from the Bureau of Radiological Health recommended that consideration be given to the quality of radiation, the total dose, overall time, underlying organs at risk and shielding factors before the institution of radiation therapy. Infants and children should be treated with ionizing radiation only in very exceptional cases and after careful evaluation of the potential risk compared with the expected benefit. Direct irradiation of the skin areas overlying organs that are particularly prone to late effects such as the thyroid, eye, gonads, bone marrow, and breast should be avoided. Meticulous radiation protection techniques should be used in all instances and the depth of penetration of the x-ray beam should be chosen in accordance with depth of the pathologic process.

The present volume is based on the American literature and the experience of American radiologists and represents a significant and important contribution in this critical and significant area of disease processes. The data indicate that radiation therapy continues to be an important part in the treatment of a large number of benign conditions where the benefits may greatly outweigh the risks which are frequently minimal.

LUTHER W. BRADY Philadelphia	HANS-PETER HEILMANN Hamburg

Contents

Prologue 1
Acknowledgement 2
Standard of Care 3
Preface, Guidelines 7

Abortion 9
Acne 9
Acromegaly with Adenoma 10
Adamantinoma (Ameloblastoma) 10
Aneurysmal Bone Cysts 14
Angiofibroma of the Nasopharynx 18
Ankylosing Spondylitis 20
Anovulation 26
Arteriovenous Malformations 26
Arthritis 28
    Rheumatoid Arthritis 28
    Arthritis Reviews 29
Astrocytoma (Grade I–II) 31

Bowen's Disease 32
Bronchial Adenomas 35
Bursitis, Synovitis and Tendinitis 43

Carcinoid 52
Complications of Treatment in Pituitary Tumors .. 55
Chemodectomas (Non-Chromaffin Paragangliomas) . 55
Chordoma 63
Choroid Plexus Papilloma 65
Craniopharyngioma 66
Cushing's Disease 67
Cystic Hygroma, Lymphangioma 67

Desmoid-Aggressive Fibromatosis 71
Dupuytren's Contracture 74

Epithelial Hemangioendothelioma 76
Erythroplasia of Queyrat 77
Extramammary Paget's Disease 79

Fibrosclerosis 83
Fungal Infections 83

Giant Cell Tumor 84
Gynecomastia (Prostate Cancer Managed with DES) . 88

Hemangioma 89
Herpes Zoster 100

Heterotopic Bone Formation ... 103
Histiocytosis ... 104
Hypersalivation in Amyotrophic Lateral Sclerosis ... 112
Hypersplenism ... 112
Hyperthyroidism ... 116
Hyperthyroid Ophthalmopathy ... 125

Immunosuppression, Lupus Nephritis, Multiple Sclerosis,
    and Organ Transplantation ... 132
Infectious Disorders ... 139
Inflammatory Conditions ... 142
    Arachnoiditis, Tendinitis, Sinusitis, Thyroiditis ... 142
Inverted Papilloma ... 147

Keloid ... 147

Lethal Midline Granuloma ... 153
    Polymorphic Reticulosis/Lymphomatoid Granulomatosis ... 153
Lymphoid Hyperplasia – Pseudotumor ... 156

Meningioma ... 157
Mikulicz Syndrome ... 158
Myasthenia Gravis and Thymus Gland Abnormalities ... 161

Neurofibroma ... 165

Optic Nerve Glioma ... 165
Osteoblastoma/Osteoid Osteoma ... 168
Otitis Media ... 169

Pancreatic Fistulae ... 170
Pancreatitis ... 170
Paraganglioma (Chromaffin Positive) ... 170
Parotitis ... 172
Peptic Ulcer ... 175
Perifolliculitis Capitis Abscedens et Suffodiens ... 179
Peyronie's Disease ... 180
Pinealoma ... 185
Pituitary Adenomas ... 186
Plantar Fibromatosis ... 188
Plasmacytoma (Solitary) ... 189
Pterygium ... 195
Pyogenic Granuloma ... 200

Salivary Gland Adenoma ... 200
Sarcoidosis ... 201
Skin Disorders ... 202

Therapeutic Castration ... 206
Thymus ... 208
Tinea ... 208
Tonsillitis ... 210
Tuberculosis ... 211

Xanthoma ... 212

Subject Index ... 213

Prologue

The purpose of this text is to provide a functional workbook for the radiation oncologist who faces on occasion rare, non-malignant disorders. The scarcity of disease incidence is reflected in the paucity of reference for these diseases in the literature. This minimal exchange of information may make research and analysis difficult, tedious and not easily directed. Through the cooperation of the American College of Radiology 834 radiation oncologists were canvassed in a national survey regarding treatment of these benign disorders. Although benign by nomenclature, benign disorders may have grave consequences, or even be malignant. Further confusion is created by more than a single nomenclature for a given disorder. For example, asked if they would treat polymorphic reticulosis, 86% of the oncologists surveyed were unwilling to treat the disorder. When asked, however, if they would treat lethal midline granuloma, only 17% of these radiation oncologists would not treat the disorder. Polymorphic reticulosis and lethal midline granuloma are the same disorder. In addition to nomenclature problems, decision making is rendered even more complicated for the radiation oncologist by the relative rarity of these benign disorders. Unfamiliarity with sarcoid, for example, leads 92% of radiation oncologists to be unwilling to treat the disorder, while the literature, in fact, indicates that in life-threatening situations, treatment may be appropriate and beneficial.

The text begins with *Standard of Care*, a discussion of guidelines for the treatment of benign disorders, especially when treatment must take into account long-term effects and risk-benefit analysis. The various benign conditions follow this introductory discussion in alphabetical order. Each disease begins with a brief resume which is followed by citations of pertinent literature both in explanatory tables and reference lists. The use of rad and Roentgen is indiscriminately designated in the literature and the reviewers indicate to readers their need to read original scripts if such distinction is necessary. An index is also provided to facilitate reference access. The results of the survey, jointly conducted by The American College of Radiology and the Inter Society Council for Radiation Oncology (ISCRO), are included for each of the disorders as they are reviewed. This book, although utilizing European literature where appropriate, represents *the view of American radiation oncology in regard to the management of benign diseases*, including the medical legal aspects of such therapy.

Many novel applications of radiation will challenge our thoughts in the future. Even as this text goes to press, consideration of early radiotherapy for treatment of paraquat poisoning, for example, has recently been discussed (*Br J Radiology* **61**: 405, 1988). These investigators conclude that controlled trials following identification of the subsets at risk should be conducted to determine the benefit of adding radiotherapy to treatment protocols. The conduct and documentation of controlled trials for benign disorders would help greatly in the radiation oncologist's decision making. A general consensus that radiation of tendinitis, bursitis and synovitis provides benefit, for example, has no substantiation in the literature and randomized trials now indicate no benefit accrues from treatment. We must insist upon controlled trials for the radiation of benign disorders where questions of efficacy arise, as we do for more conventional radiation oncology.

Acknowledgement

We wish to acknowledge the leadership provided by the American College of Radiology through the efforts of Mr. John Curry and James Diamond, Ph.D., as well as the dedicated assistance of Suzanne Bohn, who in conjunction with the Inter Society Council for Radiation Oncology (ISCRO), aided in coordinating and carrying out the extensive mailings, the collection and the preparation of data for the National Survey for the Radiation Therapy of Benign Diseases. Marvin Ellin, an outstanding malpractice lawyer, presents the *Standard of Care* section in lucid terms that should greatly aid those of us practicing radiation oncology. Two residents from Johns Hopkins, Drs. Catherine North and Clinton Leinweber, contributed sections on bronchial adenoma and extramedullary hematopoiesis, respectively. Thanks to Mrs. Laverne Fair and Mrs. Edna Maciejczyk for the continual assistance in the secretarial tasks. Finally, we extend our most sincere appreciation to William L. Clark whose editorial assistance has been invaluable.

Marvin Ellin, LLB

Marvin Ellin was born in Baltimore, Maryland. He attended college at the University of Baltimore and graduated from its Law School in 1953. He was admitted to the Bar the same year. Mr. Ellin is a specialist in medically related trials, and has represented surgeons and physicians who themselves suffered injury through professional negligence. He has written and lectured at law schools, medical associations and hospitals on professional malpractice and the prevention of patient injury. He was one of the first trial lawyers to utilize experts from outside the United States, and has secured expert witness participation from specialists in England, Italy and Canada. He is admitted to practice before the Supreme Court of the United States, the Fourth Circuit Court of Appeals, the Federal District Court of Maryland, and the Court of Appeals of Maryland. He has previously served as an officer of the Bar Association and has frequently participated as a lecturer in the continuing education series featured by the American Bar Association, the City and State Bar. In the chapter that follows, Mr. Ellin shares his opinions regarding the proper application of standards of care in the radiation therapy of benign disorders.

Standard of Care

Malpractice

The appellate courts have defined malpractice as the failure of a practitioner to give and to exercise that degree of care as would be practiced by a reasonably competent practitioner under the same or similar circumstances. Simply stated, the appellate courts have recognized the existence of standards of care followed by competent specialists in the various fields. Thus, malpractice is found where a patient's injury or death occurs as a result of a physician's failure to use diagnostic and/or treatment methods which would be followed by the majority of competent physicians in the same field.

Standard of Care

As applied to the specialty of radiation therapy, a therapist who renders radiation care must conform to the standards which generally prevail in the specialty. Hazen v. Miller F.2d 394 (D.C. Cir., 1929) is an early case that demonstrates the medical profession's establishment of standards of care. The action was brought by a patient who maintained that she suffered severe injury due to radiation overexposure. The appellate court reversed the jury's award to the patient of $15,000 and stated:
It is conceded that Dr. Hazen possessed the requisite degree of skill and ability; that x-ray treatment was the recognized treatment for tubercular glands; it clearly appears that the length of time between exposures of the same area depends upon existing conditions and the judgment of the operator; that telangiectasis may occur even if the highest skill is exercised in the treatment.
Moreover, this decision contained the following statement of law important to the issue of standards of care:
As already observed, there is no evidence upon which it reasonably may be found that Dr. Hazen did not exercise his best judgment and ability in treating the plaintiff, or that in his treatment of the plaintiff he failed to exercise the care and skill ordinarily possessed and exercised by others in the profession.
Although the Defendant was alleged to have deviated from acceptable standards by excessive radiation therapy given at too frequent intervals, the qualifications of the Defendant were not challenged by the Plaintiff. The Court found that the Defendant did conform to the requisite standards of care in the administration of radiation treatment. The Court further noted that the testimony established that even the exercise of the "highest degree of skill and care" may not avoid an adverse reaction by the patient. Thus, the Hazen case set the principle as early as 1929 that, ultimately, the medical profession establishes its own standard of care. The standard is not one able to be determined by a judge or jury, since any court and jury would require the medical expert evaluation of the treatment modality and treatment rendered in order to determine standard of care. The fact that a patient suffers injury raises no implication of negligence in most jurisdictions. Moreover, *res ipsa loquitur,* that is to say, "the injury speaks for itself," which would establish a suggestion of negligence, has been rejected, unless unusual circumstances occurred.

Negligence by Technical Error

Through error while applying 800 rad of electron beam therapy to a patient, a technician adjusted the machine to 80,000 rad. The patient manifested burns of such intensity that under those circumstances it could not be said that the patient had an adverse reaction or an idiosyncratic response to the treatment rendered. It would follow that, absent the admission that the therapy had exceeded its intended dosage by 100 times, the extent and nature of the injury in such an extreme case would indicate negligence.

Individual Standards for the Specific Patient

Although the specialist must adhere to the standards of radiation therapy that prevail across the country, he is not deprived of utilizing his own particular technique. Indeed, freedom in the exercise of treatment may be pursued so long as the specialist's approach does not violate the safeguards and the advances developed in the specialty and utilized by colleagues under the same or similar circumstances.

Negligence in Medical Judgment

Carver v. The United States of America, 587 F. Supp. 794 (N.D., Cal. 1984) provides an example of a medical malpractice action brought under the Federal Tort Claims Act. The action alleged that physicians at a U.S. Army Medical Center had negligently subjected patient Carver to radiotherapy, thereby causing brain tissue damage. The history of the case is as follows:

On April 1, 1979, the 56 year old patient was admitted to Letterman Army Medical Center with complaints of staggering gait, clumsiness, left handed weakness, slurred speech and personality change. After one inconclusive CT scan, the patient was sent to the University of California Medical Center for a second CT scan performed by a prominent neuroradiologist. The CT scan was reported to indicate that the most likely diagnosis was multiple metastatic neoplasm.

Subsequently, an extensive work-up that included liver and spleen scan, lung tomograms, an IVP, sigmoidoscopy, bronchoscopy and a bone scan, failed to reveal the primary site of the cancer. Consultations were also obtained with cardiology, hematology-oncology, nuclear medicine, radiotherapy, neurosurgery, pathology, proctology, as well as the diabetic and immunization clinics. During this period of search for the primary site, April 3 through April 23, the patient's condition steadily declined. He had attacks of nausea and dizziness that were accompanied by ECG changes. He developed diplopia which continued for three days and necessitated the use of Decadron. On April 11, the patient developed hiccups and the dose of Decadron was increased. The patient eventually received Thorazine in an attempt to control his hiccups.

From April 16 to 18, the patient continued to decline. He was considered for palliative radiotherapy; a radiotherapy consultation was requested. The radiotherapist, noting that the extensive search for the primary site had been without success, recommended a biopsy of one of the lesions, if possible. The radiotherapist noted that he would proceed with radiotherapy of 3600 rad over a period of two and one-half weeks, if the biopsy were not able to be performed. Steroids continued to be administered to control the worsening symptoms. Some evidence of improvement was noted. On April 19, a neurosurgery consultation was obtained to evaluate the patient for a brain biopsy prior to radiotherapy. The neurosurgeon recommended that radiation therapy and chemotherapy proceed without a brain biopsy:

I do not feel that the risk of biopsy is indicated in this patient in that there is no chance for surgical cure and bilateral multiple lesions are likely metastasizing, though primary RCS [reticulum cell sarcoma] of the brain is a reasonable differential. Multiple abscesses would likely be very positive on brain scan, as well as show surrounding inflammatory edema and shift.

Prior to radiotherapy a third CT scan was performed on April 24. That scan was interpreted to show progression of the metastases observed on the prior scan. Radiotherapy was begun the same day. By April 26 the patient had improved. Radiation was completed on May 9 and another CT scan that date showed improvement. The patient was discharged on May 12, 1979.

Following his discharge the patient lived at home. He gradually grew weaker. In late 1979 and early 1980 he was again admitted to Letterman Army Medical Center. In 1980 he was diagnosed as possibly having multiple sclerosis. His physical and mental condition continued to deteriorate and he was eventually placed in a convalescent home.

The United States District Court of Appeals for the Northern District of California held that the Plaintiff failed to sustain the burden of proof by a preponderance of the evidence that the physicians failed to conform to the standard of care in prescribing and administering radiotherapy. As this was a Federal Tort Claims case, the physicians individually were not Defendants in the suit. The Plaintiff in Federal Tort Claims cases is limited to a court trial by judge without a jury.

The Appeals Court held that the physicians exercised judgment involving a serious disease process. Further, when weighing the possible benefits against the possible risks, the suit amounted to nothing more than an *ex post facto* attack on the exercise of medical judgment. The case was dismissed.

Informed Consent

The explanation and information for informed consent must be stated in clear, unambiguous language understandable to a lay patient. To presume a patient's knowledge of the subject matter would possibly deprive the individual of the right to have this information reduced to lay comprehension, and could contribute to his confusion regarding his disease and its possible treatment.

The radiologist's task to explain complicated aspects of radiotherapy such as dosimetry is a difficult one. The radiologist would be doing himself and the patient a favor by reducing verbal explanations to written form, and then making this explanation part of the patient's record. This would avoid the possibility of later contention of patient misunderstanding or claims that language used to gain consent was not simple enough to allow truly informed consent to radiation therapy. Informed consent consists of the following: the patient is given a full explanation of the disease from which he or she suffers, the necessity for the radiation treatment, the approximate number of treatments to be rendered, the probable length of each treatment and the risks, side effects and/or possible idiosyncratic reaction(s) likely to occur from such treatment.

The obligation of the physician to inform the patient of the possible risk of treatment does not require inclusion of risks which are regarded as slight. Nor does the informed consent require the radiation therapist to cover every conceivable aspect of risk attendant to treatment. The probable risks are those which the law requires for patient notification, not every possible, though improbable, risk that might exist.

Informed Consent and Standard of Care

The North Carolina court in 1985 stated in the case of Nelson v. Patrick 326 se 2d 45, (N.C. App., 1985) that:

The court properly instructed that one of the things Plaintiff had to prove in order to prevail was that Defendant Patrick did not obtain Plaintiff's informed consent to the treatment.

And:

In order to prove . . . that the Defendant did not obtain the Plaintiff's informed consent, the Plaintiff must prove that the Defendant failed to provide information to the Plaintiff which would, under the same or similar circumstances, have given a reasonable person a general understanding of the procedures and treatments to be used and the usual and most frequent risks and hazards inherent in the treatments as recognized by other therapeutic radiologists in the same or similar communities.

The decision involves a standard of care based on the so-called locality or similar community rule. The locality rule exists in very few states today, as a national standard of care is recognized to prevail across the country. This national standard of care is established by widespread dissemination of radiation therapy knowledge through routine publication of ongoing improvements and discoveries in the field, by presentation of clinical and laboratory data at national meetings, and by the activity of the National Institutes of Health which serves as a national forum for identifying needs and supporting advancements in the science. In the treatment of benign disease, however, this becomes more restrictive. The national survey by the American College of Radiology and the enclosed reviews have been written so that, taken in conjunction with new treatment, an accurate estimate of standard of care may be established by the radiation oncologist.

The all purpose, standard hospital informed consent sheet with blanks for the names of the physician and the patient may not best serve the needs of the radiation oncologist. A separate, individual memorandum signed by the patient should be made part of the patient's record. This document, simply dictated by the radiologist or the resident assisting with the patient present, would explain the disease being treated, the purpose of the radiation to be rendered, and the possible side effects that might result from the treatment. Such individually directed and specially dictated acknowledgement would prove of great use in the event of future litigation.

Radiation Therapy Informed Consent Check List

The written consent form should be stated in simple, lay terminology.

1. Inform the patient about the benign disease or tumor and the region of the body to be irradiated. Make certain that the patient understands the other options of treatment and the desired benefit of the radiation to be given. Do not assume that the patient has any prior understanding of the medical and/or surgical history of the disease or the reason for referral to the radiation therapist.
2. Explain the desired goal of the planned radiation.

3. Explain the number of treatments contemplated.
4. Describe the dose to be administered and the probable effect on the tumor as well as the general reaction to this treatment by the patient (i.e., nausea, diarrhea, hair loss, etc.).
5. Try to arrange a meeting with patient and spouse or patient and parent so that Informed Consent is understood by close family members.
6. Provide the opportunity for the patient to pose questions regarding the treatment to be given and the goals of such treatment. **Specifically ask: Do you have any questions?**
7. If the patient manifests uncertainty or confusion, strongly recommend a second opinion **prior** to starting treatment.
8. Send a letter after meeting with the patient to the referring physician, sending a copy to patients as well. Legal counsel recommends outlining the treatment contemplated.
9. If the patient has past or present psychiatric history, obtain the patient's permission to send a copy of the letter to the referring physician and to the patient's psychiatrist as well.
10. Have a nurse, secretary, or witness present while the explanation of the Informed Consent is obtained, and have that person witness the consent form.

Preface

The authors would like radiation oncologists to realize that this text represents both a survey of the practices of our nation in the radiation therapy of benign disorders as well as a compendium of the literature. The final risk/benefit ratio for the treatment of any patient should be dependent on the *"Guidelines of Treatment."*

Guidelines

1. Determine the consequence of no treatment and the natural history of the benign disease.
2. Use this text and other source material for reference to possible alternate methods of treatment and to determine the risk/benefit ratio regarding radiation treatment and other therapies.
3. Consider radiation treatment if conventional methods of treatment have not succeeded in alleviating the condition. If the risk of other therapies is greater than the risk of radiation therapy, and the potential consequences of no further treatment are unacceptable, then radiation treatment may be considered.
4. Determine the potential long-term risk of radiation treatment; consider the quality of radiation, total dose, time over which radiation is administered, the underlying organs at risk, and any underlying disease.
5. If radiation is being considered as the treatment modality, inform the patient or guardian of the potential hazardous risks.

It is our hope that this text, an alphabetically arranged compendium, will prove to be a useful, convenient resource in evaluating treatment policy.

Abortion

Although radiation has been known to cause abortion, we cannot find any justifiable reason for its use to induce abortion. In our survey, ninety-six percent of radiation oncologists would not carry out abortion with radiation.

Acne

Historically acne, particularly the more severe forms that effect deep papular structures, has responded to fractionated orthovoltage radiation. This potential benefit must be weighed against the risk of thyroid cancer, specifically, and other unknown risks for young patients. Considering the risk/benefit ratio and modern antibiotics, dietary regulation, and facial care, we have concluded that acne should not be treated with radiation. The informed physician, however, who wishes to accept a high risk, must indicate in the "informed consent" to the patient and/or patients what the risks are. Even then, the physician may find that an altered interpretation by a patient and/or family may introduce litigation. Justification of "it works" does not indicate the late risk of what we consider inappropriate treatment. The psychological distress of the teenager could be supplanted by the psychologic depression of a young adult, who now realizes that thyroid abnormalities have become a source of anxiety in his or her life. Thyroid abnormalities are 2-3% with a range in years of risk from 9 to more than 40 years and a proven 0.66% risk of thyroid cancer. These risks may be amplified by radiation technique and age at treatment, and may be larger based on these variables. Pertinent literature is cited for such a review (1,3). In recent times only the dermatologist has been willing to carry out such treatments. The challenge in such management is objective demonstration of degree of psychological distress, thorough knowledge of best radiation technique and "fully informed consent."

Finally, it must be mentioned that salivary gland abnormalities and tumors, as well as the breast, should be analyzed in reference to acne treatment as proper data are not available. It also needs to be mentioned that best care in follow up examination of such previously treated patients includes thyroid palpation and scan with technetium^{99} if a nodule has been felt upon examination.

The most careful review of radiation techniques and possible thyroid risk is that of Goldschmidt for those who feel impelled to such treatments, and who accept questionable threshold doses and other extrapolations of data for risk versus treatment of this benign disorder. Of the radiation oncologists surveyed nationally, 96% would not treat acne.

References

1. Thomson DB, Grammes CF, Starkey RH, Monsarert RP, Sunderlin FS (1984) Thyroid abnormalities in patients previously treated with irradiation for acne vulgaris. Arch Dermatol South Med J 77: 21-23.
2. Goldschmidt H, Gorson RO, Lassen M (1983) Dermatologic radiotherapy and thyroid cancer. Arch Dermatol 119: 383-390.
3. Paloyan E, Lawrence AM (1978) Thyroid neoplasms after radiation therapy for adolescent acne vulgaris. Arch Dermatol 114: 53-55.
4. Albright EC, Allday RW (1967) Thyroid carcinoma after radiation. JAMA 199: 280-281.

Acromegaly with Adenoma

Eight hormones may be associated with benign pituitary tumors, including growth hormones and corticotropin hormones, the former being associated with acromegaly. Acromegaly requires treatment, being potentially fatal. Bromocriptidine has played a role in the management of hormonal problems associated with these tumors and radiation techniques are similar to chromophobe adenoma. Dose response relationships have been reported, a growth hormone reduction following surgery and radiation therapy of 73% of GH less than 10mg/ml being an expected response rate. Standard texts and references should be reviewed.

References

1. Sheline GE and Tyroll JB (1983) Pituitary adenomas. In: Phyllips TL and Pistenmaa DA (eds) **Radiation Oncology Annual**, Raven Press:New York, pp 1-35.
2. Eastman RC, Gorden P and Roth J (1979) Conventional supravoltage irradiation is an effective treatment for acromegaly. *J Clin Endocrino Metab* **48**: 931.
3. Pistenmaa DA, Goffinet DR and Bagshaw MA (1976) Treatment of acromegaly with megavoltage radiation therapy. *Int J Rad Oncol Biol Phys* **1**: 885.
4. Sheline GE, Goldberg MB and Feldman R (1961) Pituitary irradiation for acromegaly. *Radiology* **76**: 70-82.

Adamantinoma (Ameloblastoma)

This rare tumor which is often treated with limited surgery and radiation seems to offer the probability of local control following surgery. Scientific data are not available for an in-depth evaluation. In the national survey fifty-seven percent of radiation oncologists will not treat this disorder.

Adamantinoma (Ameloblastoma)

Author, Year	Total # Patients	Treatment	Results	Notes
Chaudhuri, 1975	1	Local excision. Recurrence treated with partial excision of the maxilla.	Recurrences three years later at a margin of original excision.	All were cases of ameloblastoma of the maxilla.
	1	Excision followed by radiotherapy, 6000r/21 days.	No recurrence.	
	1	Radiotherapy, 4500r/20 days.	Almost complete resolution six months after treatment.	
Gall et al, 1975	1	Segmental resection of the body of the mandible. The margins of the resected mandible were free of tumor.	Patient was well until four years later when pulmonary metastases were discovered. Patient was placed on chemotherapy but there was no measurable tumor regression.	Ameloblastoma of the mandible. Author provides a review of eleven cases in the literature of ameloblastoma with metastasis.
Hartman, 1974	15	1. Enucleation (4). 2. Curettage (4). 3. En bloc excision (3). 4. Partial resection (2). 5. External irradiation (2).	1. 4/4. 2. 4/4. 3. 1/3. 4. 0/2. 5. 2/2.	All were cases of granular cell ameloblastoma of the mandible.
Huffman, 1974	4	Curettage via an intraoral approach followed by either electrocauterization of the tumor bed or removal of surrounding bone with a large burr.	Follow up of 15 months - 15.5 years. No recurrences.	All were cases of ameloblastoma of the mandible.

Adamantinoma (Ameloblastoma) (Continued)

Author, Year	Total # Patients	Treatment	Results	Notes
Keaton, 1974	1	Marginal resection.	Some bone apposition at surgical site at six month follow up.	Both were cases of ameloblastoma of the mandible.
	1	Partial mandibulectomy. Patient free of disease at 10 month follow up.		
Sehder et al, 1974	92	Lesions of the mandible (72): 1. External radiotherapy (9). 2. Curettage (32). 3. Resection (31). Lesions of the maxilla (20): 4. External radiotherapy (2). 5. Curettage (11). 6. Resection (7).	Recurrences (following initial treatment) mandibular lesions: 1. 9/9(100%). 2. 29/32(90%). 3. 5/31(22%) Maxillary lesions: 4. 2/2(100%). 5. 11/11(100%), seven of these are dead or alive with massive local recurrences. 6. 0/5, one died of pneumonia, one lost to follow up.	Authors conclude that it may not be disastrous to try curettage initially in ameloblastoma involving the mandible, it should be vehemently condemned for ameloblastoma of the maxilla where a prompt adequate resection should be carried out. Mandibular resection may control the recurrence after currettage in most patients, but maxillary resection for recurrence is usually ineffective or impossible.
Seymour et al, 1974	1	Curettage.	No complications and healing satisfactory at two years post-op.	Adenoameloblastoma. This is a histologic variant of ameloblastoma. The author provides a review of reported cases of this neoplasm and recommends a conservative surgical approach as the treatment of choice.
Shaw and Katsikas, 1973	1	Second recurrence following surgical excision was treated with radiotherapy, 6000r total dose, Co^{60}.	Patient was free of disease nine years later.	All were cases of ameloblastoma of the maxilla.
	1	Radiotherapy, 5048r/36 days, Co^{60}.	Good local improvement. Patient died 1.5 months later of unknown but probably unrelated causes.	
	1	Radiotherapy, 6250r total tumor dose, Co^{60}. This was followed by surgical excision of residual tumor. Recurrence treated surgically.	Fair response to radiotherapy, but still some slight swelling. Recurrence 7.5 years later. This was treated by surgical excision. No further recurrence at 15 month follow up.	
	1	Total left maxillectomy.	No recurrence at five year follow up.	

Adamantinoma (Ameloblastoma) (Continued)

Author, Year	Total # Patients	Treatment	Results	Notes
Melisch et al, 1972	126	Primary treatment (36): 1. Cautery only (10). 2. Curettage plus cautery in some cases (8). 3. Excision plus cautery in some cases (6). 4. Resection and cautery (1). 5. Resection en bloc (2). 6. Segmental resection. Secondary treatment (90): 1. Cautery only (25). 2. Curettage plus excision in some cases (20). 3. Excision plus cautery in some cases (13). 4. Resection and cautery (8). 5. Resection en bloc. 6. Segmental resection.	Recurrences: 1. 5/10. 2. 5/8. 3. 2/6. 4. 0/1. 5. 0/2. 6. 2/6. Subsequent recurrences: 1. 15/20(75%) (5 died of tumor). 2. 18/20(90%). 3. 10/13(77%). 4. 1/8. 5. 0/1. 6. 0/8.	All were cases of ameloblastoma of the mandible or maxilla.
Pandya and Stuteville, 1972	74	Primary cases: Mandibular lesions (40): 1. Enucleation with cauterization (4). 2. Intra-oral local excision (5). 3. Primary oral resections and bone grafts (30). 4. Palliative resection (1). Maxillary lesions (10): 5. Maxillectomy Radiation was used as an adjunct to surgery in three patients, all of whom responded to the radiotherapy. Secondary cases (23): 6. Wide extra-oral segmental resection plus bone graft.	Recurrences: 1. 1/4(25%). 2. 1/5(20%) 5/39(12.8%) 3. 3/30(10%). 4. 1/1. 5. 0/10. 6. 2/23(9%)	Authors state that radiation alone does not significantly affect this tumor but it may have a place in conjunction with surgery in the management of selected cases.
Zand et al, 1972	1	Radiotherapy: 6200r/42 days, Co^{60}.	At 2.5 years follow up x-rays showed the lesion to be healed with no evidence of recurrence. No recurrence at nine years. At 8.5 years right humerus was 2 inches shorter than the left humerus.	Adamantinoma of the humerus in a seven year old boy.
Sugimura et al, 1969		Mandibular ostectomy followed by chemotherapy (cyclosphophamide) and radiotherapy, 3900r/15 days.	Patient lost to follow up until three years later. At that time metastases to the lumbar vertebra were noted. Initially these responded to Co^{60} radiotherapy. Patient died seven years after onset of primary lesion.	Malignant ameloblastoma of the mandible.
Hoffman et al, 1968	38	1. Local removal. 2. Wide resection as primary treatment. 3. Wide resection following recurrences.	Recurrences: 1. 23/24(96%). 2. 0/2. 3. 6/14.	All were cases of ameloblastoma of the mandible (37). Maxilla (1).
Taylor, 1968	25	1. Curettage (10). 2. Wide resection (13).	1. 5/8(63%) recurred. 2. 1/9(11%) recurred.	All were cases of ameloblastoma of the mandible.

Adamantinoma (Ameloblastoma) (Continued)

Author, Year	Total # Patients	Treatment	Results	Notes
Ward and Brandeburg, 1968	3	Surgical excision (maxillectomy, or hemimandibulectomy).	Follow up of six months – twenty-one years. 0/3 recurrences.	Maxillary lesion (2). Mandibular lesion (1).
Moon, 1965	61	1. Irradiation only (1). 2. Local excision with or without graft (24). 3. Amputation (36).	1. 1/1 recurred. 2. 2 recurrences: 19 well, 0–10 years. 5 died, 0–10 years. 3. 1 recurrence: 25 well, 0–10 years. 11 died, 0–10 years.	All were cases of adamantinoma of the appendicular skeleton. Review of reported cases of adamantinoma of the appendicular skeleton plus ten new cases reported by the author.
Shatkin and Hoffmeister, 1965	22	Primary cases: 1. Curettage (13). 2. Radiotherapy (2). 3. En bloc excision (7).	Recurrences: 1. 11/13(86%). Four later died of tumor. 2. 2/2(100%). One later died of tumor. 3. 1/7(14%).	All were cases of ameloblastoma of the mandible or maxilla, the mandible being the more common site.
Goldwyn et al, 1963	32	Primary cases: 1. Local excision (14). 2. Wide resection (3). 3. Palliative irradiation. 4. Local excision plus irradiation (1). Secondary cases: 5. Local excision (4). 6. Wide resection (9). 7. Palliative irradiation (1).	1. 8/13 recurred (two died from disease). One patient lost to follow up. 2. 0/3 recurred. 3. 1/1 recurred and died from disease. 4. 1/1 recurred and died from disease. 5. 4/4 recurred. 6. 0/7 recurred. Two patients lost to follow up. 7. 1/1 recurred and died from disease.	Ameloblastoma of the mandible (27). Ameloblastoma of the maxilla (3).
Hair, 1963	1	Radiotherapy, 3750r/45 days.	External swelling gradually diminished. X-rays showed recalcification.	Ameloblastoma of the maxilla.
Smith, 1960	30	Surgical excision.	4/30(13%) recurred.	Location of lesion: Mandible (24). Maxilla (3). Palate (2). Cheek (1).
Small and Waldron, 1955		1. Local excision or curettage, including chemical cautery or irradiation in some cases. 2. Irradiation alone (18).	Recurrences: 1. 89/193(46%). 2. 13/18(72%).	Statistical survey of the literature. Only cases of ameloblastoma of the maxilla and mandible were included.

References

1. Chandhuri P (1975) Ameloblastoma of the upper jaw. *J Laryngol & Otol* **89**: 457–465.
2. Gall JA, Sortiano GP and Shreiner DP (1975) Ameloblastoma of the mandible with pulmonary metastasis. *Oncology* **32**: 118–126.
3. Hartman KS (1974) Granular cell ameloblastoma. *Oral Surg Oral Med & Oral Path* **38**: 241–253.
4. Huffman GG and Thatcher JW (1974) Ameloblastoma – the conservative surgical approach to treatment: Report of four cases. *J Oral Surg* **32**: 850–854.
5. Keaton WM, Kolodny SC, Roche WC and Koutnik AW (1974) Ameloblastoma: Report of two cases. *J Oral Surg* **32**: 382–385.
6. Sehdev MK, Huvos AG, Strong EW, Gerald FP & Willis GW (1974) Ameloblastoma of maxilla and mandible. *Cancer* **33**: 324–333.
7. Seymour RL, Funke FW and Irby WB (1974) Adenoameloblastoma. Report of a case and review of the literature. *Oral Surg Oral Med & Oral Path* **38**: 860–865.
8. Shaw HJ and Katsikas DK (1973) Ameloblastoma of the maxilla. A clinical study with four cases. *J Laryngol & Otol* **87**: 873–884.

9. Mehlisch DR, Dahlin DC and Masson JK (1972) Ameloblastoma: A clinicopathalogic report. *J Oral Surg* **30**: 9–22.
10. Pandya NJ and Stuteville OH (1972) Treatment of ameloblastoma. *Plast & Reconstr Surg* **50**: 242–248.
11. Zand A, Chambers GH and Street DM (1972) So-called: Adamantinoma of long bone. *Clin Orth* **86**: 178–182.
12. Sugimura M, Yamauchi T, Yashikawa K, Sakita M and Miyazaki T (1969) Malignant ameloblastoma with metastasis to the lumbar vertebra: Report of a case. *J Oral Surg* **27**: 350–357.
13. Hoffman PJ, Baden E, Rankow RM and Potter GD (1968) The fate of the uncontrolled ameloblastoma. *Oral Surg Oral Med & Oral Path* **26**: 419–426.
14. Taylor BG (1968) Ameloblastoma of the mandible: A clinical study of 25 patients. *Am Surg* **34**: 57–62.
15. Ward RH and Brandenburg JH (1968) Ameloblastoma - a report of three cases. *Laryngoscope* **78**: 2025–2032.
16. Pennis VR, Young A, Anlyan J and Grisez JL (1966) Ameloblastoma with long standing pulmonary metastases. *Plast & Reconstr Surg* **38**: 534–540.
17. Moon NF (1965) Adamantinoma of the appendicular skeleton. A statistical review of reported cases and inclusion of 10 new cases. *Clin Orth* **43**: 189–213.
18. Shatkin S and Hoffmeister FS (1965) Ameloblastoma: A rational approach to therapy. *Oral Surg Oral Med & Oral Path* **20**: 421–435.
19. Goldwyn R, Constable J and Murray J (1963) Ameloblastoma of the jaw. A clinical study. *New Eng J Med* **269**: 126–129.
20. Hair JA (1963) Radiosensitive adamantinoma. *Br Med J* **1**: 105–106.
21. Smith JF (1960) Ameloblastoma. Report of thirty cases. *Oral Surg Oral Med & Oral Path* **13**: 1253–1257.
22. Small IA and Waldron CA (1955) Ameloblastoma of the jaws. *Oral Surg Oral Med & Oral Path* **8**: 281–297.

Aneurysmal Bone Cysts

This benign disorder may be aided in local control when surgery cannot be executed or complete. Fifty-one percent of radiation oncologists would treat this disorder according to the national survey.

Aneurysmal Bone Cysts

Author, Year	Total # Patients	Treatment	Results	Notes
Marks et al, 1976	3	Radiotherapy: 4000r (midline dose)/18–20F/ 3.5 weeks. Megavoltage irradiation was used.	Recalcification with no evidence of recurrence in all three patients at follow ups of 2–7 years.	Age range of the patients was 11–16 years. All three lesions were in the pelvis.
Delorit and Summers, 1975	1	Radiotherapy: 3800r (tumor dose) followed by surgical removal.	Objective improvement of the XI and XII nerve palsies but no changes were evident on the cerebral arteriogram. It was then decided to surgically remove the tumor. Six month follow up showed almost complete resolution of the cranial nerve palsies.	Lesion of the sphenoid sinus. The patient presented with bilateral VIth, IXth, Xth, XIth and XIIth palsies. Patient was 23 years of age.
Habermann et al, 1974	1	Curettage followed by radiotherapy, 1000r in divided doses using a Co^{60} source followed four weeks later by a second course of 1000r.	Increased size of the lesion was demonstrated one month after surgery. There was a slight decrease in the size of the lesion following the first course of radiotherapy but symptoms and clinical findings were unchanged. Following the second course of radiotherapy the patient had improved range of motion and no pain. Ten months later the cyst cavity had ossified and the patient had full range of motion of both hips without pain.	Lesion of the ischium. Age of patient was seven years.

Aneurysmal Bone Cysts (Continued)

Author, Year	Total # Patients	Treatment	Results	Notes
Clough and Price, 1973	21	1. Curettage (19 patients, 16 also had a graft). 2. Resection (5 patients). 3. Radiotherapy plus curettage (2). 4. Radiotherapy (2).	Recurrences (includes treatment of both initial and recurrent lesions): 1. 11/19 2. 0/5 3. 0/2 4. 0/2	Minimum follow up of two years.
Prakash et al, 1973	4	Surgical removal followed by a course of radiotherapy 800–2000r.	3/4 moderately quick recovery of spinal cord function which was maintained at follow ups of 1.5–7 years. One case was quadriplegic at presentation and showed only partial neurological recovery.	All four were aneurysmal bone cysts of the spine. Age range: 17–48 years.
Biesecker et al, 1970	44	Primary treatment: 1. Curettage (44). 2. Radiotherapy, 1200–3200r (tumor dose) (4). 3. Cryosurgery. 4. Block excision. 5. Amputation.	Recurrences: 1. 26/44 (60%) 2. 1/4 3. 1/7 4. 0/8 5. 0/1	Fifty-nine percent of the lesions were of long bones. Data based on total treatment (including recurrences) showed a significant difference in the recurrence rate between radiation therapy and curettage and between cryosurgery and curettage. There was no significant difference between radiation therapy and cryosurgery.
Stevens and Weaver, 1970	1	Excision and spinal fusion.	Good recovery.	Lesion of the spine. Patient was eleven years of age.
	1	Excision followed one month later by radiotherapy, 2000r.	Patient free of pain and no complaints at three month follow up.	Lesion of the spine. Patient was eighteen years of age.
Dabska and Buraczewski, 1969	13	1. Surgical excision (radical or partial). (4) 2. Excision or curettage plus radiotherapy (3500–5000r). (4) 3. Radiotherapy alone (2500–4428r). (4)	1. Condition satisfactory at 1–7 year follow up. 2. Condition satisfactory at 1–3 year follow up. 3. Condition satisfactory at 4–10 year follow up in three patients. Malignant change requiring amputation in one fourth patient.	Age range: 14–44 years.
Nobler et al, 1968	33	1. Surgery initially (26). 2. Surgery for recurrence (5). 3. Irradiation initially (6). 4. Irradiation for recurrence (5). 5. Irradiation plus surgery (1). Details of radiotherapy: 1200–3160r (tumor dose)/9–18 days with 250 Kv, 100 Kv or Co^{60}.	Recurrences: 1. 8/26 (31%) 10/31 (32%) 2. 2/5 (40%) 3. 1/6 (16%) 4. 0/5 1/12 (8%) 5. 0/1	20/33 (61%) were 19 years of age or younger. Sixty percent of the lesions were in the pelvis and lower extremities.
Slowick et al, 1968	13	1. Resection (4). 2. Curettage plus bone grafts (5). 3. Radiotherapy, 1400–2000r (tumor dose) (4). All had lesions of the spine.	Recurrences: 1. 0/4 2. 1/5 3. 0/4	12/13 were twenty years of age or younger.

Aneurysmal Bone Cysts (Continued)

Author, Year	Total # Patients	Treatment	Results	Notes
Tillman et al, 1968	15	1. Curettage alone or in combination with cautery and/or graft (34). Six patients also received radiotherapy. 2. Resection and graft (11). 3. Excision (9) plus radiotherapy (6). 4. Amputation plus radiotherapy (1). 5. Radiotherapy (1).	Recurrences: 1. 0/6 with radiotherapy. 8/28 without radiotherapy. 2. 0/11 3. 1/6 with radiotherapy. 2/9 without radiotherapy. 4. 0/1 5. 1/1 Overall results: 2/14 recurred with radiotherapy. 11/48 recurred without radiotherapy.	All were cases of aneurysmal bone cyst. Sarcoma developed in 3/95. Irradiation had been used in all three cases. Authors suggest reservation of radiotherapy only for cases in which surgical removal is not feasible.
Garnjobst and Hopkins, 1967	1	Radiotherapy: 2470r (tumor dose) followed by excision and curettement two years later.	At presentation the tumor was massive and highly vascular. Following irradiation the growth of the tumor ceased and calcification increased. Following surgery the cavity in the pubis and ischium healed. There was no recurrence at eight year follow up.	Lesion of the left superior pubic ramus. Patient was seventeen years of age. The irradiation was not curative, but it may have reduced the vascularity of the tumor, making the surgical approach less hazardous.
Parrish and Pevey, 1967	3	Excision followed by radiotherapy. Tumor dose: 1500r/10F/12 days or 3000-3800r/20-25F/4-5 weeks.	2/3 cysts healed and there was no evidence of recurrence at two year follow up. In one patient the cyst recurred and was excised twice. There was filling in the sacral mass and no recurrence six months following the last excision.	All were lesions of the vertebral column. Age range of 13-30 years.
Verbiest, 1965	2	Surgery alone (1) or radiotherapy followed one year later by surgery (1) but doubt as to the exact diagnosis.	Recovery from neurological disturbances in both patients. No evidence of recurrence at six years and 21 year follow up.	Both cases were lesions of the spine. Ages 15 and 44 years.
Donaldson, 1962	6	1. Excision followed by radiotherapy 1150-2250r (tumor dose) post-op (2). 2. Excision or curettage and packing (4).	1. No evidence of recurrence at three year and six year follow up. 2. 3/4 no recurrence at 3-7 year follow ups. Recurrence in one patient following curettage and packing treating by excision. No recurrence at four year follow up.	Age range 2-19 years.
MacCarthy et al, 1961	11	1. Excision or curettement (4). 2. Excision or curettage followed by radiotherapy (6). 3. Radiotherapy followed two months later by surgical removal (1).	1. No recurrences at three month - eight year follow up. 2. 5/6 patients well at 3-18 year follow up. 3. Healing at site of graft, but extension into lamina and spinous process. Lesion was again removed. Patient well at three year follow up.	All were lesions of the spine, sacrum or occipital bone. Age range 10-25 years.

Aneurysmal Bone Cysts (Continued)

Author, Year	Total # Patients	Treatment	Results	Notes
Godfrey and Gresham, 1959	5	1. Excision (4). 2. Curettage and grafting followed by radiotherapy (1500r tumor dose) (1).	1. Recovery in all four patients. 2. Gradual recalcification and no further extension of the cyst at one year follow up.	Age range 3-43 years.
Beeler et al, 1957	7	1. Radiotherapy only (2). 2. Radiotherapy plus surgery (5). In both groups radiotherapy was usually 1200-1600r in air/2 weeks. Two courses two months apart were given.	1. Complete recovery in one case. Satisfactory recovery with some residual deformity in the other case. 2. 4/5 complete recovery. 1/5 satisfactory recovery (less than complete regression at 2 year follow up).	Age range 13-28 years.
Barnes, 1956	5	Excision or curettage.	5/5 good recovery.	Age range 8-20 years.
Cruz and Coley, 1956	20	1. Surgery alone (13). 2. Radiotherapy alone (5). One received radium treatment. 3. Surgery plus radiotherapy (2). Radiotherapy: 500-2320r total air dose.	Follow up of four months - 32 years. 1. 13/13 cured. 2. 5/5 cured. 3. 2/2 cured.	Age range 9-44 years.
Taylor, 1956	3	1. Surgery alone (1). 2. Biopsy and partial removal followed by radiotherapy (1). 3. Radiotherapy alone (1).	1. Patient free from symptoms and no recurrence at one year follow up. 2. Patient free from symptoms and no recurrence at three year follow up. 3. Patient free from symptoms and no recurrence at nine year follow up.	Age range 4-16 years.

References

1. Marks RD, Scrugg HJ, Wallace KM and Fenn JD (1976) Megavoltage therapy in patients with aneurysmal bone cysts. *Radiology* 118: 421-424.
2. Delorit GJ and Summer GW (1975) Aneurysmal bone cyst of the spenoid sinus. *Trans Am Acad Opth & Otol* 80: 438-443.
3. Haberman ET, Cabot W and Smith HS (1974) Aneurysmal bone cyst of the pelvis. An unusual case presentation. *Bull Hosp Joint Dis* 35: 151-157.
4. Clough JR and Price CHG (1973) Aneurysmal bone cyst: Pathogenesis and long term results of treatment. *Clin Orth* 97: 52-63.
5. Prakash B, Bareji AK and Tandon PN (1973) Aneurysmal bone cyst of the spine. *J Neurol Neurosurg & Psych* 36: 112-117.
6. Daugherty JW and Eversole LR (1971) Aneurysmal bone cyst of the sphenoid sinus. *Trans Am Acad Opth & Otol* 80: 438-443.
7. Biesecker JI (1970) Aneurysmal bone cysts. A clinicopathologic study of 66 cases. *Cancer* 26: 615-625.
8. Stevens WW and Weaver EN (1970) Giant cell tumors and aneurysmal bone cysts of the spine: Report of four cases. *S Med J* 63: 218-221.
9. Dabska M and Buraczewski J (1969) Aneurysmal bone cyst. *Cancer* 23: 371-389.
10. Nobler MP, Higinbotham NL and Phillips RF (1968) The cure of aneurysmal bone cyst. Irradiation superior to surgery in an analysis of 33 cases. *Radiology* 90: 1185-1192.
11. Slowick FA, Campbell CJ and Kettelkamp DB (1968) Aneurysmal bone cyst. An analysis of thirteen cases. *J Bone & Joint Surg Am* 50: 1142-1151.
12. Tillman BP, Dahlin DC, Lipscomb PR and Stewart JR (1968) Aneurysmal bone cyst: An analysis of ninety five cases. *Mayo Clin Proc* 43: 478-495.
13. Granjobst W and Hopkins R (1967) Aneurysmal bone cyst of pubis. *J Bone & Joint Surg Am* 47: 971-975.
14. Parrish F and Povey JK (1967) Surgical management of aneurysmal bone cyst of the vertebral column. A report of three cases. *J Bone & Joint Surg Am* 49: 1597-1604.
15. Verbiest H (1965) Giant cell tumors and aneurysmal bone cysts of the spine. *J Bone & Joint Surg Br* 47: 699-713.
16. Donaldson WF (1962) Aneurysmal bone cyst. *J Bone & Joint Surg Am* 44: 25-40.
17. MacCarty CS, Dahlin DC, Doyle JB Jr, Lipscomb PR

and Pugh DG (1961) Aneurysmal bone cysts of the neural axis. *J Neurosurg* **18:** 671-677.
18. Godfrey LW and Gresham GA (1959) The natural history of aneurysmal bone cyst. *Proc Roy Soc Med* **52:** 900-918.
19. Beder JW, Helman CH and Campbell JA (1957) Aneurysmal bone cysts of the spine. *JAMA* **163:** 914-918.
20. Lichenstein L (1957) Aneurysmal bone cyst. Observations of fifty cases. *J Bone & Joint Surg Am* **39:** 873-882.
21. Barnes R (1956) Aneurysmal bone cyst. *J Bone & Joint Surg Br* **38:** 301-311.
22. Cruz M and Coley BL (1956) Aneurysmal bone cyst. *Surg Gyn & Obst* **103:** 67-77.
23. Taylor FW (1956) Aneurysmal bone cyst. Report of three cases. *J Bone & Joint Surg Br* **38:** 293-300.
24. Lichenstein L (1953) Aneurysmal bone cyst. *Cancer* **6:** 1228-1237.

Angiofibroma of the Nasopharynx

Radiation therapy is an alternative treatment to surgical resection. Most authors recommend doses of 3000-3500 cGy in three weeks using megavoltage radiation. Whereas extracranial angiofibroma may be approached by either surgical resection or radiotherapy, intracranial angiofibromas are often non-resectable and associated with recurrence. As surgical resection carries untoward morbidity, in such cases of intracranial angiofibroma radiation is an attractive alternative.

Nasopharyngeal Angiofibroma

Author, Year	Total # Patients	Treatment	Results	Notes
Cummings et al, 1984	55	3000-3500 cGy in 3 weeks	Extracranial: 37/46 (80%) controlled by initial treatment course none died. Intracranial: All 9 controlled, although two required a second course of radiation.	Nasopharynx, 9-30 years. Median 15 years.
Vadivel et al, 1980	7	3000 rad in 3 weeks. 6480 rad in 8 weeks.	6 of 7 patients receiving doses of > 3000r/3 weeks rendered free of disease	Follow up 2-9 years. Nasopharynx 13-22 years.
Jafek et al, 1979	15	Surgery with resection, radiation of 3000-4000 rad of residual tumor 3 months postoperatively.	60% no evidence of disease 3-14 years post-treatment	Intracranial nasopharyngeal masses 5-18 years.
Sinha and Azia, 1978	7	3000-3600 rad in 3 weeks.	Good results, no side effects.	Nasopharynx 15-20 years.
Biller et al, 1974	43	Surgery, if persistence through radiotherapy.	61% of cases revealed persistence following surgery alone. A planned treatment course with surgery and radiotherapy controlled 93% of patients.	Nasopharynx 6-20 years.
Kadin et al, 1974	1	Radiotherapy: 4500 rad/ 10F/4.5 weeks. 6 Mev, parallel opposed lateral fields.	Follow up at 8 months revealed little visible tumor. Angiograms showed residual mass to be smaller and less vascular. Also extension into the orbit and middle cranial fossa was no longer evident. No significant regrowth at 2 year follow up.	Patient had extensive nasopharyngeal fibroma with extension into the left intratemporal space, left orbit, the sphenoid sinus, and the floor of the middle (left) cranial fossa. Patient was 14 years of age.

Historical Data: Nasopharyngeal Angiofibroma

Author, Year	Total # Patients	Treatment	Results	Notes
Fitzpatrick and Rider, 1973	37	Radiotherapy: 3000–3500 rad/14–16F/3 weeks with supervoltage irradiation in the majority of cases.	31/37 control – usually early symptomatic relief. Objective tumor regression often took many months.	18/37 had previous surgery. Of the 6 who were not controlled by surgery, 2 were controlled after a second course of irradiation, two by subsequent surgery and radiotherapy, and two by subsequent surgery alone.
Jafek, 1973	25	Surgical removal.	18/25 no recurrence following one procedure (two more controlled by a 2nd procedure). The five patients with residual tumor following one or more attempts at resection all had intracranial extension.	36% received pre-op estrogen therapy. Age range of 10–14 years. Side effects: Marked to moderate rhinolalia aperta which improved gradually over several months.
English et al, 1972	12	Surgical excision.	Follow up of 2 years or more. 9/9 no evidence of recurrence. Follow up of 6–18 months. 3/3 no evidence of recurrence.	83% had tumor invasion of surrounding areas. Age range of patients was 10–20 years.
Wilson et al, 1972	2	Surgical resection.	No recurrences at 2.5 years post-op.	Both patients were over 13 years of age.
Thomsen, 1971	8	Surgical resection.	7/7 no recurrences at follow up of 2–4.5 years.	Age rage of 13–23 years.
Jereb et al, 1970	69	1. Surgery only (3) 2. Radiotherapy (pre-op) and surgery (2) 3. Surgery, radiotherapy for recurrence (14) 4. Radiotherapy alone (50) The majority of patients receiving radiotherapy received 2000–6000 rad.	57/63 free of disease for 5 years or more.	Radiation damage: Atrophic changes in skin or nasal mucosa (31) Cataract (2) Osteonecrosis (1)
Wang, 1970	3	Radiation (pre-op) followed by surgery. Dose: 4500–5000 rad/31–37 days. Co^{60} or supervoltage. One patient received two courses of radiotherapy prior to surgery.	No recurrences 4–8 years after treatment.	Age range of patients was unusual: 31–58 years.
McGauran et al, 1969	30	1. Transnasal piecemeal avulsion primary (15) after recurrences (14). 2. Transpalative excision primary (10) after recurrences (5). 3. Caldwell-Luc excision or lateral rhinotomy primary (4) after recurrences (10). 4. Radiation primary (1) after recurrences (3).	Recurrences: 1. 10/15 primary 12/14 after previous recurrences 2. 4/10 primary 3/5 after previous recurrences 3. 2/4 primary 6/10 after previous recurrences 4. 1/1 primary 0/3 after previous recurrences.	

Historical Data: Nasopharyngeal Angiofibroma (Continued)

Author, Year	Total # Patients	Treatment	Results	Notes
Conley et al, 1968	38	1. Radiation (4) 2. Radiation (pre-op) and surgery (3) 3. Surgery alone (34)	1. 2/4 control 2. 3/3 free of tumor 3. 17/34 tumor remaining Total of 55 operative procedures were done.	1. Radionecrosis of the maxilla (1) and squamous cell epithelioma of the face and orbit developed 18 years after irradiation (1). Completion in 1/3 of the patients: Osteomyelitis Severe post irradiation bleeding Severe bleeding following biopsy Persistent palatal fistulas (2) Hypotension and hypovolemia leading to cardiac arrest (2) Meningeal irritation (2) Dacrocystitis (1) Hepatitis and nephritis (2) Post-op death (1)

References

1. Cummings BJ, Blend R, Keane T, Fitzpatrick P, Beale F, Clark R, Garrett P, Harwood A, Payne D and Rider W (1984) Primary radiation therapy for juvenile nasopharyngeal angiofibroma. *Laryngoscope* **94**: 1599–1605.
2. Vadivel SP, Bosch A and Jose B (1980) Juvenile nasopharyngeal angiofibroma. *J Surg Oncol* **15**: 323–326.
3. Jafek BW, Krekorian EA, Kirsch WM and Wood RP (1979) Juvenile nasopharyngeal angiofibroma: Management of intracranial extension. *Head Neck Surg* **2**: 119–128.
4. Sinha PP and Aziz HI (1978) Juvenile nasopharyngeal angiofibroma. A report of seven cases. *Radiology* **127**: 501–505.
5. Biller HF, Sessions DG and Ogura JH (1974) Angiofibroma: A treatment approach. *Laryngoscope* **84**: 695–706.
6. Kadin MR, Thompson RW, Bentson JR, Ward PH and Calcetena TC (1974) Angiographic evaluation of the regression of an extensive juvenile nasopharyngeal angiofibroma after radiation therapy. A case report with therapeutic implications. *Br J Rad* **47**: 902–905.
7. Fitzpatrick PJ (1967) The nasopharyngeal angiofibroma. *Clin Rad* **18**: 62–68.
8. Jafek BW, Nahum AM, Butler RM and Ward PH (1973) Surgical treatment of juvenile nasopharyngeal angiofibroma. *Laryngoscope* **83**: 707–720.
9. English GM, Hemenway WG and Cundy RL (1972) Surgical treatment of invasive angiofibroma. *Arch Otol* **96**: 312–318.
10. Wilson WR, Miller D, Lee KJ and Yules RB (1972) Juvenile nasopharyngeal angiofibroma. *Laryngoscope* **82**: 985–997.
11. Thomsen KA (1971) Surgical treatment of juvenile nasopharyngeal angiofibroma. *Arch Otol* **94**: 191–194.
12. Jereb B, Anggard A and Baryd I (1970) Juvenile nasopharyngeal angiofibroma. A clinical study of 69 cases. *Acta Radiol (Ther) Stockholm* **9**: 302–310.
13. Wang CC (1970) Management of vascular tumors of the nasal cavity by combined irradiation and surgery. *EENT Monthly* **49**: 90–92.
14. McGauran MH, Serssions DG, Dorfman RF, Davis DO and Ogura JH (1969) Nasopharyngeal angiofibroma. *Arch Otol* **90**: 94–104.
15. Conley J, Hearley WV, Blaugrund SM and Perzin KH (1968) Nasopharyngeal angiofibroma in the juvenile. *Surg Gyn & Obst* **126**: 825–837.
16. Fitzpatrick PJ (1967) The nasopharyngeal angiofibroma. *Clin Rad* **18**: 62–68.

Ankylosing Spondylitis

Perhaps a classic in risk/benefit ratios is the contrast of the report of Brown and Doll (22) showing a 9.5 times incidence of leukemia in irradiated patients with the report of Radford, Doll and Smith (3) showing the severity of the underlying pathology without irradiation. It is our opinion that treatment of this disorder would be experimental and would require institutional approval. There are many unexplained features such as orthovoltage versus supervoltage, as well as total dose, but these belong in a research setting rather than in practice. The accompanying list of references should serve the reader with appropriate caution. In our national survey, 68% of radiation oncologists would not treat ankylosing spondylitis.

Radiotherapy: Ankylosing Spondylitis

Author, Year	Total # Pts.	Technical Details	Time/Dose	Results	Complications/Comments
Belcourt, 1973	533	1948 to 1960 1960 to 1971		60% patients treated with radiotherapy 20% improved 20% deteriorated 11% patients treated with radiotherapy 50% improved 10% deteriorated	There were significantly more cases of leukemia in the first period than in the second
Sinclair, 1971	195	None given	157 patients received full treatment to whole spine and sacroiliac regions.		
Kinsella et al, 1966	50	200 Kv, HVL 1mm Cu, FSD, 50cm Eight ports: 15 x 15cm port for each sacroiliac joint. 10 x 15cm port for each lumbar, thoracic and cervical area.	1000r depth dose/15 days to epiphyseal and costovertebral joints followed by a second course 3-4 months later. Third course given 6-8 months later.	spinal joints: 88-96% clinically active lesions peripheral joints: 23-33% clinically active lesions	Acute leukemia and aplastic anemia (2 pts). The disease showed no evident decrease in activity in the irradiated patients based on the patient's subjective response, physical exam, lab tests and radiological indices. There was, however, a symptomatic relief of spinal arthralgia which lasted for approximately 2 years in those pts. able to tolerate the initial radiation sickness.
	22	No treatment		spinal joints: 90% clinically active lesions. peripheral joints: 12-14% clinically active lesions	
Parry, 1966	170	Deep x-ray therapy or physiotherapy and drugs (salicylates and oxyphenylbutazone).	not given	X-ray therapy: 7/40 (42%) progression of the disease Physiotherapy and drugs: 31/130 (24%) progression of the disease	
Mason, 1964	250	Radiotherapy or drug treatment (phenylbutazone and oxyphenylbutazone)		*Radiotherapy:* 93/189 (49%) marked symptomatic relief 3 mos later. 13/23 (57%) marked symptomatic relief 1-5 yrs later. 57/166 (34%) marked symptomatic relief more than 5 yrs later. *Drug therapy:* 46/61 (75%) marked symptomatic relief 3 mos later. 33/43 (77%) marked symptomatic relief 1-5 yrs later. 12/18 (67%) marked symptomatic relief more than 5 yrs later.	

Historical Data: Ankylosing Spondylitis Radiotherapy

Author, Year	Total # Pts.	Technical Details	Time/Dose	Results	Complications/Comments
Sambrook, 1963	108	250 Kv, HVL, 1.5mm Cu	Average incident dose to the spine of 1400r. Average incident dose to peripheral joints of 900r.	*Stage 1 pts. (44):* 83% symptomatic relief. 75% objective improvement (range of motion). 50% needed further treatment within 10 yrs.	
Fulton, 1961	573	None given. Four methods of irradiation: a) trunk baths b) whole spine c) limited portion of spine d) isolated joints of muscle insertions.	1. *High dose:* a) 2000r or more/2 wks to skin of back; b) 750r single treatment to a local area. 2. *Low dose:* a) 1500r or less 2 wks to skin of back; b) long-protracted treatment.	*5 year results* *High dose:* 112/149 (75%) Stage I improved. 108/194 (56%) Stage II improved. 76/157 (49%) Stage III improved. *Low dose:* 6/18 (33%) Stage I, improved. 13/33 (39%) Stage II, improved. 5/22 (23%) Stage II, improved.	Aplastic anemia (1) subacute myeloid leukemia (1) Improvement rate at 5 yrs in high dose group was twice that of low dose group.
Wilkinson and Bywaters, 1958	200	200–500 Kv, 1mm Cu plus 1mm Al filtration FSD 5cm.	1000–2000r (total skin dose) 3 weeks to each of 4–5 spinal fields.	*Relief of pain:* 134/200 good 42/200 moderate symptomatic relapse of 67.4% at one yr, 90% at 10 yr follow up.	Only 43% of patients were not requiring regular analgesics within one year after treatment. Myeloid leukemia (1) Possible activation of pulmonary tuberculosis.
Howard, 1957	455	200 Kv, HVL, 2.3mm Cu, FSD, 50 cm. *Fields:* 1 sacroiliac field: 16 x 12 cm or 10 x 15 cm. 3 spinal fields: 16 x 15 cm or 6 x 20 cm.	1500r skin dose/ 8–10F. Two fields treated daily. Total length of treatment 3–4 weeks.	*Stage I pts (138):* 115/138 (83%) good 19/138 (14%) moderate *Stage II pts (156):* 121/156 (78%) good 32/156 (20.5%) moderate *Stage III pts (103):* 80/103 (77%) good 11/103 (10%) moderate *Stage IV pts (58):* 45/58 (78%) good 11/58 (19%) moderate	198 (43%) relapses 144 retreated at a later date.
Ward, 1955	93	Deep x-rays. 17 pts received more than one course of treatment.	Not given.	39/93 well 28/93 moderately well	
Hair, 1954	118	Deep x-rays. Spine is treated in sections, the sacroiliac joints first.	Not given.	91 pts symptom free after 5 yrs. 27 pts still under treatment.	

Historical Data: Ankylosing Spondylitis Radiotherapy (Continued)

Author, Year	Total # Pts.	Technical Details	Time/Dose	Results	Complications/Comments
Sharp and Easson, 1954	275	250 Kv, HVL 1.6mm Cu, FSD, 50 cm.	1500r (skin dose) 10F/10 wks. Whole spine and sacroiliac joints treated through rectangular applications, 7.5cm in width. Peripheral joints treated through parallel opposing fields.	178/275 (65%) much improved. 68/275 (25%) slightly improved.	Extensive haemochromatosis 2 1/2 yrs after treatment (1). Reactivation of pulmonary tuberculosis.
Desmarais, 1953	70	220 Kv, 15ma, 1mm Cu plus 1mm Al filters, HVL, 1.5Cu, FSD, 50cm. *or* 140 Kv, 5ma, .25mm Cu plus 1mm Al filtration, HVL, 7.5mm Al, FSD, 25cm.	*High voltage:* a) 500r (spine, hip); b) 1000r (spine, hip); c) 1500 (spine) 2000 (hip) Spine and sacroiliac joints divided into 5 fields, each field received approximately 300r/2F/1 week. Total length of course: 4-6 weeks. *Low voltage:* 300r skin dose/6F/3 weeks. Fields: 10cm strip over sacrum and sacroiliac joints.	Marked improvement: 7/14 (50%) Technique a. 13/17 (76%) Technique b. 7/19 (89%) Technique c. 3/11 (27%) low voltage. 4/9 (44%) controls.	Similar results in cases where treatment was directed to areas other than the spine.
Toone, 1949	29	190Kv, 20ma, 0.5mm Cu plus 1mm Al filtration, FSD 50cm. *Four fields:* a) sacroiliac, 20 x 20 b) lumbar, 10 x 15 c) dorsal, 10 x 15 d) cervical, 10 x 10	600r/4F to each field.	19/29 (67.9%) good-excellent results	
Hilton, 1943	47	Small field, local irradiation.	Not given.	7/47 completely free of pain. 38/47 improved (free from continuous pain).	
Smyth et al, 1941	52	200Kv, .5mm Cu plus 1mm Al filtration, HVL .9mm Cu, FSD 50cm.	600r/3F/5 days. Three series given at monthly intervals. No more than 300r/series over female pelvis.	37/52 (72%) significant improvement, subjective. 26/52 (50%) significant improvement, objective.	12/13(92%) with early disease improved significantly. Leukopenia in 3 pts - dosage reduced.
Hare, 1940	35	150-200 Kv, 20ma, .25-.5mm Cu plus 1mm Al filtration. FSD, 50cm. 6 portals (300 sq. cm. each)	300r to each portal. Repeated in 3 wks if necessary.	80% relief of pain. 33/35 are now able to work.	

Historical Data: Ankylosing Spondylitis Alternate Modes of Treatment

Investigator, Year	# Cases	Treatment	Results	Notes
Hill and Hill, 1975	36	Naproxen	35/36 reported naproxen to be as effective or better than previous therapy.	Previous therapy: Phenylbutazone (17) Indomethacin (10) Other analgesics or no treatment (9) No serious side effects.
Calin and Grahame, 1974	17 18	Flurbiprofen Phenylbutazone	Approximately equal results shown by both drugs in subjective assessments of day/night pain. Phenylbutazone more effective in reducing morning stiffness.	Headaches, vertigo and hot flashes while undergoing flurbiprofen therapy (1).
Sturrock and Hart, 1974	20	Indomethacin, flurbiprofen and placebo	Flurbiprofen and indomethacin equal in improving spinal movement. Analgesic properties of flurbiprofen significantly greater than those of indomethacin.	
McMaster and Coventry, 1973	17	Spinal osteotomy	All patients were pleased with results of the operation. Degree of correction remained constant in the lumbar spinal region once the osteotomy had fully united, but recurred in thoracic and cervical regions in patients whose disease was still active.	
Arden et al, 1972	2	Total hip replacement (three bilateral procedures).	*Clinical Status:* Pre-op: 2 fair, 8 poor Post-op: 4 excellent, 4 good, 2 fair *Functional Status:* Pre-op: 2 walking, 4 crutches/cane, 1 chair bound Post-op: 5 walking normally, 1 crutches/cane.	Patients followed for 1 year or more. Evaluation of clinical status is based on degree of pain.
Welch and Charnley, 1970	20	Total hip replacement (13 bilateral procedures).	All patients free of pain at follow up. No case in which hip re-ankylosed about the arthroplasty.	38.7% of the hips were not painful pre-op, but were clinically ankylosed.
Calabro and Amante, 1968	28	Indomethacin	*Functional class:* Prior to treatment: 1 (I) 21 (II) 5 (III) 1 (IV) Post treatment: 21 (I) 5 (III) 2 (IV)	Side effects (headache, nausea, dizziness) were usually transient. American Rheumatism Association Classification: I. Ability to carry on all usual duties without handicap. II. Adequate for normal activities despite handicap or discomfort or limited motion of one or more joints. III. Limited only to little or none of the duties of usual occupation or self-care. IV. Bedridden or confined to a wheelchair, little or no self-care.

Historical Data: Ankylosing Spondylitis Alternate Modes of Treatment (Continued)

Investigator, Year	# Cases	Treatment	Results	Notes
Emneus, 1968	5	Wedge osteotomy	All 5 patients were satisfied with results of the operation.	Post-op immobility is long (7-15 weeks in plaster cast, followed by plaster corset for 5-9 months). Pseudoarthritis at the site of osteotomy developed in one patient, requiring reoperation.
Rothermich, 1966	22	Indomethacin: initiated in small doses and gradually increased.	15/22 excellent results. 4/22 good results.	
Hart and Boardman, 1965	14	Indomethacin.	9/14 marked relief, thought indomethacin was more effective than phenylbutazone.	6/14 - side effects (headache, giddiness, faintness, nausea, vomiting, diarrhea, drowsiness, blurred vision, mental change, *etc.*); 3 patients withdrew from the study.
Toone and Irby, 1954	50	Phenylbutazone. *N.B.* Phenylbutazone treatment has been linked with development of acute leukemia; *cf.* Woodliff and Dougan (24).	No complete remissions. 27/50(54%) major improvement 8/50(16%) minor improvement. 15/50(30%) failure.	17/50(34%) toxic reactions: Skin rash (5) Hematuria (4) Fluid retention (4) G.I. reactions (3) Stomatitis (1) Drug was withdrawn in three cases

References

1. Hart FD and Boardman PL (1965) Indomethacin and phenylbutazone: a comparison. *Br Med J* **27**: 1281-1284.
2. Sturrock RD and Hart FD (1974) Double-blind crossover comparison of indomethacin, flurbiprofen and placebo in ankylosing spondylitis. *Ann Rheum Dis* **33**: 129-131.
3. Radford EP, Doll R and Smith PG (1977) Mortality among patients with ankylosing spondylitis not given x-ray therapy. *N Eng J Med* **297**: 572-576.
4. Hill HF and Hill AGS (1975) Ankylosing spondylitis: Open long term and double blind crossover studies with naproxen. *J Clin Pharm* **15**: 355-362.
5. Calin A and Grahame R (1974) Double-blind cross-over trial of flurbiprofen and phenylbutazone in ankylosing spondylitis. *Br Med J* **4**: 496-499.
6. Belcourt JJ (1973) 533 patients with ankylosing spondylitis seen and followed in the period 1948 to 1971. *Ann Rheum Dis* **32**: 383-385.
7. Edgar MA and Robinson MP (1973) Post-radiation sarcoma in ankylosing spondylitis. *J Bone and Joint Surg Br* **55**: 183-188.
8. McMaster MJ and Coventry MB (1973) Spinal osteotomy ankylosing spondylitis. Technique, complications and long-term results. *Mayo Clin Proc* **48**: 476-486.
9. Arden GP, Ansell BM and Hunter MJ (1972) Total hip replacement in juvenile chronic polyarthritis and ankylosing spondylitis. *Clin. Orthop.* **84**: 130-136.
10. Golding JR (1972) The treatment of ankylosing spondylitis. *Practitioner* **208**: 57-63.
11. Sambrook DK (1972) Ankylosing spondylitis. *Br Med J* **3**: 46.
12. Calabro JJ, Maltz BA and Sussman P (1971) Ankylosing spondylitis. *Am Fam Physician GP* **2**: 80-89.
13. Gardner-Thorpe C and Neophytou M (1971) Chloroma following irradiation in ankylosing spondylitis. *Med J Aust* **1**: 1121-1122.
14. Sinclair RJG (1971) Treatment of rheumatic disorders with special reference to ankylosing spondylitis. *Proc Roy Soc Med* **64**: 1031-1038.
15. Welch RB and Charnley J (1970) Low friction arthroplasty of the hip in rheumatoid arthritis and ankylosing spondylitis. *Clin Orthop* **72**: 22.
16. Calabro JJ and Amante CM (1968) Indomethacin in ankylosing spondylitis. *Arth and Rheum* **11**: 56-64.
17. Emneus H (1968) Wedge osteotomy of spine in ankylosing spondylitis. *Acta Orthopscand* **39**: 321-326.
18. Hart FD (1966) Lessons learnt in a twenty-year study of ankylosing spondylitis. *Proc Roy Soc Med* **59**: 456-458.
19. Kinsella TD, MacDonald FR and Johnson LG (1966) Ankylosing spondylitis: A late re-evaluation of 92 cases. *Canada Med Assoc J* **95**: 1-9.
20. Parry CBW (1966) Management of ankylosing spondylitis. *Proc Roy Soc Med* **59**: 619-623.
21. Rothermich NO (1966) An extended study of indomethacin II. Clinical therapy. *JAMA* **195**: 1102-1106.
22. Brown WMC and Doll R (1965) Mortality from cancer and other causes after radiotherapy for ankylosing spondylitis. *Br Med J* **2**: 1327-1332.

23. Mason RM (1964) Spondylitis. *Proc Roy Soc Med* **57**: 533–540.
24. Woodliff HJ and Dougan L (1964) Acute leukemia associated with phenylbutazone treatment. *Br Med J* **1**: 744–746.
25. Hart FD and Boardman PL (1963) Indomethacin: A new nonsteroid anti-inflammatory agent. *Br Med J* **2**: 965–970.
26. Sambrook DK (1963) Radiotherapy for ankylosing spondylitis. *Rheumatism* **19**: 30–40.
27. Fulton JS (1961) Ankylosing spondylitis. *Clin Radiol* **12**: 132–135.
28. Graham DC (1960) Leukemia following x-ray therapy for ankylosing spondylitis. *Arch Int Med* **105**: 51–59.
29. Wilkinson M and Bywaters EGL (1958) Clinical features and course of ankylosing spondylitis. *Ann Rheum Dis* **17**: 209–228.
30. Howard N (1957) The value of irradiation in ankylosing spondylitis. *Br J Radiol* **30**: 371–374.
31. Abbott JD and Lea AS (1956) The incidence of leukaemia in ankylosing spondylitis treated with x-rays. *Lancet* **2**: 1317–1320.
32. Brown WMC and Abbott JD (1955) The incidence of leukaemia in ankylosing spondylitis treated with x-rays. A preliminary report *Lancet* **1**: 1283–1285.
33. VanWaay H (1955) Aplastic anaemia and myeloid leukemia after irradiation of the vertebral column. *Lancet* **2**: 225–227.
34. Ward WR (1955) Discussion of some aspects of ankylosing spondylitis. Review of 93 service cases. *Proc Roy Soc Med* **48**: 210.
35. Hair JAG (1954) Treatment of ankylosing spondylitis by radiotherapy. *J Bone and Joint Surg Br* **36**: 671–672.
36. Sharp J and Easson EC (1954) Deep x-ray therapy spondylitis. *Br Med J* **1**: 619–623.
37. Toone EC and Irby WK (1954) Evaluation of phenylbutazone (Butasolidin) in the treatment of rheumatoid spondylitis: Report of 50 cases. *Ann Int Med* **41**: 70–78.
38. Desmarais MHL (1953) Radiotherapy in arthritis. *Ann Rheum Dis* **12**: 25–28.
39. Toone EC (1949) Rheumatoid spondylitis: Observations on the incidence and response to therapy among veterans of the recent war. *Ann Int Med* **30**: 733–739.
40. Hilton G (1943) Some observations on the x-ray treatment of ankylosing spondylitis. *Proc Roy Soc Med* **36**: 608–610.
41. Smyth CJ, Freyberg RH and Lampe I (1941) Roentgen therapy for rheumatoid arthritis of the spine. *JAMA* **116**: 1995–2001.
42. Hare EH (1940) The diagnosis of Marie-Strumpell arthritis with certain aspects of treatment. *N Eng J Med* **223**: 702–705.

Anovulation

To use radiation therapy in attempts to induce ovulation is unreasonable. Ninety-six percent of the radiation oncologists participating in our national survey would not use radiation in the treatment of anovulation.

Reference

1. Shearman RP (1969) Progress in the investigation and treatment of anovulation. *Amer J Obst and Gyn* **103**: 444–463.

Arteriovenous Malformations

The rise of radiosurgery with the original gamma knife or with Bragg peak helium ion therapy has had a significant response rate in the treatment of CNS arteriovenous malformations (AVM). Linear accelerators are now being used in investigations with new techniques and hold equal promise. Technical advances in stereotactic placement have facilitated this therapy. There is a close margin of safety relative to total dose delivered and treatment volume. Vascular obliteration takes several months to occur. The series reported to date document shrinkage of AVMs and partial to complete obliteration of lesions with associated symptomatic relief without excessive complications. Fifty-three percent of radiation oncologists in the national survey would treat AVM.

Arteriovenous Malformations

Author, Year	Total # Pts.	Site and Age	Treatment	Results	Notes
Poulsen, 1987	6 Ages: 12–38	Arteriovenous malformations of brain	4500–7500r using linear accelerator	One of six had complete clearing of AVM. None had recurrent bleeding.	No treatment complications. Minimum follow-up 17 mos.

Historical Data: Arteriovenous Malformations

Author, Year	Total # Pts.	Site and Age	Treatment	Results	Notes
Greitz et al, 1986	29	Cerebral tumors and AVM.	Stereotactic radiation therapy using 6 MV photons from linear accelerator 42 Gy or 70 Gy, with fractions of 3.5 Gy and 5.0 Gy twice a week for volumes < 90 cm^3.	Too preliminary	6-beam techniques for three-dimensional treatment. Emphasis is upon methodology.
Solomon and Stein, 1986	12	Brain stem Age: 18–65 years	9 patients treated surgically. 1 patient treated with embolization therapy 2 patients treated with radiotherapy: (3000r of conventional RT in 1, and gamma-beam irradiation in 1)	Of the irradiated group: 1 had 75% reduction of AVM @ 5 years, but suffered a hemorrhage @ 6 years. 1 had no change 6 months after treatment.	Emphasis on surgical aspect of managing AVMs of brain stem.
Zeilstra et al, 1986	52	Intracranial AVMs	Linear accelerator therapy in a semi-stereotactic fashion.	25% of the patients achieved a reduction of more than 50% of the volume of the AVM. In 3 of 25, the AVM was completely obliterated.	Smaller lesions had better results. No side effects.
Fabrikant et al, 1985	130	Intracranial vascular disorder.	Bragg peak radiosurgery using helium ions. Maximum range of the helium-ion beam is 230 MeV/u. Total doses: 25, 35 or 45 Gy equivalent to volumes 120–25000mm^3 via 3–5 entry portals.	Clinical symptoms: 68% improved neurologically 24% no change 7% worsened FU angiography: 18% complete obliteration 60% partial obliteration 21% no change	Follow-up is short (update of Fabrikant 1984 paper).
Tognetti et al, 1985	1	Intracranial AVM 27 years	4500r/6 weeks in 150r fractions gamma irradiation	Angiography 2 years after treatment revealed minor residue lesion. Decrease in headaches, no seizures.	Mechanism of AVM obliteration – endarteritis with coarctation of vessels and late necrosis.
Fabrikant et al, 1984	55	Inoperable or inaccessible deep arteriovenous malformations and carotid artery – cavernous sinus fistulas.	Stereotactic helium ion Bragg peak radiosurgery 0.6–4.0 cm beam diameter. 45 Gy equivalent to treatment volumes of 25000mm^3.	Significant decreases in size of AVM in the 7 patients followed.	Initial observations only, short follow-up.
Kjellberg et al, 1983	439	AVM of brain. Mean age 31 years.	Stereotactic Bragg peak proton therapy. Dose used = < 1% for brain injury, ie: < 50 Gy for 7mm beam to 10.5 Gy for 50mm beam.	Hemorrhage rate = 2.4%/year. Seizures improved in one-half. One-third had neurologic deficit improved. Two-thirds had lessening of headaches. 87% had reduction of AVM.	Follow up on 244 of 439 patients (55%). Complication was amplified later by subsequent letters to the editors in the NEJM.

Historical Data: Arteriovenous Malformations (Continued)

Author, Year	Total # Pts.	Site and Age	Treatment	Results	Notes
Leksell, 1983	204	AVM	Stereotactic radiosurgery gamma unit using Cobalt ^{60}.	Total obliteration of the pathological vessels in 83% cases, partial obliteration in 10.5%, and no change in 6%. 6-18 months time before obliteration occurs.	A review article.

References

1. Poulsen MG (1987) Arteriovenous malformations – a summary of 6 cases treated with radiation therapy. *Int J Radiation Oncol Biol Phys* **13**: 1553-1557.
2. Greitz T, Lax I, Bergstrom M, Arndt J, Berggren BM, Blomgren H, Boethius J, Lindqvist M, Ribbe T and Steiner L (1986) Stereotactic radiation therapy of intracranial lesions – methodologic aspects. *Acta Radiol Oncol* **25**: 81-89.
3. Solomon RA and Stein BM (1986) Management of arteriovenous malformations of the brain stem. *J Neurosurg* **64**: 857-864.
4. Zeilstra D, Bettag W and Makoski H (1986) Radiotherapy of intracranial AVM's. *J Neurosurg* **64**: 525.
5. Fabrikant JI, Lyman JT and Frankel KA (1985) Heavy charged particle Bragg peak radiosurgery for intracranial vascular disorders. *Radiat Res Suppl:* 244-258.
6. Tognetti F, Andreoli A, Cuscini A and Testa C (1985) Successful management of an intracranial arteriovenous malformation by conventional irradiation. *J Neurosurg* **63**: 193-195.
7. Fabrikant JI, Lyman JT and Hosobuchi Y (1984) Stereotactic heavy ion Bragg peak radiosurgery for intracranial vascular disorders: Method for treatment of deep arteriovenous malformations. *British J Radiol* **57**: 479-490.
8. Kjellberg RN, Davis KR, Lyons SL, Butler W and Adams RD (1983) Bragg peak proton beam therapy for arteriovenous malformations of the brain. *Clin Neurosurg* **31**: 248-290.
9. Kjellberg RN, Hanamura T, David KR, Lyons SL and Adams RD (1983) Bragg peak proton-beam therapy for arteriovenous malformations of the brain. *N Engl J Med* **309**: 269-274.
10. Leksell L (1983) Stereotactic radiosurgery. *J Neurol Neurosurg Psych* **46**: 797-803.

Arthritis

Any value gained for painful degenerative and inflammatory musculoskeletal disease from direct external radiation of tendonitis is equivalent to the value of a powerful placebo. Three studies critically examined radiation for arthritis, comparing control non-irradiated patients to irradiated patients, and observed no differences between the patient groups. Until a clinical investigator demonstrates benefit from direct irradiation in a new randomized trial, the "myth" of radiation treatment benefit should be relinquished. No further treatment of this disorder should be undertaken except in research studies.

Goldie et al. reported in a double blind study of 399 patients equivalent subjective and objective results for a variety of tendonitis, arthritis, etc. These researchers observed 45% objective improvement for placebo compared to 43% objective improvement for radiation. No statistical difference in the chi square test was observed between external irradiated and non-irradiated patients. Similarly, Valtonen conducted a double blind trial in 104 patients who had painful degenerative and inflammatory musculoskeletal conditions and observed 59% improvement in irradiated patients, compared to 65% improvement in the placebo group. Plenk also reported no difference between treated and non-treated patients with calcific tendonitis of the shoulder. Sixty-five percent of the radiation oncologists responding to our national survey would not treat arthritis with external radiation.

Rheumatoid Arthritis

It seems clear that the pathogenesis of rheumatoid arthritis itself is variable. The potential for different responses in light of the nature of this disorder must be considered when viewing the most recent experience with total lymphoid irradiation. Total lymphoid irradiation (TLI) treatment, similar to that applied in Hodgkin's disease, is an experimental therapy yet to be fully defined. The rationale for TLI therapy is the potential reduction of total lymphocyte numbers (OK T3) and the increased repopulation of suppressor T-lymphocytes, Leu 2 (OK T8) versus Leu 3 (OK T4) helper cells. Although immunologic suppression is established, the antibody titer to rheumatoid factor was not altered by TLI, nor was antibody to pneumococcal polysaccharide. In contrast, antibody to tetanus and diphtheria was reduced. In further contrast, autoantibody to nuclear DNA in lupus nephritis following treatment with TLI was decreased both experimentally and clinically. The finding in rheumatoid arthritis that autoantibody was not reduced despite arthritis reduction, implied that cellular immunity was necessary for arthritis progression, and that autoantibody was not an integral part of the important pathogenic mechanisms.

An additional and inadequately explored question remains whether the ideal dose of TLI has been established definitively. In a randomized study from Ireland published in 1986, 750 rad was as adequate in remission induction as 2000 rad. Additional differences in total dose of TLI, e.g., 2000 rad (Stanford) versus 3000 rad (Harvard), seems to imply a more sustained immunosuppression with the lower dose. This, combined with increased infection and complications following the higher dose, raises the issue of whether repeated modest doses of TLI distributed over fractional courses, quite unlike present schedules, might not prove superior. Finally, it has been interesting to note no increased potential for leukemia, unlike experience with orthovoltage radiation in a younger population with ankylosing spondylitis. Practitioners are recommended not to treat with TLI, but to refer patients to centers where investigative studies are underway.

References

1. Hanley JF, Hassan J, Morantz M, Barny C, Molony, J, Casey E. Whelan A, Fergeny C and Breshnian B (1986) Lymphoid irradiation in intractable rheumatoid arthritis. *Arthritis and Rheum* **29**: 16-25.
2. Tanaz A, Schiffman G and Strober S (1986) Effect of total lymphoid irradiation on levels of serum autoantibodies in systemic lupus erythematosus and in rheumatoid arthritis. *Arthritis and Rheum* **29**: 26-41.
3. Nusslein JG, Herbst M, Manger BJ, Gramatzki M, Burmester GR, Fritz H, Sauer R and Kalden JR (1985) Total lymphoid irradiation in patients with refractory rheumatoid arthritis. *Arthritis and Rheum* **28**: 1205-1210.
4. Brahn E, Helfgott SM, Bell JA, Anderson RJ, Reinherz EL, Schlossman SF, Austen KF and Trentham DE (1984) Total lymphoid irradiation therapy in refractory rheumatoid arthritis. *Arthritis and Rheum* **27**: 481-488.
5. Kotzin BL, Strober S, Engleman EG, Calin A, Hoppe RT, Kansas GS, Terrell CP and Kaplan HS (1981) Treatment of intractable rheumatoid arthritis with total lymphoid irradiation *N Eng J Med* **305**: 969-976.
6. Trentham DE, Belli JA, Anderson RJ, Buckler JA, Goetzl EJ, David JR and Austen KF (1981) Clinical and immunologic effects of fractionated total lymphoid irradiation in refractory rheumatoid arthritis. *N Eng J Med* **305**: 976-982.
7. Valtonen EJ, Lilivis HG and Malmio K (1975) The value of roentgen irradiation in the treatment of painful degenerative and inflammatory musculoskeletal conditions. *Scand J Rheum* **4**: 247-249.
8. Goldie I, Rosengren B, Bomerg E and Hedelin E (1970) Evaluation of radiation treatment of painful conditions of the locomotor. *Acta Radiol* **9**: 311-322.
9. Plenk HP (1952) Calcifying tendenitis of the shoulder. A critical study of the value of x-ray therapy. *Radiol* **59**: 384-389.
10. Tanay A, Strober S, Logue GL and Schiffman G (1984) Use of total lymphoid irradiation (TLI) in studies of the T-cell dependence of autoantibody in rheumatoid arthritis. *J Immunol* **132**: 1036-1040.

Arthritis Reviews

Rheumatoid, osteo, and chronic phosphate arthritis will be referred to by specific review articles. Essentially, however, treatments include immunosuppressive irradiation, total lymphoid irradiation (TLI), local field external radiation, and isotope irradiation. As an experimental modality, TLI should be studied only by protocols approved through institutional committee review. Local field irradiation for treatment of arthritis should be abandoned. Radioactive isotopes, predominantly used in Europe for correcting joints, require formal randomized prospective study prior to acceptance in the U.S.A. Finally, risk exists for radiation dermatitis, neuritis, and probably, of tumors as well. Appropriate articles are reviewed to allow the practitioner to evaluate these varied treatments.

Radioactive Colloids in Arthritis

Author	# Patients	Treatment	Results	Notes
Spooren et al, 1985	33 27 rheumatoid 6 osteoarthritis	5mCi 90Y silicate flush 2ml 1% lidocaine	35–41% improvement. Mean 16 months. Side effect: severe arthritis	Temporary postradiation arthritis. Radiographic abnormalities do not correlate with treatment
Sledge, 1985	53 rheumatoid 77 synovitis	dysprosium 165Iron colloid 250–300mCi half-life 2.3hr	80% improved. 1 year.	3 half-lives to minimize leakage
Onetti et al, 1981	111 rheumatoid arthritis 217 joints	0.3mCi–6mCi 32P	84% improved. 1–10 year FU	Details for varied joint doses and stages given.
Doherty and Dieppe, 1981	15 random double blind bilateral symmetrical chronic pyrophosphatase arthropathy	5mCi 90Yttrium + steroid versus saline + steroids	$p = < 0.01$ for range of movement; $p = < 0.05$ for joint circumference treatment 90Yttrium $p = < 0.01$	No complications in this study
Tubiana, 1979	rheumatoid hands	Brief review article, doses for varied joints	66% response in rheumatoid hands	Synovitis without deformity
Szanto, 1977	33 patients bilateral randomized 18 rheumatoid 5 polyarteritis 6 psoriatic 4 pelvic spondylitis	3–4mCi 90Yttrium resin colloid most patients	52% 90Yttrium 26% steroids 2.5 yrs FU	Rheumatoid response good. Psoriatic therapy does not work. Severe articular destruction does not respond.
Rekonen et al, 1976		4–6mCi 90Yttrium silicate 3ml 2% lidocaine 50mg hydrocortisone	82.8% activity restored in knee	0.5–2% into lymph nodes 3/5 patients

Potential Complications of Radioactive Isotopes In the Treatment of Arthritis

Author	# Patients	Treatment	Results	Comments
Doyle et al, 1977	30 patients 27 rheumatoid 1 psoriatic	5mCi 90yttrium silicate	40% response	chromosome aberrations 0.33–0.8% $p = < 0.02$
Wick and Grossner, 1983	1531 patients 267 not treated ankylosing spondylitis	224Radium	3 bone tumors	cataract, speculative not used anymore, but historically interesting
Bertrand et al, 1978	60 ankylosing spondylitis 80 rheumatoid joints	560–1680mCi of 224Radium intravenous 28–616mCi of 224Radium intraarticular	65% improved ankylosing 35% CR in rheumatoid arthritis	no bone sarcomas or soft tissue cancer up to 10 years

References

1. Harbert J (ed.) (1987) Radiocolloid Therapy in Joint Disease, Nuclear Medicine Therapy. Thieme Medical Pub Inc: New York NY, pp. 169-186.
2. Boerbooms AM, Buys WC, Daner M, and vande Putte LB (1985) Radio-synovectomy in chronic synovitis of the knee joint in patients with rheumatoid arthritis. *Eur J Nuc Med* **10**: 446-449.
3. Gordon RS (1985) Radionuclide therapy for arthritic knees. *JAMA* **253**: 744-745.
4. Revard GE, Girard M, Lamane C, Jutras M, Danias S, Gudy JP and Belanger RD (1985) Synovitis with colloidal 32P chromic phosphate for hemophiliac arthopathy: clinical follow up. *Arch Phys Med Rehab* **11**: 753-756.
5. Sledge C (1985) Radionuclide therapy for arthritic knees. *JAMA* **253**: 744-745.
6. Spooren PFMJ, Rasker JJ and Arens RPJH (1985) Synovectomy of the knee with 90Y. *Eur J Nucl Med* **10**: 441.
7. Fernandez-Palazzi R, DeBosch NB and DeVaegas AF (1984) Radioactive synovectomy in haemophilic haemarthrosis. Follow-up of fifty cases. *Scand J Haematol* **40**: 291-300.
8. Sledge CB, Atcher RW, Shortkoff S, Anderson RJ, Bloomer WD and Hurson BJ (1984) Intraarticular radiation synovectomy. *Clin Orthop* **182**: 37-40.
9. Wilson APR, Prouse PJ and Gumpel JM (1984) Listeria monocytogenes septic arthritis following intraarticular Yttrium-90 therapy. *Ann Rheum Dis* **3**: 518-519.
10. Kyle V, Hazelman BL and Wraight EP (1983) Yttrium-90 therapy and 99m TC pertechnetate knee uptake measurements in the management of rheumatoid arthritis. *Ann Rheum Dis* **2**: 132-137.
11. Wick RR and Gossner W (1983) Follow up study of late effects in 224 Ra treated ankylosing spondylitis patients. *Health Phys* **44**: 187-195.
12. Onetti CM, Gutierrez E, Hiba E and Aguirre CR (1982) Synovitis with 32P colloidal chromic phosphate in rheumatoid arthritis - clinical, histopathologic and arthrographic changes. *J Rheumatol* **9**: 229.
13. Stojanovic I, Roksanda S and Davoslava G (1982) A controlled study of the effect of radiation synovectomy of the knee joint in rheumatoid arthritis. *Rheumatologia* **20**: 182-187.
14. Wiss DA (1982) Recurrent villonodular synovitis of the knee: successful treatment with 90-Yttrium. *Clin Orthop* **169**: 139-144.
15. Doherty M and Dieppe PA (1981) Effect of intraarticular Yttrium-90 on chronic pyrophosphate arthropathy of the knee. *Lancet* **2**: 1243.
16. Daker MG (1979) Prospective chromosomal study of 30 patients undergoing 90-Y synovectomy. *Rheumatol Rehab Suppl* **4**: 1-4.
17. Gumpel M, Matthews SA and Fisher M (1979) Synovitis with Erbium-169: a double blind controlled comparison of Erbium-169 with corticosteroid. *Ann Rheum Dis* **4**: 341-343.
18. Tubiana R (1979) Intraarticular injection of radioisotopic beta-emitters. *Rheumatol Rehab Suppl* **4**: 7-9.
19. Winfield J and Gumpel JM (1979) An evaluation of repeat intraarticular injections of Yttrium-90 colloids in resistant synovitis of the knee. *Ann Rheum Dis* **2**: 145-147.
20. Bertrand A, Legras B and Martin J (1978) Use of Radium-224 in the treatment of ankylosing spondylitis and rheumatoid arthritis. *Hlth Phys* **35**: 57-60.
21. Doyle DV, Glass JC, Gow PJ, Baker M and Graham R (1977) A clinical and prospective chromosomal study of 90-Yttrium synovectomy. *Rheumatol Rehab* **16**: 217-222.
22. Szanto E (1977) Long term follow up of 90-Yttrium treated knee joint arthritis. *Scand J Rheumatol* **6**: 209.
23. Rekonen A, Kuikka J and Oka M (1976) Retention and extra-articular spread of intraarticularly injected 90-Yttrium silicate. *Scand J Rheumatol* **5**: 47.

Astrocytoma (Grade I-II)

High dose post-operative radiotherapy to limited volumes has been assumed to improve survival, although there are no randomized studies of partially or completely excised astrocytomas grade I-II to critically evaluate the value of post-operative irradiation. The principle of using high dose to reduced volumes, as applied in treatment of more malignant grades of astrocytoma, has been the generally accepted standard. Although a definitive statement regarding these so-called benign astrocytomas cannot be made, considering the risk benefit ratio, treatment is favored. Ninety-seven percent of radiation oncologists in the national survey would treat grade I-II astrocytoma.

Astrocytoma (Grade I-II)

Author, Year	Total Cases	Site and Age	Treatment	Results	Notes
Rutter et al, 1981	27	Brain, average age - 32	Partial resection followed by XRT. Local irradiation to tumor site 400-4000r.	5-year actuarial survival 11/27(44%).; median survival of 63.7 mos.	Grade II tumors only

Astrocytoma (Grade I-II) (Continued)

Author, Year	Total Cases	Site and Age	Treatment	Results	Notes
Scanlon and Taylor 1979	134	Intracranial; mean age – 26.5. Grade I – 26.5 years Grade II – 28.3 years	Surgery (Biopsy, partial or complete resection), followed by XRT. Doses > and < 1400rets were used.	Survival at 5 yrs. Grade I – 76% Grade II – 58%	Young patients have greatly improved survival over older patients. Patients receiving less than 1400rets have longer survival than those receiving more than 1400rets. Patients with limited volume treatment had better survival than those receiving whole brain treatment.
Fazekas, 1977	68	Brain, all ages	Surgery and post-operative XRT Doses: 850–1450rets	10 year survival 20–30% regardless of treatment and prognostic parameters. For incompletely excised cases, adjacent radiotherapy improved survival.	12 grade I, 56 grade II tumors. 45 irradiated, 23 non-irradiated.
Salazar et al, 1976	44	Intracranial, all ages.	Surgery ± post-operative XRT 5000r/6.5 weeks to tumor bed with margin.	54% survival 5 years from diagnosis	7 grade I, 37 grade II
Leibel et al, 1975		Intracranial, all ages.	Surgery ± post-operative irradiation 5000–5500r/5.5–6 weeks to tumor plus margin.	5 year survival Grade I – (58%) Grade II – (25%)	Survival improved with post-operative irradiation with those incompletely excised.

References

1. Rutter EHJM, Kazem I, Sloof JL and Walder AHD (1981) Post operative radiation therapy in the management of brain astrocytomata - retrospective study of 142 patients. *Int J Radiation Oncology Biol Phys* **7**: 191–195.
2. Scanlon PW and Taylor WF (1979) Radiotherapy of intracranial astrocytomas: Analysis of 417 cases treated from 1960 through 1969. *Neurosurgery* **5**: 301–308.
3. Fazekas JT (1977) Treatment of grades I and II brain astrocytomas. The role of radiotherapy. *Int J Radiation Oncology Biol Phys* **2**: 661–666.
4. Salazar OM, Rubin P, McDonald JV, and Feldstein ML (1976) Patterns of failure in intracranial astrocytomas after irradiation: Analysis of dose and field factors. *Am J Roentgenol* **126**: 279–292.
5. Leibel SA, Sheline GE, Wara WM, Boldrey EB and Neilsen SL (1975) The role of radiation therapy in the treatment of astrocytomas. *Cancer* **35**: 1551–1557.

Bowen's Disease

Bowens' disease is often described as an intraepithelial carcinoma. There are so many methods of treating the disease that in our reference out of 125 verified lesions, only 19 were treated with grenz rays. We conclude that alternate methods of therapy are the treatment methods of choice. Fifty-three percent of radiation oncologists would not treat Bowen's disease according to the national survey.

Bowen's Disease

Author, Year	Total # Patients	Treatment	Results	Notes
Scoma and Levy, 1975	2	Complete excision.	Wound healed completely and there has been no evidence of recurrence.	Lesions of the anus. Authors state that the preferred method of treatment is complete surgical excision with multiple frozen section examination at the time of operation.
Mikhail, 1974	4	Mohs chemosurgery technique.	No recurrences at six months to two years.	All four patients had a primary histological diagnosis of Bowen's disease of the nail bed, but all four patients were subsequently discovered to have invasive squamous cell carcinoma of the nail bed.
Hausmen, 1974	7	Topical 5-fluorouracil.	Severe response in one patient. Treatment was stopped. Subsequent partial clearing. A second treatment produced little response. Patient lost to follow up. Marked inflammatory response in the second patient. Treatment discontinued after three weeks. One month later the lesion had clinically resolved.	Bowen's disease of the hand.
Sharma and Majumdar, 1972	1	Local excision.	No recurrence one year later when patient died of sudden heart failure.	Invasive Bowen's disease of the flank, lesion had been present for 16 years.
Bensaude and Parturier-Albot, 1971	1	Recurred twice following excision and coagulation. Recurred after radio-contact therapy. Second course of contact therapy was given.	No recurrence at 3 years after second course of contact therapy.	Bowen's disease of the anus. Precancerous (3) Invasive or cancerous (2) Both precancerous and invasive (1)
	2	Electrocoagulation	No recurrence at 4 years; one patient required a second treatment.	
Bensaude and Parturier-Albot, 1971	1	Contact therapy.	No recurrence at 3 years.	
	1	Electrocoagulation followed by contact therapy.	No recurrence at 7 years.	
Yaffee, 1970	1	Topical 5-fluorouracil followed by excision.	5-fluorouracil caused significant inflammation and discomfort so therapy was discontinued. Uneventful recovery following excision and no recurrence at date.	Multicentric pigmented Bowen's disease of the groin.
Fulton et al, 1968	1	Topical 5-fluorouracil.	Within 12 days the lesion had sloughed and by one month the lesion had returned to normal.	Lesion of the thigh.

Bowen's Disease (Continued)

Author, Year	Total # Patients	Treatment	Results	Notes
Janson et al, 1967	13	Topical 5-fluorouracil.	9/13 lesion cleared and remained clear up to three years after treatment. 3/13 small recurrent areas but good resolution followed a second application. 1/13 treatment stopped subsequent vulvectomy.	Bowen's disease of the skin. The majority of lesions were on the ear, face and neck.
Blank and Schnyder, 1985	73 Ages 50-60. Preponderantly Male.	3200-5000 roentgens. Author recommends 4000-5600 roentgens.	100% responses in extra-genital. 88% response in ano-genital.	2-10 years follow-up.
Stevens et al, 1977	16 Ages 46-80 years. 9 Females and 7 Males.	Grenz rays 5000 roentgens 500r x 10 fractions.	10% recurrence.	Follow up 1.5-12.5 years.

References

1. Blank AA and Schnyder VW (1985) Soft x-ray therapy in Bowen's disease and erythroplasia of Queyrat. *Dermatologica* **171**: 89-94.
2. Stevens DM, Kopf AW, Gladstein A and Bart RS (1977) Treatment of Bowen's disease with grenz rays. *Int J Dermatol* **16**: 329-339.
3. Scoma JA and Levy EI (1975) Bowen's disease of the anus: Report of two cases. *Dis Colon & Rectum* **18**: 137-140.
4. Hausmen JE (1974) Cryotherapy for treatment of intra-oral leukoplakia and the morbus Bowen. *Minerva Medica* **65**: 3715-3717.
5. Mikhail GR (1974) Bowen's disease and squamous cell carcinoma of the nail bed. *Arch Derm* **110**: 267-270.
6. Wagers LT, Shapiro L and Kroll JJ (1973) Bowen's disease of the hand. *Arch Derm* **107**: 745-746.
7. Sharma K and Majumdar M (1972) Invasive Bowen's disease. *Med J Aust* **1**: 376-377.
8. Bensaude A and Parturier-Albot M (1971) Anal localization of Bowen's disease. *Proc Roy Soc Med* **64**: 1190-1191.
9. Lloyd KM (1970) Multicentric pigmented Bowen's disease of the groin. *Arch Derm* **101**: 48-51.
10. Yaffee HS (1970) Renal vasculitis and Bowen's disease. *Arch Derm* **101**: 372-373.
11. Fulton JE, Caeter DM and Hurley HJ (1968) Treatment of Bowen's disease with topical 5-fluorouracil under occlusion. *Arch Derm* **97**: 178-180.
12. Janson GT, Dillaha CJ and Honecutt WM (1967) Bowenoid conditions of the skin: Treatment with topical 5-fluorouracil. *Southern Med J* **60**: 185-188.
13. Edwards M (1965) Bowen's disease: A case report. *Dis Colon & Rectum* **8**: 297-299.
14. Michaelides P and Hyman AB (1964) Bowen's disease of the palm. Report of a case. *Dermatologica* **128**: 239-244.
15. Graham JH and Helwig EB (1959) Bowen's disease and its relationship to systemic cancer. *Arch Derm* **80**: 133-159.

Bronchial Adenomas

The term "adenoma" is a misnomer. Bronchial adenomas are neoplasms arising from the mucous glands and ducts of the tracheobronchial tree. They comprise several types: 1) *Bronchial carcinoids* were named by Hamperl because of their histological similarity to intestinal carcinoids; they have the capacity to produce carcinoid syndrome in 8% of the series reported here, and they account for 75-80% of all adenomas. 2) *Cylindromas (adenoid cystic carcinomas)* comprise 8-10% of all adenomas and resemble salivary gland tumors in their high propensity for local invasiveness and metastasis to regional lymph nodes. 3) *Mucoepidermoid carcinomas* are exceedingly rare, constituting only 1-3% of adenomas. Unlike mucoepidermoid carcinoma of the salivary glands, which is usually a low grade, indolent malignancy, the bronchial counterpart behaves in an aggressive fashion with a 0% 5-year survival reported in some series. These tumors have the capability to metastasize distantly in 23-44% of patients. Although the incidence of metastasis appears to be similar for different cell types, adenoid cystic carcinoma behaves more aggressively than the carcinoid. The former has an average survival rate of 50%, whereas the carcinoids have a survival rate in excess of 90%. Patients with bronchial adenomas may survive for many years following the development of distant metastases; surgical resection is sometimes warranted. Although the metastatic rate is high and there is a very high rate of metastasis to local lymph nodes, local recurrence is the most common mode of failure.

Surgical resection is the treatment of choice, with a very high cure rate ranging from 50-100% in cylindromas and carcinoids. Radical resection is generally preferred (pneumonectomy or lobectomy), even though lesser surgical procedures such as wedge resection or bronchoplasty (resection and reconstruction of the involved bronchus or trachea) have not been shown conclusively to be less effective.

Treatment with radiotherapy has been reserved for medically inoperable patients or for patients with unresectable tumors. Since no uniform method of treatment has been established, determination of radiotherapeutic efficacy is difficult to assess. Dosages have varied from 3000 Roentgen in air to 23,200 Roentgen with orthovoltage therapy, and 3000cGy to 7000cGy with supervoltage therapy. Dosages that attain at least 5500cGy are also effective, and intrabronchial radiation has been used with varying success. Several long term survivors and excellent palliation of obstructed bronchi have been reported. Presumably, failure results when tumors extend beyond the region treated; local recurrence is the rule.

In designing a radiation portal, careful consideration should be given to the natural history of bronchial adenomas, i.e., their high rate of local recurrence and the incidence of local lymph node metastasis. Generous margins should encompass the tumor and local, draining lymph nodes. Dosages should be above 5500cGy.

In the national survey 68% of radiation oncologists would not treat bronchial adenomas.

Bronchial Adenoma

Author, Year	Total # Patients	Treatment	Results	Notes
Simpson et al, 1974	25	Surgical excision (approx. 50% were lobectomies).	23/25 alive and well (6 months to 18 years post-op) 2/25 died – one from widespread tumor	Distribution of Disease: Carcinoid (19) Cylindroma (2) Spindle cell (2)
Walker, 1974	1	Lung resection for adenoma 4 years previously. Presented with lesions in both eyes. Right eye: 2.50mc radon seed secured to sclera over lesion for 10 hours. Second treatment 15 months later. Left eye: 7.50mmCo60 plaque applied for a week.	No recurrence of the primary adenoma. Right eye: Lesion steadily decreased in size. Left eye: Lesion disappeared. Patient is alive 13 years following the lung resection.	Medial rectus of right eye had to be detached.

Historical Data: Bronchial Adenoma

Author, Year	Total # Patients	Treatment	Results	Notes
Turnbull et al, 1972	58	Carcinoid: 1. Endoscopic excision plus radon seed implants in 2 and chemotherapy in 1. 2. Resection. 3. Radiation (3175–7800r) plus supplemental chemotherapy in 2. 4. Supportive treatment (6) or systemic chemotherapy (2). Cylindroma: 1. Resection. 2. Radiation. 3. Endoscopic excision plus radon seed implant. 4. No treatment. Mucoepidermoid: 1. Resection (plus radiation in 3). 2. Radiation.	5 year Survival: Carcinoid: 1. 3/3 2. 17/24 3. 4/6 4. 0/8 Cylindroma: 1. 1/1 2. 2/2 3. 0/1 4. 0/1 Mucoepidermoid: 1. 0/4 2. 0/6	The only patients undergoing radiation treatment were those with nonresectable tumors. Carcinoid: 1. Two are alive at 14 years and 19 years. One died at 15 years of unknown causes. 2. Two died of post-op complications. 3. Two are free of disease at 13 years and 14 years. 4. All had far advanced disease. Cylindroma: 1. Free of disease at 13 years. 2. One – no recurrence at 12 years. One – died at 9 years, metastatic disease. Mucoepidermoid: Two patients had terminal disease when first seen and are not included.
Tolis et al, 1972	24	Peripheral lesions (9 pts) Pulmonary resection: 3 wedge resections, 6 lobectomies. Central lesions (15 pts) Bronchoscopic removal (2) Pneumonectomy (3). Bilobectomy (2). Wedgectomy (5). Rt. basilar sigmentectomy (1). Exploratory thoracotomy (1).	Peripheral lesions 8/9 survived 1–12 years post-op without a recurrence. 1/9 recurrence at 5 years, the patient died 9 years after diagnosis. Central lesions 10/13 alive 3–13 years after initial treatment (2 patients lost to follow up). 1/13 died of disseminated tumor. 1/13 died post-op after attempted removal of recurrence 33 years after initial treatment. 1/13 died of recurrent pneumonia after 2 years with no evidence of recurrent tumor.	Distribution of disease: Carcinoid (18) Cylindroma (4) Mucoepidermoid (2) Central tumors-arising in a major bronchus. Peripheral tumors – arising in the pulmonary parenchyma. Five cases had lymph node involvement.
Meffert, 1970	35	30/35 underwent resection.	Carcinoid: 23/28 good-excellent health at average of 11 years, three months follow up. Five patients known dead (3) from this disease. Four patients lost to follow up. Cylindroma: Two alive at 4 1/3 years and 18 years. One died at 13 years 9 months with recurrent disease.	Carcinoid (32) – Twenty-one of these showed no extra-bronchial extension. Cylindroma (3) – One was a mucoepidermoid variant.

Historical Data: Bronchial Adenoma (Continued)

Author, Year	Total # Patients	Treatment	Results	Notes
O'Grady et al, 1970	33	Pulmonary resection. Bronchoscopic resection (one also had a pulmonary resection 4 years later). Radiation (tumor was nonresectable).	5 year survival 28/29 2/3 0/1 (tumor was of the cylindroid type).	88% carcinoid (29 pts). 12% cylindroma (4 pts). 5 year survival rate was 95% (28/29) in the carcinoid group. All four patients with the cylindroid tumor died (two at 4 years, one at 6 years, one at 11 years)
Smith, 1969	16	Surgical excision.	9/16 alive and well.	All were carcinoid tumors. Deaths: 1 post-op, 5 from disease at 3 mos, 4 mos, 1 year, 10 years and 12 years.
Donahue et al, 1968	35	1. Resection (33). 2. Radiation (1). 3. No treatment (1).	1. 5 year survival (excluding operative deaths and death from other causes): 28/30 2. No evidence of endobronchial lesions at 3 months follow up. 3. Died of pneumonia due to obstruction by bronchial adenoma.	Distribution of Disease: Carcinoid (31) Cylindromas (4) Cumulative 10 year survival is 63.6%.
Baldwin and Grimes, 1967	56	1920-1940: 1. Lobectomy or pneumonectomy. 2. Drainage of empyema spaces. 3. Intensive irradiation. 4. Bronchoscopic removal. 1940-1965: 1. Thoracotomy with resection. 2. Bronchoscopic removal. (Thoracotomy was contraindicated because of associated illness).	1920-1940: 1. 5/6 alive at 20 year follow up (one post-op death) 2. 2/2 alive at 10 year follow up. 3. 3/3 alive at 15 year follow up. 4. 2/7 alive at 10 years but most had recurrences necessitating further removal. 1940-1965: 1. 22/27 alive (4 died of unrelated causes, one died of metastatic disease).	Distribution of Disease: Carcinoid (49) Cylindroma (2) Mixed (5) 1940-1965: 6 lost to follow up.
Brindley and Bannet, 1967	12	1. Pneumonectomy (5), one patient also had lymph adenectomy. 2. Lobectomy (7), one patient also had 5FU intra-arterial x-rays to the liver, and cyclophosphamide.	1. One patient died of coronary infarction. Other four alive at 3 1/2, 9, 13 and 15 years post-op. 2. All patients alive at 3, 16, 14 months, 2 1/2, 5 1/2, 10 1/2 and 13 years post-op.	All were cases of carcinoid tumors.
Reichle and Rosemond, 1966	2	Pneumonectomy or lobectomy.	No evidence of disease at 1 1/2 years and 13 years post-op.	Both were mucoepidermoid tumors. Author provides a summary of reported mucoepidermoid tumors.
Batson et al, 1966	43	Surgical excision (27 lobectomies, 9 pneumonectomies, 4 bilobectomies, 1 bronchotomy with local resection, 1 multiple segmental resection).	30/43 alive without evidence of recurrence at 2 1/2 to 22 year follow up. 5 year survival (excluding operative deaths): 94%.	Distribution of Disease: Carcinoid (36) Cylindroma (6) Mucoepidermoid (1) Five patients had hilar and mediastinal involvement at surgery, two are still alive. Deaths: 4 post-op/operative mortality of 11.2% 4 from unrelated causes. 4 from tumor at 16, 24, 66 and 72 months post-op.

Historical Data: Bronchial Adenoma (Continued)

Author, Year	Total # Patients	Treatment	Results	Notes
Bower, 1965	28	Resectional surgery (23) Radiation (radon seeds-1)	Surgery: 21/23 alive and normal post-op chest films at 1-11 year follow ups (one operative death). Radiation: Patient died but tumor may have been metastatic adenocarcinoma from breast tumor removed 5 years previously.	Distribution of Disease: Carcinoma (21) Cylindroma (1) Mixed oncocytoid carcinoid (1) Unclassified (5) 3 patients lost to follow up; 1 patient not treated - died at 5 years from unrelated causes.
Markel et al, 1964	5	Partial endoscopic resection followed by 3000-6100r x-rays or Co60 radiation, 4 patients. Endoscopic resection only (1 patient). Each patient was followed for 6.8-13 years and repeat irradiation and/or endoscopic resections were performed.	5 year survival: 5/5 Three deaths occurred during the follow up period at 8 years, 12 1/2 years and 13 years following initial treatment. All were either directly or indirectly attributable to recurrent neoplasm. Two patients are still alive at 6.8 year and 8 year follow ups.	All were cases of adenocystic carcinoma of the trachea.
Markel et al, 1964	61	Carcinoid: 1. Pneumonectomy. 2. Lobectomy. 3. Local (electron coagulation, fulgaration, radium implants, resection of bronchial stump. 4. No treatment. Cylindroma: 1. Radiation (3). All were considered to have inoperable disease. 2. Pneumonectomy (2). Mucoepidermoid: (2) Lobectomy	Carcinoid: 5 year survival 10 yr survival 1. 18/19(95%) 15/16(94%) 2. 18/18(100%) 10/10(100%) 3. 3/3 2/3(67%) 4. 3/4(75%) 3/4(75%) Cylindroma: 1. 2/3 died within 2 years, third is still alive at 41 months. 2. One died 7 months later. The other died 10 years later from other causes. Mucoepidermoid: 1. All are alive at 3 1/2, 5, and 16 1/2 years after treatment.	Distribution of Disease: 53/61(86.9%) Carcinoid 5/61(8.2%) Cylindroma 3/61(4.9%) Mucoepidermoid Cylindroma: All three were considered to have inoperable disease.
Wilkins et al, 1963	82	1. Resections (67) 2. Radiation only (2) 3. Endoscopy (11) 4. No treatment (2)	1. 3 operative deaths and 13 subsequent deaths (8) from unrelated causes. 2. 1 subsequent death. 3. 2 operative deaths and 8 subsequent deaths. 4. 2 subsequent deaths. Total cumulative survival of 70% at 10 years.	Distribution of Disease: 84% Carcinoid (69) 9% Cylindroma (7) 7% Mucoepidermoid (6) 5 year survival of 98.1% cumulative 5 year survival of 75%.
Zellos, 1962	40	1. Resection (38) 2. Radiotherapy (1)	1. 32/38 alive (30 after more than three years). 2. Patient alive at 13 years following treatment.	Distribution of Disease: Carcinoid (33) Cylindroma (6) Mixed (1)
Weisel et al, 1961	42	Surgical excision.	41/42 normal exam at follow up	Respiratory tract tumors: Distribution of Disease: Carcinoid (35) Cylindroma (4) Mixed (3)

Historical Data: Bronchial Adenoma (Continued)

Author, Year	Total # Patients	Treatment	Results	Notes
Goodner et al, 1961	32	Carcinoids: 1. Exploratory operation or no treatment (6). 2. Bronchoscopic removal of tumor (twice) plus cauterization of the tumor once (1). 3. Radium element pack plus external irradiation (1) or radon seeds (18mc, 2410mc-hr-30mc, 3.924mc-hr) (2) 4. External irradiation 3000-23,200r air dose (200-250Kv) (4). 5. Pulmonary resections (13). Cylindromas: 1. External irradiation (3000-7,800r air dose, 250-100Kv) (3). 2. Lobectomy (1). 3. Patient presented with multiple skin and skull metastases. Treated only by irradiation to the metastases.	Carcinoids (26 patients): 1. 6/6 dead within 5 months. 2. Alive with persistent carcinoid 16 years after first treatments. 3. Alive at 13, 19, and 7 years respectively, following treatments. 4. 3/4 dead at 3 months, 3 months and 2 years. All 3 had extensive tumors when first seen. 5. Average survival 6.6 years. Cylindromas (5 patients): 1. 2/3 alive after 5 years (one at 12 years, the other at 9 years). 2. Alive at 13 years, 8 months post-op. 3. Died 2 months later.	Distribution of Disease: Carcinoids (27) Cylindroma(5) Carcinoids: 1. One patient had radiation pre-op (2850r) and pleural recurrences (7000r) and is alive at 19 years follow up. Cylindromas: 1. One patient had also received multiple fulgurations prior to irradiation. Another patient received radon seed implants (58.92mc) plus additional external irradiation (3,900r, 250Kv to recurrences).
Weiss and Ingram, 1961		1. Lobectomy (2) 2. Bronchotomy (2) 3. Pneumonectomy (1)	1. Alive at 5 and 6 year follow up. 2. Alive at 3 month and 5 year follow up. 3. Alive at 3 year follow up.	The only cases included here are those for which the authors provided adequate follow up data.
Ricketts et al, 1955	1	Radiotherapy (2000r) A second course of radiotherapy (2,604r) given at 3 month follow up when nodules on the tracheal and bronchial walls were noted.	Patient became asymptomatic following first treatment. Patient was asymptomatic after second treatement. One month later metastases to the eye were found (rapid growth necessitated enucleation).	Tumor was adenoid cystic carcinoma type.
Vieta and Maier, 1957	1	Bronchoscopic fulgurations followed approximately 8 months later by radiotherapy (3900r x 2/1 month, 1000Kv, two anterior-posterior portals).	Marked improvement at one year follow up. Patient died 5 years after initial treatment.	Adenoid cystic carcinoma.
	1	2900r (air) to each of two portals (250Kv) to the larynx. Palliative irradiation to lungs and skull.	The laryngeal lesion showed excellent regression but patient died approximately 3 years after initial observation due to widespread disease.	Patient had lung metastases when first seen.
		A selective review of bronchial adenomas treated by surgery and/or radiation is provided by the authors: Radiation With or Without Additive Endoscopy: 11/24 dead of disease 1 month - 10 years after treatment.		

Historical Data: Bronchial Adenoma (Continued)

Author, Year	Total # Patients	Treatment	Results	Notes
		6/24 alive without evidence of recurrence 5 years or more. 3/24 living with recurrence or residual disease 1 month - 5 years or more. 4/24 living without recurrence 1 month - 5 years. <u>Surgery:</u> 11/29 dead of disease 1 month - 10 years after treatment. 5/29 alive without evidence or recurrence 5 years or more. 5/29 living with recurrence or residual disease 1 month - 5 years or more. 8/29 living without recurrence 1 month - 5 years.		

Historical Data: Bronchial Adenomas Cell Type

Author, Year	Total # Pts.	Cell Type	Treatment Type	Results	Complications/ Comments
Aberg and Blondal, 1981	313	All carcinoids (literature review)	All surgical resection 179 lobectomies 76 pneumonectomies 31 wedge resections 27 bronchoplasties	Survival % 5y 10y 20y >20y 90 90 80 (5 at risk) 90 80 - (0 at risk) 90 67 20 (5 at risk) 90 72 - (0 at risk) Of 255 patients with radical surgery, 10.6% recurred or are DOD. Of 58 patients wedge or bronchoplasty, 22% recurred or are DOD.	No multivariate analysis; patients with lesser surgery may have been older or in poor condition. No conclusion about optimum surgical therapy can be answered from this study.
de Gruneck and Naef, 1977	24	19 Carcinoid 2 Adenoid cystic 3 Mucoepidermoid	All surgical resection 10/19 pneumo/lobectomy 4/19 wedge resection 5/19 bronchoplasty 1 lobectomy 1 unresectable-XRT Co60,5500cGy 3/3 pneumo/lobectomy	Survival % 100% 19/19 NED 50% 1/1 DOD at 3y 1/1 NED at 3y 0% 3/3 DOD	Mucoepidermoid behaved like a high grade malignancy. Many series report similar results; see Burchart and Turnball. 0% carcinoid syndrome.
Marks and Marks, 1977	28	24 Carcinoid 3 Adenoid cystic 1 Mucoepidermoid	All surgical resection 9/28 pneumonectomy 8/28 lobectomy 7/28 biopsy only 4/28 autopsy dx	8/28 deaths- 1 brain Mets -1 operative -6 intercurrent ds	Survival by treatment unclear because numbers do not add to total. No correction with survival by cell type is done. No actuarial survival is calculated. 2/24 carcinoids had syndrome. 3/17 radical surg had limited mets. Incidence distant mets is not addressed, but 1 pt died of brain mets (4%)

Historical Data: Bronchial Adenomas Cell Type (Continued)

Author, Year	Total # Pts.	Cell Type	Treatment Type	Results	Complications/Comments
Vieta and Maier, 1957	31	All adenoid cystic	All radiotherapy No uniform XRT Ext beam (orthovoltage) Radon seeds No doses mentioned	10 NED 1mo to >5y (5 NED >5y) 3 AWD 1mo to >5y (1 AWD >5y) 11 DOD 1mo to >5y (5 DOD >5y)	No conclusions can be ordered about the effectiveness of XRT from this paper. Actuarial survival not given.
Vieta and Maier, 1957 (continued)	35	All adenoid cystic	All surgical resection Types of surgery unspecified.	13 NED 1mo to >5y (6 NED >5y) 5 AWD 1mo to >56 (1 AWD >5y) 11 DOD 1mo to >5y (5 DOD >5y) 5 no follow up 1 operative mortality	No actuarial survival curve was calculated. Extent of disease is unspecified and patient characteristics are unknown. Overall, survival is approximately 50% if pts lost to follow up are considered dead.
Goodner et al, 1961	32	27 Carcinoid	RADIOTHERAPY -1 radon seeds (6 implants over 4 months/total 18mc or 2410mc-h) -1 radon and ext beam (19 tx's but dose unknown), radon dose unknown. -4 orthovoltage, 198-250Kv dose ranged 3000R in air to 23,200R in air. 13 SURGERY -1 wedge resection -6 lobectomy -6 pneumonectomy 5 NO SURGERY OR XRT -3 no tx -1 autopsy dx -2 very ill -3 explored not resectable -1 tx'd nitrogen mustard -2 unknown tx -1 bronchoplasty x 2	NED at 19y post tx Died intercurrent ds at 15y post tx-original symptoms never resolved but no mets developed. AWD, locally at 13y. 3/4 DOD at 3mo, 3mo and 2y (all with massive ds) 1/4 DOD at 14y, pt NED 9y 1/6 operative mortality 1/6 preop XRT (2850R in air) pt recurred-7000R, NED at 19y. 4/6 average survival=5y. 1/6 op sort 1/6 NED < 1y 4/6 NED 4-9y DOD at 10 days and 1mo No response and DOD at 5 mo DOD at 1 day and 5mo post dx AWD at 16y post dx	Incidence of Metastasis 12/27(44%) -8/12 mediastinal nod -2/12 diffuse mets Conclusions: 58% of pts surviving 5y had radical surgery, whereas, 86% of pts surviving NED received radical surgery. It would appear that surgery is the tx of choice; however, pts receiving XRT alone had larger, unresectable and less favorable tumors. Only 1 of 3 pts tx's with radon seeds was cured. XRT doses should be higher, namely 6-6500cGy, similar to HEENT tumors. Complications: Not mentioned, but each pt described individually mentioned.
Goodner et al, 1961 (continued)		5 Adenoid cystic	4 RADIOTHERAPY -1 mets at dx, xrt top mets -1 unresectable (250Kv-3000 in air to chest) -1 unresectable (1000Kv-420 in air) -1 post mult fulgurations (XRT-7800R in air) 1 Lobectomy	DOD at 2 mo NED at 12y Recurred at 7y-radon seeds 58.92mc and ext beam (250Kv-3900R), DOD at 96 post tx, local and distant sites. DOD at 3y 6mo NED at 14y	

Historical Data: Bronchial Adenomas Cell Type (Continued)

Author, Year	Total # Pts.	Cell Type	Treatment Type	Results	Complications/Comments
Donahue et al, 1968	33	31 Carcinoid 4 Adenoid cystic	Surgery and 1 XRT 16 Pneumonectomy 13 Lobectomy 2 Bilobectomy 2 Segmental Total = 33 1 radiotherapy (dose??) (supravoltage) 1 no therapy (old age)	23/33 NED (follow up time?) 2/33 operative mortality 2/33 died intercurrent ds 2/33 alive with mets (liver/bone) 4/33 died diffuse mets (at 1, 4, 6 and 7 years) unresectable adenoid cystic of carina, NED at 3 mo. DOD at 4y from obstructive pneumonia.	Survival curve at 10y (63.6%) flattens, suggesting cure at 10y. No mention of follow up times or numbers of pts at risk. 1 pt controlled for 20y by radon seeds, then recurred locally and had pneumonectomy. 2 pts had carcinoid syndrome and 1 had hepatic mets (DOD at 6mo follow up of the 2nd pt not mentioned)
Rowe and Jafek, 1979	1	Carcinoid	1 Radiotherapy and Chemotherapy −4000cGy in 4 wks −Cytoxan 20mg/kg x 3d, then 50 mg po thereafter.		
Price et al, 1979	1	Adenoid cystic of trachea unresectable	1 Radiotherapy −4700 Co60, AP/PA −3y later, true recurrence 3000cGy ext beam and Ir implant (2300cGy)	DOD at 20mo	
Boedker and Hald, 1982	1	Adenoid cystic of trachea unresectable	1 Radiotherapy −6000cGy ext beam plus Hydrea in 1975 (Hydrea continued x 3y)	Recurred locally 3y later Mainsteam bronchus tx'd twice with intrabronchial XRT x 4 tx's Right bronchus 1800cGy total Left bronchus 1400cGy total.	DOD in 1980, 5y post ext beam. Pt was palliated well with intrabronchial RT.

Key: DOD = dead of local disease unless otherwise specified. AWD = alive with local disease, either from local persistence or recurrence. NED = no evidence of disease. XRT = radiotherapy. Tx = treatment. Bronchoplasty = resection or reconstruction of the involved bronchus or trachea, similar to local excision.

Bronchial Adenomas Radiotherapy and Surgery

Ref	Operative Mortality	RADIOTHERAPY ALONE				SURGERY ALONE			
		Adenoid	Carcinoid	Mucoepiderm	All types	Adenoid	Carcinoid	Mucoepiderm	All types
1							90% 5y		
	0/23(0%)	1/2(50%,5y)				0/1(0%,3y)	19/19(100%)	0/3(0%,8mo)	83%, 5y
4	1/24(4%)								71%
28					42%				
28	1/35(3%)					18/35(51%)			
	2/23(6%)	1/1(100%)							85%, 5yr
24		2/4(50%,5y)	4/7(57%,5y)		55%,5y	1/1(100%,5y)	10/13(77%,5y)		79%

References

1. Boedker A and Hald A (1982) A method for selective endobronchial and endotracheal irradiation. *J Thorac Cardiovasc Surg* **84:** 59-61.
2. Aberg T, Blondal T, Nou E, et al (1981) The choice of operation for bronchial carcinoids. *Ann Thorac Surg* **1:** 19-22.
3. Price JC Lt Col, Percarpio B, Murphy PW, et al (1979) Recurrent adenoid cystic carcinoma of the trachea: Intraluminal radiotherapy. *Otolaryngol Head Neck Surg* **5:** 614-623.
4. Rowe LD and Jafek BW (1979) Bronchial adenoma: A malignant misnomer. *The Laryngoscope* **12:** 1991-1999.
5. deGruneck JM and Naef AP (1977) Adenomas bronchiques. *Schweiz Med Worchenschr* **107:** 259-266.
6. Marks C and Marks M (1977) Bronchial adenoma. *Chest* **3:** 376-380.
7. Goldstraw P, Lamb D, McCormack RJM and Walbaum PR (1976) The malignancy of bronchial adenoma. *J Thorac Cardiovasc Surg* **72:** 309.
8. Simpson JA, Smith F, Mutz LR and Hodge AJ (1974) Bronchial adenoma: A review of 26 cases. *Aust & New Zealand J Surg* **44:** 10-116.
9. Walker C (1974) Bilateral choroidal metastases from "adenoma: of bronchus." *Br J Opth* **58:** 625-629.
10. Burchart F and Axelsson C (1972) Bronchial adenomas. *Thorax* **27:** 442-449.
11. Tolis GA, Fry WA, Head L and Shields TW (1972) Bronchial adenomas. *Surg Gynec & Obstet* **134:** 605-610.
12. Turnbull AD, Huvos AG, Doodner JT and Beattie, EJ (1972) The malignant potential of bronchial adenoma. *Ann Thoracic Surg* **14:** 453-464.
13. Meffert WG and Lindskog GE (1970) Bronchial adenoma. *J Thoracic and Cardiovasc Surg* **59:** 588-602.
14. O'Grady WP, McDivitt RW, Holman CW and Moore SW (1970) Bronchial adenomas. *Arch Surg* **101:** 558-561.
15. Smith RA (1969) Bronchial carcinoid tumors. *Thorax* **24:** 43-50.
16. Donahue JK, Weichert RF and Ochsner JL (1968) Bronchial adenoma. *Ann Surg* **167:** 873-885.
17. Baldwin JN and Grimes OF (1967) Bronchial adenomas. *Surg Gynec Obstet* **124:** 813-818.
18. Brindley Jr GV and Bannet JD (1967) Bronchial adenoma and the carcinoid syndrome. *Ann Surg* **165:** 670-680.
19. Batson JF, Gale JW and Hickey RC (1966) Bronchial adenomata. *Arch Surg* **92:** 623-630.
20. Reichle FA and Rosemond GP (1966) Mucoepidermoid tumors of the bronchus. *J Thoracic and Cardiovas Surg* **51:** 443-448.
21. Bower G (1965) Bronchial adenoma. *Am Rev Resp Dis* **92:** 558-563.
22. Markel SF and Abell MR (1964) Adenocystic basal cell carcinoma of the trachea. *J Thoracic & Cardiovas Surg* **48:** 211-225.
23. Markel SF, Abell MR, Haight C and French AJ (1964) Neoplasms of bronchus commonly designated as adenomas. *Cancer* **17:** 590-608.
24. Wilkins EW, Darling RC, Soitter L and Sniften RC (1963) A continuing clinical survey of adenomas of the trachea and bronchus in a general hospital. *J Thoracic & Cardiovasc Surg* **46:** 279-291.
25. Zellos S (1962) Bronchial adenoma. *Thorax* **17:** 61-68.
26. Goodner JT, Berg JW and Watson WL (1961) The nonbenign nature of bronchial carcinoids and cylindromas. *Cancer* **14:** 539-546.
27. Weisel W, Lepley Jr D and Watson RR (1961) Respiratory tract adenomas: A ten year survey. *Ann Surg* **154:** 898-902.
28. Weiss L and Ingram M (1961) Adenomatoid bronchial tumors. *Cancer* **14:** 161-178.
29. Payne WS, Ellis FH, Woolner LB and Moersch HJ (1959) The surgical treatment of cylindroma (adenoid cystic carcinoma) and mucoepidermoid tumors of the bronchus. *J Thorac Cardiovasc Surg* **38:** 709.
30. Vieta, JO and Maier HC (1957) The treatment of adenoid cystic carcinoma (cylindroma) of the respiratory tract by surgery and radiation therapy. *Dis Chest* **31:** 493-511.
31. Ricketts MM, Price T and Thomas M (1955) Choroidal metastasis of bronchial adenoma. *Am J Opth* **39:** 33-36.
32. Muller H, Quoted by Engelbreth-Holm J (1945) Benign bronchial adenomas, *Acta Chir Scand* **90:** 383.

Bursitis, Synovitis and Tendinitis

Bursitis, synovitis and tendinitis are inflammatory discomforts having ill-defined natural histories. Although some experience in the literature exists for radiotherapy, the evidence does not convincingly demonstrate therapeutic benefit. The national survey of radiation oncologists indicates 65% would not treat tendinitis and 48% would not treat bursitis. The 30% of respondents who favor treatment for bursitis would do so only under the most stringent of criteria. Three randomized studies cited below (cf. Plenk, Goldie and Valtonen) conclude there is "no benefit" derived from treatment. Treatment with radiation for these disorders is not recommended.

Bursitis Radiotherapy

Author, Year	Total # Pts.	Technical Details	Time/Dose	Results	Complications/Comments
Milone and Copeland, 1961	136	250Kv, 15ma, 1.95mm Cu filtration, FSD 50cm Field size: 10 x 10cm Three fields: anterior, posterior and lateral.	450r(air)/3F/3 days alternating between the three portals.	Immediate results (3 days-4 weeks) Acute cases: 49/54(90.7%) favorable response Subacute cases: 11/14(78.6%) favorable response Chronic cases: 15/24(62.5%) favorable response Chronic cases with acute exacerbation: 34/44(77.3%) favorable response	Roentgenographic evidence of tissue calcification was present in all cases. Acute: A few days to 2 weeks. Subacute: 3-8 weeks. Chronic: 3 or more months.
Arner et al, 1958	80	None given	700r/10 days	Late results Acute cases: 45/45(100%) good results Chronic cases: 11/12 (91.7%) good results Chronic with acute exacerbation: 15/23(65.2%) good results.	Calcific deposits in all cases.
Shoss and Otto, 1955	153	140Kv, 15ma, 0.25mm Cu plus 1mm Al filtration. HVL 0.5mm Cu, FSD 50cm. Two 15 x 15cm ports to the shoulder, one anterior, one posterior	450r(air)/3F/5 days to each port. Anterior and posterior ports treated on alternate days.	Immediate Results Acute cases: 84/88(95.4%) favorable results Chronic cases: 56/65(86.1%) favorable results.	64.4% of those x-rayed showed calcium deposits. Acute: 10 days or less Chronic: Longer than 10 days.
King and Mahaffey, 1953	456	200Kv, 0.5mm Cu plus 1mm Al filtration, FSD 50cm Field Size: 10 x 15 to 15 x 20cm	125-150r(air) may be repeated in 24-48 hrs. Third treatment, if necessary, given 2-3 days following 2nd treatment. Fourth treatment may be given 1 week later.	83% completely relieved of pain and function re-established 14% recurrences	8% involvement of sites other than the shoulder
Garber, 1952	111	200Kv, 0.5mm Cu plus 1mm Al filtration, FSD 50cm One portal, 10 x 10cm to the anterior-lateral aspect of the shoulder	450r(air)/3F/1 week, repeated for chronic cases.	92.8% good results	57.6% had calcification.
Kratzman and Frankel, 1952		200Kv, 15ma, 0.5mm Cu plus 1mm Al filtration, FSD 50cm.	450-600r(air)/3-4F/3-4 days	Immediate results (220 cases) Acute cases: 98.1% favorable results. Subacute cases: 95.6% favorable results. Chronic cases: 75.5% favorable results. Late Results 80.6%	87.3% of those x-rayed showed calcification. Acute: 1 week or less. Subacute: 1-4 weeks. Chronic: Longer than 4 weeks.

Historical Data: Bursitis Radiotherapy

Author, Year	Total # Pts.	Technical Details	Time/Dose	Results	Complications/Comments
Mann, 1952	52	200Kv, 0.25mm Cu	75-150r/treatment usually 2-6 treatments are given. Treatments given every 2-5 days.	47/52(90%) satisfactory response	No calcium in only 2 patients.
Plenk, 1952	38	400Kv, 5mm 2mm Cu plus 1mm Al filtration, HVL 3.75mm Cu, FSD 70cm Field size: 10 x 10 or 10 x 15cm	450r(air)/3F/5 days.	15/21 definite improvement Controls (no treatment) 15/17 definite improvement	Calcification in 82% of controls, 81% of the treated group.
Witt and Titterington, 1952	50	1. Deep therapy (37 pts): 200Kv, 15ma, 1mm Cu plus 1mm Al filtration. 2. Superficial therapy (17 pts): 100Kv, 5ma, 1-3ma Al filtration. Portal size: 100-225 sq cm	225-450r/3F/1 week. Additional treatments (75-150r) at weekly intervals up to a total of 6 treatments may be given.	Acute cases (17): 96.2% good results Chronic cases (33): 85.8% good results. Little significant difference between the deep and superficial therapy	Acute: Less than 1 month. Chronic: Longer than 1 month.
Steen and McCullough, 1951	300	200Kv, 0.5mm Cu. plus 1mm Al filtration, FSD 50cm Field size: 10 x 10cm	600r(air)4F/4 days to the point of maximum tenderness. A further course given if necessary.	251/300(83.6%) favorable results.	68% of those x-rayed had evidence of calcium.
O'Brien, 1950	78	200Kv, 0.5mm Cu plus 1mm Al filtration, FSD 50cm Field size: 15 x 15cm	200r/treatment four to six treatments 4 days apart.	The majority reported relief after the second treatment.	
Lattomus and Hunter, 1949	235	1. Low voltage: 120Kv, 10ma, 4mm Al filtration at FSD 30cm 2. Deep therapy: 200Kv, 15ma, 0.5mm Cu plus 0.5mm Al filtration, FSD 50cm Field Size: Circular, 10cm diam.	1. 400R/2-4F 2. 600R/3F/5 days	1. Low Voltage: Acute cases: 41/45(90.9%) good results. Subacute cases: 50/61(82%) good results Chronic cases: 43/77(55.8%) good results 2. Deep therapy: Acute cases: 4/4 good results 6/10 (60%) good results Chronic cases: 18/38(47.4%) good results.	Acute: Up to 1 week Subacute: Up to 2 months. Chronic: Longer than 2 months.
Hodges and Boyer, 1948	200	120Kv, 0.5mm Cu plus 0.5mm Al filtration, FSD, 25cm	600-800r/3-4F/3-4 days divided between anterior and posterior fields. If the response is slow, an additional 250r to the posterior cervical spine is given.	Acute cases: 89% relief of symptoms. Subacute cases: 75% relief of symptoms.	
Allen, 1947	40	200Kv, 10ma, 0.5mm Cu plus 1mm Al filtration, FSD 50cm Field size: three 3.5 x 7cm or one 10 x 10cm.	400-800r to each of three fields or 800-1000r/4-5F/4-5 days to one field.	27/40(67.5%) complete relief of pain. 31/40(77.5%) complete use of arm.	

Historical Data: Bursitis Radiotherapy (Continued)

Author, Year	Total # Pts.	Technical Details	Time/Dose	Results	Complications/Comments
Gelber, 1947	15	180Kv, 0.5mm Cu plus 1mm Al filtration, FSD 80cm	800–1000r(air)/4–5F of this total dose, approximately 300r are given anteriorally, 300r posteriorally, and 200–300r laterally.	13/15 showed improvement.	
Pohle and Morton, 1947	33	200Kv, 0.5mm Cu plus 1mm Al filtration, HVL 1.05mm Cu, FSD 50cm, or 400Kv, 1.75mm Cu filtration, HVL 2.4mm Cu, FSD 50cm	450r(air)/3F/3 days or 600r(air)/3F/5 days	80% moderate to complete relief.	
Young, 1947	87	180Kv, 8ma, 0.5mm Cu plus 1mm Al filtration, FSD 50cm Portals: 10 x 15 or 15 x 15cm	150r(air)/treatment. One to four treatments were given.	Acute cases: 14/16 complete relief Subacute cases: 19/23 complete relief Chronic cases: 16/48(33%) complete relief.	43.6% incidence of calcification.
Klein, 1946	100	125–200Kv, 5–7ma, FSD 30–40cm	750–1000r/6–8F/7–14 days.	Acute cases (61): 69% reduction in calcification. Subacute cases (11): 36% reduction in calcification. Chronic cases (28): 32% reduction in calcification.	Acute: Less than 1 month. Subacute: 1–2 months. Chronic: Longer than 2 months.
Nobre and De Araujo Cintra, 1944	18	None given	150–200r/treatment Six or more treatments with 2–3 days between treatments	15/18(85%) favorable results	
Baird, 1941	18	200Kv, 18ma, 1mm Cu plus 1mm Al filtration, FSD 50cm Field size: 15 x 15cm angled over the anterior-lateral portion of the shoulder	300r(air) Repeated at intervals of 3–4 weeks if necessary.	16/18 completely cured.	Calcification present in all cases. Acute: 9 cases Subacute: 5 cases Chronic: 5 cases
Pendergrass and Hodes, 1941	90	120Kv, 5ma, 5mm Al filtration or 0.25mm Cu plus 1mm Al filtration, FSD, 30–40cm Or 50 Kv, 0.2mm Cu filtration, FSD 3–5cm	300–450r/3F/ # days	64% benefited.	
Weinberg, 1940	24	180Kv, 4ma, 0.5mm Cu plus 1mm Al filtration, FSD 50cm Field size: 10 x 10cm to 15 x 20cm	100–250r given 2–3 times weekly. Total of 3–12 treatments given.	15/24 complete relief.	

References

1. Milone FP and Copeland MM (1961) Calcific tendinitis of the shoulder joint. *Am J Roent Rad Ther Nucl Med* **85**: 901–913.
2. Arner O, Lindvall N and Rieger A (1958) Calcific tendinitis (tendinitis calcarea) of the shoulder joint. *Acta Chir Scand* **114**: 319–331.
3. Schoss M and Otto TG (1955) Roentgen therapy of subdeltoid tendinitis and bursitis. *Missouri Med* **52**: 855–863.
4. King JC and Mahaffey CK (1953) Bursitis and peritendinitis: the diagnosis and treatment. *South Med J* **56**: 469–474.
5. Garber RL (1952) Some observations on roentgen therapy of bursitis and peritendinitis calcarea of the shoulder. *Ohio State Med J* **48**: 918–919.
6. Kratzman EA and Frankel RS (1952) Roentgen therapy of peritendinitis calcarea of the shoulder. *Radiology* **59**: 826–830.
7. Mann LS (1952) Treatment of subdeltoid bursitis with roentgen therapy. *J Int Coll Surg* **18**: 385–388.
8. Plenk HP (1952) Calcifying tendinitis of the shoulder. *Radiology* **59**: 384–389.
9. Steen OT and McCullough JAL (1951) Supraspinatus tendinitis. *Am J Roent Rad Ther Nucl Med* **65**: 245–254.
10. Witt CM and Titterington PF (1951) Roentgen therapy in bursitis of the shoulder. *J Missouri Med Assoc* **48**: 870–873.
11. O'Brien FW (1950) Roentgen therapy and the relief of pain. *Radiology* **54**: 1–9.
12. Lattomus WW and Hunter LM (1949) Roentgen therapy of subdeltoid bursitis. *Delaware State Med J* **21**: 115–117.
13. Hodges FM and Boyer RA (1948) Roentgen therapy of bursitis. *Virginia Med Monthly* **75**: 547–549.
14. Allen ML (1947) X-ray therapy in the treatment of para-arthritis of the shoulder. *Rocky Mountain Med J* **44**: 621–625.
15. Gelber LJ (1947) X-ray therapy of arthritis and bursitis. *Medical Record* **160**: 344–350.
16. Pohle EA and Morton JA (1947) Roentgen therapy in arthritis, bursitis, and allied conditions. *Radiology* **49**: 19–25.
17. Young BR (1947) The roentgen treatment of bursitis of the shoulder. *Am J Roent Rad Ther Nucl Med* **56**: 626–630
18. Klein I (1946) Treatment of peritendinitis calcarea of the shoulder joint by roentgen irradiation. *Am J Roent Rad Ther Nucl Med* **56**: 366–375.
19. Nobre MOR and de Araujo Cintra RR (1944) Radiotherapy in Duplay's disease. *Am J Roent Rad Ther Nucl Med* **52**: 415–422.
20. Baird LW (1941) Roentgen irradiation of calcareous deposits about the shoulder. *Radiology* **37**: 316–324.
21. Klein I and Klemes IS (1941) Treatment of peritendinitis calcarea in the shoulder joint. *Radiology* **37**: 325–330.
22. Pendergrass EP and Hodes PJ (1941) Roentgen irradiation in the treatment of inflammations. *Am J Roent Rad Ther Nucl Med* **45**: 74–106.
23. Weinberg TB (1940) Arthritis and para-arthritis treated with the roentgen ray. *Am J Roent Rad Ther Nucl Med* **43**: 416–424.

Synovitis Radiotherapy

Author, Year	Total # Knees	Treatment	Results	Notes
Gumpel and Roles, 1975	20	Intra-articular injection of ^{90}Y (resin, citrate, or silicate). Dose: 5mCi Particle size: not stated or surgical synovectomy	Two year follow-up: Irradiation: 3/10 relapses Surgery: 2/10 relapses. Irradiation was superior in terms of side effects, complications, hospital stay, nurse dependency, and rehabilitation.	Patients expressed slightly higher symptomatic improvement with synovectomy than with irradiation, but there was little difference in the objective results. Of four patients who underwent both methods of treatment (one in each knee), all preferred irradiation.
Oka, 1975	48	Intra-articular injection of ^{90}Y resin colloid. Dose: 3–6mCi Particle size: 30–50mm	60% good-excellent results at one year follow up. 46% good-excellent results at 2 years. 33% good-excellent results at 3 years. 17% good-excellent results at 4 years. Leakage to the inguinal lymph nodes reduced from 1600–2090r by recommending 3 days of bedrest following injection.	Rheumatoid knees. Average follow up of 39 months. Crystal synovitis one month after isotope injection (2). Definite correlation between the clinical result and the pretreatment x-ray grading.
Bowen et al, 1975	14	Intra-articular injection of ^{90}Y citrates colloid. Dose: not stated. Particle size: 5–15mm	Subjective improvement in pain, stiffness and swelling and objective improvement in size of infusion and range of motion of the knee in all patients.	Follow up of at least 6 months Procedure was restricted to patients over the age of 40 years due to possible chromosome damage

Historical Data: Synovitis Radiotherapy

Author, Year	Total # Knees	Treatment	Results	Notes
Gumpel et al, 1974	16	Intra-articular injection of ^{90}resin (resin in one knee, citrate in the other).	Greater uptake in regional nodes on the citrate side occurring much earlier than the resin side.	
Bridgman et al, 1973	44	Intra-articular injection of ^{90}Y resin colloid or intra-articular saline injection. (Study was double-blind) Dose: 3mCi, calculated to give approx. 10,000 rads at 1mm and 3,000r at 2mm thickness of tissue. Particle size: 40-50 mm	One year follow up: 13/23(57%) significant sustained improvement in joint range. 8/23(35%) significant sustained improvement of knee circumference. 7/23(30%) the joint effusion completely resolved. ^{90}Y treatment did not prevent worsening of the x-ray appearance of the joint.	All of the patients had undergone other forms of therapy. One third of the patients developed general and local reactions to the ^{90}Y injection.
Jalava, 1973	67	Intra-articular injection of ^{90}Y resin colloid Dose: 6mCi Particle size: 20-50mm	Rheumatoid arthritis: 23/63(36.5%) remission. 24/63(38.2%) partial remission. 16/63(25.3%) no response. Traumatic effusion: 4/4 poor results. All were later operated on. Slight leakage of radioactivity from the knee in 2/22.	Rheumatoid arthritis (63). Traumatic effusion (4). Follow up of 7-19 months.
Winston et al, 1973	9	Intra-articular ^{32}p-chromic phosphate. 100mCi ^{32}P (2 patients) 500mCi ^{32}P (5 patients) 1mCi ^{32}P (2 patients) Particle size: 500-1000mm	No clinical results given; only one case of migration of radioactivity to the inguinal nodes.	Authors suggest that ^{32}p-chromic phosphate has greater stability than materials previously used.
Prichard et al, 1970	10	^{90}Y resin or ^{90}Y silicate 300mCi.	Silicate leaks from the knee joint in the first 24 hours and considerable localization takes place, especially in the liver region. No significant leakage in 3 days with resin.	Based on these results the resin is considered to be a more satisfactory preparation.
Topp and Cross, 1970	18	Intra-articular injection of colloidal ^{198}Au. Dose: 48mC Particle size: 30mm	12/18 complete disappearance of effusion. Percentage escape of radioactivity of the inguinal nodes of 0-37% of injected dose.	All patients had knee effusion persisting for at least 6 months and not controlled by conventional methods. The effusion usually disappeared within 3 months of treatment. There was temporary increased pain and swelling during the first week in 5 cases (2 required aspiration of the joint).
Graham et al, 1970	15	Intra-articular injection of colloidal ^{198}Au. Dose: 12mCi Particle size: Up to 0.02u	11/15 pain relief 11/15 reduction in size of effusion. 4/13 cyst disappeared. Average loss of approx. 0.5mCi from the joint.	The chronic synovial effusion had been resistant to other measures in all patients. Underlying disease was rheumatoid arthritis in the majority of patients. 13/15 had a popliteal cyst. Local reaction requiring aspiration and instillation of prednisone in 3 patients.

Historical Data: Synovitis Radiotherapy (Continued)

Author, Year	Total # Knees	Treatment	Results	Notes
Goldie et al, 1970	4	Radiotherapy: 3 x 200r (knees) 4 x 150r (metatarsophalangeal) 170Kv, HVL 1mm Cu, FSD 40cm	Synovitis genus: 3/3 improved (subjective evaluation) 2/2 improved (objective evaluation) Synovitis metatarsophal: 1/1 same or worse condition (subjective evaluation) 1/1 same (objective evaluation)	
Ahlberg et al, 1969	44	Intra-articular injection of colloidal ^{198}Au Dose: 5mCi in 20ml Particle size: Not stated. Five knees received a second injection 2 months-2 years after first injection.	28/44 no signs of recurrence of effusion. 10/44 improved. 6/44 unchanged. None became worse. Leakage to the liver and lymph nodes was small.	Rheumatoid arthritis (22) Degenerative arthritis (15) Idiopathic arthritis (4) Psoriatic arthritis (3) Average follow up of 3.2 years. Treatment was interrupted in one patient due to pain; the joint later had to be evacuated.
Makin and Robin, 1968	41	Intra-articular injection of colloidal ^{198}Au Dose: 10mCi (knees) 3mCi (ankles) Particle size: 70mm	31/41 cured of their chronic effusion. 3/41 relief for long periods before recurrence (18 months-5 years) 7/41 failures (3 of these had massive effusion, 2 had villonodular synovitis, 2 had loculated effusions). Surface scintillation counts showed only a small degree of centripetal lymph spread.	Normal conservative therapy had failed in all of the patients and the effusion had persisted for at least 6 months. Osteoarthritis (19) Idiopathic hydrops (14) Rheumatoid arthritis (4) Villonodular synovitis (2) Tabetic neuropathy (2)
Fine et al, 1967	11	Intra-articular injection of colloidal ^{198}Au Dose: 10mCi in 10ml Particle size: Not stated.	8/11 improvement in pain and/or effusion.	All patients had rheumatoid arthritis with synovitis and effusion of the knee persisting for at least 6 months and not controlled by usual measures.
Virkkunen et al, 1967	85	Intra-articular injection of colloidal ^{198}Au Dose: 5-10mc Particle size: 20mm	28/85 hydrops disappeared. 39/85 hydrops and tenderness decreased. 18/85 no effect. Considerable diffusion from the joint cavity in 36%. 5/27 radiation dose over 5,000r to the lymph nodes. Liver radiation dose was insignificant.	Rheumatoid hydrops (83) Osteoarthritis (2) Joints other than the knees (shoulder, elbow, metacarphophalangeal and interphalangeal) were also treated but there were too few cases to make conclusions.
Johnson and Christian, 1967	12	Intra-articular colloidal chromic phosphate ^{32}P	Treatment is beneficial for large effusions where little joint destruction has occurred. No significant benefit in effusions associated with moderate or severe joint destruction.	

Historical Data: Synovitis Radiotherapy (Continued)

Author, Year	Total # Knees	Treatment	Results	Notes
Ansell et al, 1963	30	Intra-articular injection of colloidal ^{198}Au Dose: To give calculated dose of 600-800r to the surface of the effusion volume. Particle size: Not stated.	At one year follow up: 16/30 good results 7/30 some benefit 7/30 no effect Results of bilateral knee effusions: 10/14 no effusion (treated knees). 4/14 no effusion (control knees)	Dx: Rheumatoid arthritis (12) Knees/sacroiliac joints affected (5) Juvenile rheumatoid arthritis (5) Knee effusion (4) Psoriatic arthritis (2) Ankylosing spondylitis (2)

Synovitis Alternate Modes of Treatment

Author, Year	Total # Knees	Treatment	Results	Notes
Anttinen and Oka, 1975	19	Intra-articular injection of triamcinolone hexacetonide.	At 1 year follow up: 36% excellent results. 6% moderate results. 58% failure.	All patients had definite or classical rheumatoid arthritis with chronic knee effusions.
	24	Intra-articular injection of triamcinolone-osmic acid.	All 1 year follow up: 39% excellent results. 4.5% good results. 8.5% moderate results. 48% failures.	Calcification of the joint capsule (3)
Nissila, 1975	52	Intra-articular injection of osmic acid and hydrocortisone acetate.	Six month follow up: 35/52(67%) dry.	
	47	Intra-articular injection of hydrocortisone acetate only.	Six month follow up: 20/47(43%) dry.	Statistically significant results.
	48	24 patients with synovitis in both knees. Osmic acid and hydrocortisone acetate was given to the knee more seriously affected, methylprednisolone acetate to the "better" knee.	Six month follow up: Osmic acid and corticosteriod: 16/24(67%) dry. Corticosteriod only: 11/24(46%) dry.	Results not statistically significant
Pilgaard et al, 1974	55	Surgical synovectomy	Patients' assessment of results: 42 good-excellent 11 fair 2 poor Improvement of joint movement in only 25%. Swelling decreased in approximately 66%.	Rheumatoid arthritis (23) Synovitis chronica non specifica (15) Villonodularis pigmentosa (6). Average follow up of 4.2 years.
Ranawat et al, 1972	60	Surgical synovectomy and debridement.	73% improvement in pain and function. This figure diminished with longer follow up due to recurrence of disease, development of valgus and varus deformities, and involvement of the hips.	All had rheumatoid arthritis. Average follow up of 2.8 years.

Historical Data: Synovitis Alternate Modes of Treatment

Author, Year	Total # Knees	Treatment	Results	Notes
Goldie et al, 1970	4	Radiotherapy: 3 x 200r (knees) 4 x 150r (metatarsophalangeal) 170Kv, HV L 1mm Cu, FSD 40cm	Synovitis genus: 3/3 improved (subjective evaluation) 2/2 improved (objective evaluation) Synovitis metatarsophal: 1/1 same or worse condition (subjective evaluation) 1/1 same (objective evaluation)	
Greens et al, 1969	31	Surgical synovectomy and debridement.	79% improvement (rated by the patient). 65% improvement (rated by the examiner). 46.5% definite or probable recurrence.	All had rheumatoid arthritis. Thrombophlebitis (1). Separation of patellar tendon (1).
Stevens and Whitefield, 1966	102	Surgical synovectomy.	93/102 relief of pain. 63/89 improvement of joint motion. 18/89 decrease in joint motion.	Rheumatoid arthritis (100). Psoriatic arthritis (2).
Hurri et al, 1963	36	Intra-articular injection of osmic acid and hydrocortisone acetate.	23/36 still in remission at end of observation period (1-24 months).	All had rheumatoid arthritis. Mean period of remission 7.5 months.

References

1. Anttinen J and Oka M (1975) Intra-articular triamcinolone hexacetonide and osmic acid in persistent synovitis of the knee. *Scand J Rheum* **4**: 125-128.
2. Bowen BM, Darracott J, Garnett ES and Tomlinson RH (1975) Yttrium 90 citrate colloid for radioisotope synovectomy. *Am J Hosp Pharm* **32**: 1027-1030.
3. Gumpel JM, Beer TC, Crawley JCW and Farran HEA (1975) Yttrium 90 in persistent synovitis of the knee - a single centre comparison. The retention and extra-articular spread of four 90Y radiocolloids. *Br J Rad* **48**: 377-381.
4. Gumpel JM and Roles NC (1975) A controlled trial of intra-articular radiocolloids versus surgical synovectomy in persistent synovitis. *Lancet* **1**: 488-489.
5. Nissila A (1975) Osmic acid treatment for rheumatoid synovitis. *Ann Clin Res* **7**: 202-204.
6. Oka M (1975) Radiation synovectomy of the rheumatoid knee with Yttrium 90. *Ann Clin Res* **7**: 205-210.
7. Gumpel JM (1974) The role of radiocolloids in the treatment of arthritis. *Rheum & Rehab* **13**: 1-9.
8. Gumpel JM, Farran HEA and Williams ED (1974) Use of Yttrium 90 in persistent synovitis of the knee. II. Direct comparison of yttrium colloid resin and yttrium citrate. *Ann Rheum Dis* **33**: 126-128.
9. Pilgaard S, Kolind-Sorensen V and Munck J (1974) Synovectomy of the knee. *Acta Orth Scand* **45**: 241-244
10. Ansell BM (1973) Early studies of 198 Au in the treatment of synovitis of the knee. *Ann Rheum Dis* **32**: Supple 1.
11. Bridgman JJ, Bruckner F, Eisen V, Tucker A and Bleehen NM (1973) Irradiation of the synovium in the treatment of rheumatoid arthritis. *Qrtly J Med* **42**: 357-367.
12. Gumpel JM, Williams ED and Glass HI (1973) Use of yttrium 90 in persistent synovitis of the knee. I. Rentention in the knee and spread in body after injection. *Ann Rheum Dis* **32**: 223-227.
13. Ingrand J (1973) Characteristics of radioisotopes for intra-articular therapy. *Ann Rheum Dis* **32**: Suppl 3-9.
14. Jalava S (1973) Irradiation synovectomy: clinical study of 67 knee effusions intra-articularly irradiated with 90 Y resin. *Curr Ther Res* **15**: 395-401.
15. Stevenson AC (1973) Chromosomal damage in human lymphocytes from radioisotope therapy. *Ann Rheum Dis* **32**: Suppl 19-22.
16. Stevenson AC, Bedford J, Dolphin GW, Purrott RF, Lloyd DC, Hill AGS, Hill HFH, Gumpel JM, Williams D, Scott JT, Tamsey NW, Bruckner FE and Fearn CBD (1973) Cytogenetic and scanning study of patients receiving intra-articular injections of gold 198 and yttrium 90. *Ann Rheum Dis* **32**: 112-123.
17. Winston MA, Bluestone R, Cracchiolo A and Bland WH (1973) Radioisotope synovectomy with P 32 chromic phosphate kinetic studies. *J Nuc Med* **14**: 886-889.
18. Hazelman BL (1972) The painful stiff shoulder. *Rheum Phys Med* **11**: 413-421.
19. Ranawat CS, Ecker ML and Straub LR (1972) Synovectomy and debridement of the knee in rheumatoid arthritis (a study of 60 knees). *Arth & Rheum* **15**: 571-581.
20. Oka M, Rekonen A, Ruotsi A and Seppala O (1971) Intra-articular injection of Y-90 resin colloid in the treatment of rheumatoid knee joint effusions. *Acta Rheum Scan* **17**: 148-160.
21. Goldie I, Rosengren B, Moberg E and Hedlin E (1970) Evaluation of radiation treatment of painful conditions of

the locomotor system. A double blind study. *Acta Rad (Ther)* **9**: 311-322.
22. Graham R, Ramsey NW and Scott JT (1970) Radioactive colloidal gold in chronic knee effusions with Baker's cyst formation. *Ann Rheum Dis* **29**: 159-163.
23. Prichard HL, Bridgman JF and Bleehen NM (1970) An investigation of radioactive yttrium (90Y) for the treatment of chronic knee effusions. *Br J Rad* **43**: 466-470.
24. Topp JR and Cross EG (1970) The treatment of persistent knee effusions with intra-articular radioactive gold: Preliminary report. *Canad Med Ass J* **102**: 709-714.
25. Ahlberg A, Mikulowski P and Odelberg-Johnson O (1969) Intra-articular injection of radioactive gold in treatment of chronic synovial effusion in the knee. *Acta Rheum Scand* **15**: 81-89.
26. Greens S, Clayton ML, Leidholt JD, Smyth CJ and Bartholomew BA (1969) Synovectomy and debridement of the knee in rheumatoid arthritis. *J Bone & Joint Surg Am* **51**: 626-642.
27. Makin M and Robin GC (1968) Radioactive colloidal gold in the treatment of chronic synovial effusions. *Proc Roy Soc Med* **61**: 908-910.
28. Fine PH, Farrer PA, Albrecht M and Jacox RF (1967) Intra-articular radioactive gold (198Au) in the treatment of rheumatoid synovitis of the knee. *Arth Rheum* **10**: 278
29. Johnson PM and Christian CC (1967) Colloidal chromic phosphate P32 for treatment of chronic synovial effusions. *J Nuc Med* **8**: 274
30. Virkkunen M, Krusius FE and Heiskanen T (1967) Experiences of intra-articular administration of radioactive gold. *Acta Rheum Scand* **13**: 81-91.
31. Lippincott SW (1966) Radiation therapy in the treatment of bursitis. *Del Med J* **10**: 318-320.
32. Stevens J and Whitefield GA (1966) Synovectomy of the knee in rheumatoid arthritis. *Ann Rheum Dis* **25**: 214-219.
33. Makin M and Robin GC (1964) Chronic synovial effusions treated with intra-articular radioactive gold. *JAMA* **188**: 725-728.
34. Ansell BM, Crook A, Mallard JR and Bywaters EGL (1963) Evaluation of intra-articular colloidal gold Au 98 in the treatment of persistent knee effusions. *Ann Rheum Dis* **22**: 435-439.
35. Hurri L, Sievers K and Oka M (1963) Intra-articular osmic acid in rheumatoid arthritis. *Acta Rheum Scand* **9**: 20-27.

Randomized Studies
1. Valtonen EJ, Liling HG and Malmio K (1975) The value of roentgen irradiation in the treatment of painful degenerative and inflammatory musculoskeletal conditions. *Scand J Rheumatol* **4**: 247-249.
2. Plenk HP (1952) Calcifying tendinitis of the shoulder. *Radiology* **59**: 384-389.

Carcinoid

The use of radiotherapy in the control of carcinoid is related to the non-secretory tumors (5-HIAA). Local regional control with sustained survivorship may be achieved, although maximal dose for site of disease as well as normal tissue tolerance must be taken into account. The role of radiotherapy in secretory carcinoid should be restricted to situations where other modalities such as chemotherapy and 1-131 MIBG cannot palliate the tumor site. In the national survey 85% of radiation oncologists would treat carcinoid.

Carcinoids

Author, Year	Total # Patients	Treatment	Results	Notes
Samlowski et al, 1986	16 Ages 37-77 years 9 Female and 7 Males	Site dependent. 1900r whole abdomen to 5100r to mediastinum.	4/16 achieved remission (25%) Median survival of responders 46 months versus 10 months for the group as a whole.	Unresectable patients. Highest radiation dose gave highest response; carcinoid syndrome responded less frequently.
Keane et al, 1981	28 Mean Age 50 years Ages 19-69 years 13 Females and 15 Males	2000-2500r/4-5 weeks whole abdominal radiation.	5 year survival 35%, median survival 2.5 years; syndrome patients 1.7 years mean survival.	21 of 28 had carcinoid syndrome. All had metastases. 61 carcinoid tumors. 6 of 7 non syndrome patients are 5-year survivors. Minimal follow up 2.5 years.
Gapany-Gapanavicius and Kenan, 1981	1 in larynx Age 55, Male	Excised and given 8000r/90days.	Failed in six months locally, salvaged by surgical excision.	Non-secretory.

Carcinoids (Continued)

Author, Year	Total # Patients	Treatment	Results	Notes
Gaitan-Gaitan et al, 1975	10	Total abdominal irradiation 2500r/25F/5 weeks.	5/10 alive and free of disease, 18 months – 11 years later.	All patients had unresectable disease. None of the survivors had a carcinoid syndrome or elevation of HIAA.
	9	No treatment or localized palliative irradiation.	9/9 died of causes directly related to their disease.	
Robboy et al, 1975	48	45/48 operative removal of tumor (unilateral salpingo-oophorectomy in 40%, bilateral salpingo-oophorectomy with or without hysterectomy in 50%.)	31/42(74%) alive without evidence of disease 1 month – 18 years post-op. 8/12 died without evidence of disease.	All were cases of insular carcinoid of the ovary. 16/48(33%) had evidence of the carcinoid syndrome.
Ryden et al, 1975	30	Appendectomy	No recurrences with up to 24 year follow up.	All were cases of carcinoid tumor of the appendix in children.
Saylor et al, 1975	26	Resection	7.4% overall mortality due to the tumor. 13/26(50%) alive, no evidence of disease at 1–21 years post-op. 4/26 died, no evidence of disease. 2/26 post-op doing well or asymptomatic.	All were cases of bronchial carcinoid tumors.
Zakarial et al, 1975	107	Intramural tumors (45): 1. Surgical resection (26) 2. Local excision (19) Tumors extending into serosa or beyond (39): 3. Curative resection (21) 4. Palliative resection (6) 5. Radiation and/or chemotherapy (12)	1. 5/26(19%) died without disease. 21/26(81%) alive without evidence of disease. 2. 2/19(10.5%) died without disease. 17/19(89.5) alive without evidence of disease. 3. 9/21(43%) died with disease. 9/21(43%) without disease. 2/21(9.5%) alive without evidence of disease. 1/21 alive with disease. 4. 3/6 died with disease. 3/6 died without disease. 5. 12/12 died with disease.	All patients had primary gastrointestinal carcinoid tumors. Intramural tumors (45) Extension of serosa or beyond (39) Five year survival: 38/45(85%) intramural carcinoid 2/39(5%) tumors extending into serosa or beyond.
Morgan et al, 1974	135	Altogether surgery was the sole mode of therapy for 106 patients. None received adjuvant chemotherapy or palliative irradiation. Rectal: 19 biopsy only 4 biopsy and fulguration 14 resection Jejuno-Ileum: 18 resection of small bowel and mesentery Stomach and duodenum: 16 surgical therapy Colon: 8 surgical resection Appendix: 25/27 appendectomy	5 year survival by site of tumor: Rectum 46% Jejuno-Ileum 57% Stomach 50% Duodenum 66% Colon 33% Appendix 80%	All were carcinoid tumors of the gastrointestinal tract. Six patients had elevated levels of 5-HIAA.

Carcinoids (Continued)

Author, Year	Total # Patients	Treatment	Results	Notes
Dent et al, 1973	29	Simple appendectomy (17) Right hemicolectomy (8)	22/25 alive and clinically free of tumor. 1/25 operative death. 2/25 late deaths.	All were carcinoid tumors of the appendix. 8/29(28%) had coexisting tumors.
Swensen et al, 1973	56	Local excision, regional resection, hepatic lobectomy, pulmonary excision, and chemotherapy. 52/56 had some form of surgical treatment. 2/56 with advanced carcinoid syndrome were treated non-operatively. 2/56 found at necropsy.	With metastases (27): Average post-op survival of 4.6 years. 14/27(52%) died from disease 8/27(30%) alive with metastatic disease from 1–14 years. Without metastases (29): 25/29(86%) alive without evidence of disease from 1–17 years post-op.	All were carcinoid tumors of the gastrointestinal tract. Six patients presented with the clinical carcinoid syndrome. Metastatic carcinoid was found in 27 patients.
Ponka, 1973	34	Appendectomy	33/34 successful. Twenty-five patients have been followed for at least 4 years. There has been no evidence of any recurrence. Only one patient in the group died of metastatic carcinoid tumor.	All were cases of carcinoid tumors of the appendix. No patient exhibited the carcinoid syndrome.
Orloff, 1971	38	Diameter of tumor 0.1–1.90cm: 1. Local excision (21) 2. Abdominoperineal resection (2) Diameter of tumor 2.0cm or larger: 3. Local excision (1) 4. Abdominoperineal resection for cure (7) 5. Anterior resection (1) 6. Palliation (6)	1. 21/21 lived more than 5 years disease free. 2. 2/2 lived more than 5 years disease free. 3. 1/1 lived more than 5 years disease free. 4. 4/7(57%) lived more than 5 years disease free 3/7(43%) died of disease or operation. 5. 6/6 died of disease.	All were cases of carcinoid tumor of the rectum. Five year survival: 40% lesions greater than 2cm in diameter. 100% lesions less than 2cm in diameter.
Holsti, 1967	8	1. Appendectomy (4) or hemicolectomy plus extirpation of liver metastases and radiotherapy (1). 2. Laparotomy plus extirpation of liver metastases (1) and/or radiotherapy, 2800r/21 days (2).	1. 5/5 symptom free at follow up of 3–8 years. 2. 3/3 died.	All were intestinal carcinoid tumors.
Vaeth et al, 1962	1	Laparotomy followed by radiotherapy, 3800r(skin dose)/38 days. 1 Mev irradiation, 3ma, no added filtration, HVL 3.2mm Pb, FSD 70cm.	Clinically and histologically the tumor showed no response to irradiation. Patient died of disease 2.5 months later.	Carcinoid of the rectum. Patient had metastatic growths of the liver at laparotomy.

References

1. Samlowski WE, Eyre HJ and Sause WT (1986) Evaluation of the response of unresectable carcinoid tumors to radiotherapy. *Int J Rad Oncol Biol Phys* **12**: 301–305.
2. Gapany-Gapanavicius B and Kenan S (1981) Carcinoid tumor of the larynx. *Ann Otol Rhinol Laryngol* **90**: 42–47.
3. Keane TJ, Rider WD, Harwood AR, Thomas GM and Cummings BJ (1981) Whole abdominal radiation in the management of metastatic gastrointestinal carcinoid tumors. *Int J Rad Oncol Biol Phys* **7**: 1519–1521.
4. Gaitan-Gaitan A, Rider WD and Bush RS (1975) Carcinoid tumors – cure by irradiation. *Int J Rad Oncol* **1**: 9–13.
5. Godwin JD (1975) Carcinoid tumors – an analysis of 2837 cases. *Cancer* **36**: 560–569.
6. Robboy SJ, Norris HJ and Scully RE (1975) Insular carcinoid primary in the ovary. A clinicopathologic analysis of 48 cases. *Cancer* **36**: 404–418.
7. Ryden SE, Drake RM and Franciosi RA (1975) Carcinoid tumors of the appendix in children. *Cancer* **36**: 1538–1542.
8. Saylor DC, Saylor WP and Eggleston JC (1975) Bronchial carcinoid tumors. *Cancer* **36**: 1522–1537.
9. Zakarial YM, Quan SH and Hajdu SI (1975) Carcinoid tumors of the gastrointestinal tract. *Cancer* **35**: 588–591.
10. Morgan JG, Marks C and Hearn D (1974) Carcinoid tumors of the gastrointestinal tract. *Ann Surg* **180**: 720–727.
11. Davis Z, Moertel CG and McIlrath DC (1973) The malignant carcinoid syndrome. *Surg Gyn & Obst* **137**: 637–644.
12. Dent TL, Batsakis JG and Lindenauer SM (1973) Carcinoid tumors of the appendix. *Surg* **73**: 828–831.
13. Ponka JL (1973) Carcinoid tumors of the appendix. Report of thirty-five cases. *Am J Surg* **126**: 77–83.
14. Ricci C, Patrassi N, Mass R, Mineo C and Fobrizio B Jr. (1973) Carcinoid syndrome in bronchial adenoma. *Ann J Surg* **126**: 671–677.
15. Swenson SR, Snow E and Gaisford WD (1973) Carcinoid tumors of the gastrointestinal tract. *Ann J Surg* **126**: 818–822.
16. Stephens JL and Grahme-Smith DG (1972) Treatment of the carcinoid syndrome by local removal of hepatic metastases. *Proc Roy Soc Med* **65**: 444–445.
17. Orloff MJ (1971) Carcinoid tumors of the rectum. *Cancer* **26**: 175–180.
18. Martin RG (1970) Management of carcinoid tumors. *Cancer* **26**: 547–551.
19. Holsti LR (1967) Radiotherapeutic aspects of intestinal carcinoid tumors. *Rad Clin Biol* **36**: 165–177.
20. Cudmore JTP and Groesbeck HP (1964) Comparison of high dosage and low dosage – maintenance therapy with 5-fluorouracil in solid tumors. *Cancer* **17**: 230–232.
21. Groesbeck HP and Cudmore JTP (1963) Evaluation of 5-fluorouracil (5-FU) in surgical practice. *Amer Surg* **29**: 683–691.
22. Vaeth JM, Rousseau RE and Purcell TR (1962) Radiation response of carcinoid of the rectum. A case report. *Am J Roent Rad Ther & Nuc Med* **88**: 967–970.

Complications of Treatment in Pituitary Tumors

Although the risks associated with irradiation of pituitary tumors are considered acceptable, they are not eliminated in current treatment regimens. There is no benefit completely independent of risk, and the following briefly lists reported complications.

References

1. Maat-Schreman MLC, Bots GTAM, Thromeer TWM and Vielvoye GJ (1985) Malignant astrocytoma following radiotherapy for craniopharyngioma. *Brit J Radiol* **58**: 480–482.
2. Anenta C (1983) Occurrence of meningioma 36 years after treatment for craniopharyngioma without radiation therapy. *J Neurosurg* **58**: 947–948.
3. Sogg RL, Donaldson SS and Yorke CH (1978) Malignant astrocytoma following radiotherapy of craniopharyngioma. *J Neurosurg* **48**: 622–627.
4. Harris JR and Levene MB (1976) Visual complications following irradiation for pituitary adenomas and craniopharyngiomas. *Radiology* **120**: 167–171.

Chemodectomas (Non-Chromaffin Paragangliomas)

The majority of non-chromaffin paragangliomas are what is termed chemodectoma, glomus jugulare or carotid-body tumor. It is our opinion, based on modern radiotherapeutic techniques, that surgery and post-operative radiotherapy of 4500 rad, or radiation alone in the 5000 rad range, has significant probability for local control.

Chemodectomas (Non-Chromaffin Paragangliomas)

Author, Year	Total # Patients	Treatment	Results	Notes
Zinreich and Lee, 1986	15	4500-5000r brain stem limit 4500r.	Surgery alone 6/7 NED 7th Salvaged by RT 8/8 Surgery plus radiation NED 6/6 Radiation alone NED (personal communication).	No complications 2-10 years follow up.
Mitchell and Clyne, 1985	12 Ages 35-73 years. All Females. 6 Glomus juglare 4 Carotid body 2 Vagal body	Radiotherapy: 4000/6600r.	9 complete response. 1 no response.	No complications. Follow up 1.5-15 years.
Cummings et al, 1984	45 Age 17-81 years 35 Females 14 Males	Radiotherapy: 3500r/ 3 weeks.	No deaths from tumors. 3/45 not controlled; symptomatic relief achieved in majority.	3/23 years follow up. 14 references are reviewed in tabular form with 3000-6500r given.
Lybbert et al, 1984	28 Mean Age - 42 years. 6 Females 22 Males	Radiotherapy: 4000/6000r.	All patients had tumor control.	1.5-18 years follow up.
Sharma et al, 1984	42	Radiotherapy: 3000/8000r (author recommends 5000-6500r)	Tympanic (92%) 22/24 controlled. Jugular 11/16 (69%) controlled. 7 patients no local control with doses 3000-4000r.	Complications: 4 Osteoradionecrosis: (2 received > 8000r, 1 had 5000r plus radium, 1 had 4000r and infection)
Reddy et al, 1983	17 14 Females 3 Males	Surgery and/or radiotherapy.	16 patients alive and disease controlled.	All glomus jugulare tumors. Follow up 2-22 years.
Dickens et al, 1982	18	Radiotherapy: 3700/5600r.	All irradiated patients had regression. Of 8 patients with cranial nerve paralysis, 5 recovered.	3 year follow up minimum. All of temporal bone.
Hurst, 1981	12 Ages 20-80 years. 8 Females 4 Males	Radiotherapy: 2400/5200r.	4 of 12 alive > 10 years. 2 cases with tumor present. 3 died.	
Kim et al, 1980	40 Average Age 54 years. Ages 15-78 years 13 Females 1 Male	Radiotherapy with/without surgery. 4000r post-operative 5000r inoperable.	Post-operative XRT - 85% control. Definitive XRT - 88% control.	Analysis of literature 22% recurrence with < 4000r/4 weeks. 2% recurrence with > 4000r. Follow up: 5-30 years.
Gibbin and Henk, 1978	14	Radiotherapy: 4250-5500r.	2 deaths from tumor progression.	Follow up mean 8.7 years.

Chemodectomas (Non-Chromaffin Paragangliomas)

Historical Data: Chemodectomas (Non-Chromaffin Paragangliomas)

Author, Year	Total # Patients	Treatment	Results	Notes
Arthur, 1977	26 15 Females 11 Males	Radiotherapy: 4500/5000r.	2 tumor recurrences. Others - disease free. One recurrence in patient who received 3000r.	
Bundi, 1974	25	Glomus jugulare tumors (19): Radiotherapy preceded by biopsy/exploration of the ear or mastoidectomy (18 pts). One patient received no treatment. 4500-6000r/24-43 days 4 Mev in most cases. Carotid body tumors (4): Radiotherapy, 5000-6000r/26-32 days, orthovoltage or megavoltage. Aortic body tumor: Radiotherapy, 5055r/20.F/28 days, 4 Mev. Chemodectoma of the larynx Section of the IXth cranial nerve followed by right partial laryngectomy 3 years later. Recurrence treated with radiotherapy, 6000r/30 F/39 days, 4 Mev.	Glomus jugulare tumors: 3/19 died, all had cranial nerve involvement at death. Carotid body tumors: 2/4 died Aortic body tumor: Patient developed adenocarcinoma of the breast 1 year later. Histology of the breast tumor and mediastinal tumor were not the same. Chemodectoma of the larynx: Recurrence following surgery. Patient continued to deteriorate and died 2.5 years following the partial laryngectomy.	Location of chemodectoma: Glomus jugulare (19) Carotid body (4) Aortic body (1) Larynx (1)
Jackson and Koshiba, 1974	32	1. Radiotherapy at any time during treatment (i.e. pre-op., post-op., or primary treatment) 2. Radiotherapy as first treatment 3. Megavoltage x-ray therapy at any time during treatment. 4. Megavoltage x-ray therapy as first treatment. Details of Radiotherapy: 4500r/21 days.	1. 14/23(61%) primary control at 5 years. 2. 8/14(57%) primary control at 5 years. 3. 12/17(71%) primary control at 5 years. 4. 8/9(89%) primary control at 5 years.	Four patients receiving radiotherapy as primary treatment died from possible cerebral necrosis caused by high dose radiation.
Spector et al, 1974	19	1. Radiation (10) 2. Pre-op radiation and surgery (4) 3. Post-op radiation (5)	1. 8/10 tumor persistence 2. 0/4 tumor persistence 3. 3/5 tumor persistence	All were glomus jugulare tumors. This series includes some of the patients in the previously published series by Spector et al.
Spector et al, 1975	15	1. Irradiation alone (10) 4600-6000r Co^{60} tumor dose. 2. Post-operative irradiation (5) 5000-7000r Co^{60} tumor dose. 3. Pre-operative irradiation (5) 4600-6000r Co^{60} tumor dose.	1. 3/10 no visible tumor 2/10 persistent but smaller 2/10 persistent, no progression 3/10 recurrent (were later successfully treated by surgical resection). 2. 2/5 no visible tumor 3/5 recurrent 3. 4/5 no visible tumor 1/5 recurrent	All were glomus jugulare tumors. Follow up of 2-27 years.

Historical Data: Chemodectomas (Non-Chromaffin Paragangliomas) (Continued)

Author, Year	Total # Patients	Treatment	Results	Notes
Tidwell and Montague, 1975	19	1. Surgery alone (2 pts). 2. Radiotherapy (17 pts) after biopsy or partial excision. Tumor dose of 4500–5000r in 4.5–5 weeks. Technical details: Co^{60} anteroposterior or superoinferior wedged filters (16 pts) 22 Mev x-rays and 10 Mev electrons through a single lateral field (1 pt).	1. One pt. alive and free of disease at 13 years following treatment. One patient had a recurrence at 110 months for which he received radiotherapy but died with intracranial extension 18 months later. 2. 16/17 no recurrence at 4–18 year follow up. One patient died 3 years following radiotherapy. Autopsy showed encephalomalacia in the rt. temporal lobe, pons, right cerebellar lobe, and focal necrosis at the right occipital lobe.	All were chemodectomas of the temporal bone.
Alldredge et al, 1973	2	Radiotherapy: 5000r/ 22–25F/5 weeks, Co^{60}.	Symptoms have disappeared.	Glomus jugulare tumors.
Moore et al, 1973	33	Group 1 (Tympanic): 1. Total resection (8) 2. Total resection plus radiotherapy (1), 3600r/16F/ 3 weeks. 3. Subtotal resection plus radiotherapy (1) 4. Biopsy only (1) Group 2 (Tympanomastoid): 1. Total resection (3) 2. Total or subtotal resection plus radiotherapy (3), (3000r/16F/3 weeks to 6054r/30F/6 weeks). 3. Biopsy only (1) Group 3 (Petrosal-Extrapetrosal): 1. Total resection (4) 2. Total or subtotal resection plus radiotherapy (5) 3150–5500r/18–25F/3–5 weeks. 3. Radiotherapy plus biopsy in some cases (5) 3900–5500r/25–29F/5 weeks.	Group 1: 1. 7/8 no progression at 3–12 years. 1/8 recurred at 2 years. 2. No progression at 14 years. 3. Progressive disease to death 30 years later. 4. Alive at 2 years. Group 2: 1. 2/3 no progression at 2 and 12 years. 1/3 recurred. 2. 3/3 no progression at 4, 10 and 12 years. 3. Alive at 3 years. Group 3: 1. 2/3 recurred. 2. 5/5 no progression at 1–15 years. 3. 5/5 no progression at 1–9 years.	
Newman et al, 1973	20	1. Surgery only (14). 2. Radiotherapy followed by surgery (2). 3. Surgery followed by planned radiotherapy (2). 4. Radiotherapy only (2). Details of Radiotherapy: 4600–5500r/6–8 weeks.	1. 11/14 recurred (10 within three years). Recurrences treated by radiotherapy: 7/8 no clinical evidence of disease at follow up of 5 months – 10 years. 2. No recurrences at 4 and 7 years post-op. 3. No evidence of disease at 5 and 7 years post-op. 4. No evidence of disease at 18 months in one patient. Symptoms improved in the other patient but was lost to follow up at 4 months.	All were tumors of the middle ear. One lost to follow-up. Two died of other causes. Most common surgical complication was damage to the facial nerve. No findings of cerebral necrosis.

Historical Data: Chemodectomas (Non-Chromaffin Paragangliomas) (Continued)

Author, Year	Total # Patients	Treatment	Results	Notes
Rosenwasser, 1973	30	Lesions with extensive involvement of the middle ear, mastoid and temporal bone: 1. Irradiation only (10 patients). 2. Surgery plus irradiation (4 patients). 3. Surgery only (2 patients). Lesions confined to middle ear and mastoid bones. 4. Radical mastoidectomy (12 patients). 5. Radical mastoidectomy plus irradiation (2 patients).	1. 4/10 alive, no symptoms except for tinnitus in two patients. 1/10 was asymptomatic for 20 years but has trouble now. 3/10 died with persistent disease. 1/10 alive, less bleeding. 1/10 lost to follow up. 2. 1/4 well with no evidence of disease at 5 years. 2/4 symptom free at 3–10 years. 1/4 died with persistent recurrent disease. 3. 1/2 died. 1/2 doing well, but surgery involved local removal of ear. 4. 11/12 well (9 have no persistent or recurrent disease). 1/12 died. 5. 1/2 well. 1/2 recurred, 2nd course of irradiation, is now symptom free.	Glomus jugulare tumors.
Silverstone, 1973	6	1. Radiotherapy only (5 patients) 4000–5000r/5–7 weeks. 2. Excision plus radiotherapy (1 patient) 4500r/5.5 weeks.	1. Good symptomatic response in all patients. Symptoms decreased or disappeared and size of tumor decreased. 2. Patient well at 6 years after treatment.	All were glomus jugulare tumors. One patient was being treated for a recurrence.
Smith et al, 1973	1	Radiotherapy, 5000r/5 weeks, 2 Mev, to the entire nasopharynx, the posterior 4 centimeters of the nasal cavity, the sphenoid sinus, posterior ethmoid sinuses and posterior one half of the orbits. An additional 1000r was later given to the nasopharynx, posterior nasal cavity and sphenoid sinus.	Tumor no longer observed in the nasopharynx. Patient remains asymptomatic at 3 year follow up.	Chemodectomas of the nasopharynx.
Spector et al, 1973	46	1. Surgery alone (25 pts) 2. Surgery followed by radiotherapy (5 pts) 3. Radiation only (10 pts)	1. 73% no recurrence 2. 40% 3. 20%	All were tumors of the middle ear. Resectable lesions were operated on as the first choice of therapy. Unresectable lesions and patients in poor health received radiation.
Brackmann et al, 1972	7	Initial treatment: 1. Surgery plus radiotherapy (4 pts), 800–3000r. 2. Surgical removal (1). 3. Surgical removal (1). 4. Biopsy plus irradiation (1), 2900r.	1. 4/4 symptoms recurred or progressed. 2. Symptoms progressed. 3. Recurrence of symptoms at 5 years. 4. Definite decrease in the size and vascularity of the tumor, but mass resembling granuloma persisted. Therefore, radical mastoidectomy was done 9 months later. Patient free of disease at 4 years.	Glomus jugulare tumors.

Historical Data: Chemodectomas (Non-Chromaffin Paragangliomas) (Continued)

Author, Year	Total # Patients	Treatment	Results	Notes
Coleman et al, 1972	1	Radiotherapy, 4500r to base of skull and rt. petrous bone.	At presentation the tumor involved 6 cranial nerves. Radiotherapy was of no benefit.	Glomus jugulare tumor.
Glover and Block, 1972	7	1. Mastoidectomy and/or craniotomy plus radiotherapy (4 pts). 2. Tympanotomy plus radiotherapy (1). 3. Radiotherapy only (1). 4. No treatment. Radiotherapy: 3425–5500r.	Follow up of 1–18 years: 1. 3/4 no visible signs of tumor. 1/4 regression in size. 2. Regression in size. 3. No visible signs of tumor. 4. No change.	Glomus jugulare tumors (6). Glomus tympanum tumor (1).
Hatfield et al, 1972	32	1. Irradiation only (4). 2. Surgery plus post-op irradiation (12). 3. Surgery only (16). Details of radiotherapy 3000–4500r Co^{60} through one or more portals.	Recurrences: 1. 0/4 2. 3/12 3. 8/16 (seven of these received radiotherapy for recurrence).	1. All patients in this group were inoperable. 2. 10/12 were incompletely excised.
Hudgins, 1972	9	Radiotherapy: 4000–5000r/ 4 weeks (patients were treated 4 days/week). 2 Mev or Co^{60}. Wedged fields.	Follow up of 1–7 years. Pain relief and tumor shrinkage followed treatment in all cases, but two patients still have tumor masses.	All were tumors of the middle ear.
Westbrook et al, 1972	20	Resection (18 pts). One patient refused surgery. One patient was observed only.	Complications: Mortality (0). CNS damage (0). Permanent nerve damage (6). Auriculotemporal syndrome (2). Pain in temporal mandibular joint (2).	Chemodectomas of the neck – the majority were carotid body tumors. Authors stated that they would employ irradiation in patients who refuse surgery or have unresectable, residual, or metastatic disease.
Guttman, 1971	1	Radiotherapy.	Originally involvement of the 8th and 9th cranial nerves. Patient is asymptomatic and free of disease at 7 years following radiotherapy.	Glomus jugulare tumor.
Maruyama et al, 1971	1	Partial resection followed by radiotherapy, 5000r/30 days, Co^{60}.	Patient free of disease at 3 years.	All were tumors of the glomus jugulare.
	1	Attempted mastoidectomy, but profuse bleeding occurred. Radiotherapy 500r/5 weeks, Co^{60}.	Symptoms disappeared but angiographically a mass is still present.	
	1	Craniotomy. Radiotherapy 6000r/6 weeks, Co^{60}, to recurrence.	Patients improved for 6 months following surgery but then deteriorated. Excellent clinical response to radiotherapy.	
Myers et al, 1971	1	Radiotherapy, 5580r/29F/ 44 days.	Mass receded but no change in the patient's neurological deficit. Patient died one year later due to radiation necrosis of the rt. temporal lobe.	Glomus jugulare tumor.

Historical Data: Chemodectomas (Non-Chromaffin Paragangliomas) (Continued)

Author, Year	Total # Patients	Treatment	Results	Notes
Spitzer et al, 1971	1	Laparotomy – tumor was considered not resectable because it was "intimately attached to bone" Radiotherapy: 5000r/5 weeks 6 Mev. Surgery – subtotal cystectomy.	There was no palpable decrease of the mass following radiotherapy. Surgery, subtotal cystectomy, was undertaken. Tumor was found at the margin of the surgical specimen. No further follow up reported.	Functioning non-chromaffin paraganglioma (chemodectoma) of the urinary bladder. This is an unusual site for a non-chromaffin paraganglioma.
Diepeveen et al, 1969	9 Average age 58 years. All Females.	Radiotherapy: 4000r/5 weeks to 6000r/6 weeks.	2 patients had complete remission – 5 year follow up. 3 patients had no further progression – 18 months to 6 year follow up.	
Oberman et al, 1968	40	Carotid Body & Vagal Body Tumors: 1. Excision (10 patients, 7 of these had carotid body tumors, 3 had vagal body tumors). 2. Subtotal excision (6, all carotid body tumors). 3. Radiotherapy (1, carotid body tumor). Glomus Jugulare Tumors: 4. Resection through a lymphanotomy (6 glomus jugulare tumors). 5. Mastoidectomy or diagnostic biopsy plus radiotherapy (7). 6. Radical mastoidectomy (10).	Carotid Body & Vagal Body Tumors: 1. 1/10 recurred, treated by radiotherapy and was asymptomatic for the subsequent 6 years. 2. 4/6 recurred. 3. No regression. Glomus Jugulare Tumors: 4. 2/6 recurred. 5. 1/7 recurred. 6. 6/10 recurred.	Chemodectomas of the head and neck. Location: Carotid body (14). Glomus jugulare (23). Vagal body (3).
Parisier and Sinclair, 1968		Radiotherapy: 4500r/1 month, Co^{60} and 20 Mev. Subsequent excision.	Lesion did not change appreciably over the next 7 months. Lesion was then excised. No recurrences to date.	Glomus tumor of the nasal cavity.

References

1. Zinreich ES and Lee DJ (1986) Radiotherapy for the treatment of paraganglioma in the temporal bone. *Ear Nose Throat J* **65**: 54–57.
2. Mitchell DC and Clyne CAC (1985) Chemodectomas of the neck: The response to radiotherapy. *Brit J Surg* **72**: 903–905.
3. Cummings BJ, Beale FA, Garrett PG, Harwood AR, Keane TJ, Payne DG and Rider WB (1984) The treatment of glomus tumors in the temporal bone by megavoltage radiation. *Cancer* **53**: 2635–2640.
4. Lybbert ML, van Andel JG, Eijkenboom WM, deJong PC and Knegt P (1984) Radiotherapy of paragangliomas. *Clin Otolaryngol* **9**: 105–109.
5. Shama PD, Johnson AP and Whitton AC (1984) Radiotherapy for jugulo-tympanic paragangliomas (glomus jugulare tumors). *Journal of Laryngology and Otology* **98**: 621–629.
6. Reddy EK, Mansfield CM and Hartman GV (1983) Chemodectoma of glomus jugulare. *Cancer* **52**: 337–340.
7. Dickens WJ, Million RR, Cassisi NJ and Singleton GT (1982) Chemodectomas arising in temporal bone structures. *Laryngoscope* **92**: 188–191.
8. Routh A, Hickman BT, Hardy JD and Suvarna L (1982) Malignant chemodectoma of posterior mediastinum. *Southern Medical Journal* **75**: 879–881.
9. Hurst WB (1981) Glomus jugulare tumors. A review of twelve cases treated with radiotherapy. *Journal of Laryngology and Otology* **95**: 581–588.
10. Kim JA, Elkon D, Lim ML and Constable WC (1980) Optimum dose of radiotherapy for chemodectomas of the middle ear. *Int J Radiation Biol Phys* **6**: 815–819.
11. Wang CC (1980) What is the optimal dose of radiation therapy for glomus tumors? *Int J Radiation Oncol Biol Phys* **6**: 945–946.
12. Gibbin KP and Henk JM (1978) Glomus jugulare tumors

in South Wales - A twenty-year review. *Clin Radiol* **29**: 607-609.
13. Arthur K (1977) Radiotherapy in chemodectoma of the glomus jugulare. *Clin Radiol* **28**: 415-417.
14. Spector GJ, Compagno J, Perez CA, Maisel RH and Ogura JH (1975) Glomus jugulare tumors: Effects of radiotherapy. *Cancer* **35**: 1316-1321.
15. Tidwell TJ and Montague ED (1975) Chemodectomas involving the temporal bone. *Radiology* **116**: 147-149.
16. Bundi RS (1974) Chemodectomas. *Clin Radiol* **25**: 293-302.
17. Jackson AW and Koshiba R (1974) Treatment of glomus jugulare tumors by radiotherapy. *Proc R Soc Med* **67**: 267-270.
18. Spector GJ, Maisel RH and Ogura JH (1974) Glomus jugulare tumors. II. A Clinico-pathologic analysis of the effects of radiotherapy. *Ann Otol* **83**: 26-32.
19. Alldredge CB, Tabb HG and Dunlap CE (1973) Glomus jugulare tumors: Review and report of two cases. *Southern Med J* **66**: 563-567.
20. Howell A, Monasterio J and Stuteville UH (1973) Chemodectomas of the head and neck. *Surg Clin North Am* **53**: 175-177.
21. Moore GR, Robbins JP, Seale, DL, Fitz-Hugh GS and Constable WC (1973) Chemodectomas of the middle ear. *Arch Otolaryngol* **98**: 330-335.
22. Newman H, Rowe JF and Phillips TL (1973) Radiation therapy of the glomus jugulare tumor. *Am J Roent* **118**: 663-669.
23. Rosenwasser H (1973) Long-term results of therapy of glomus jugulare tumors. *Arch Otolaryngol* **97**: 49-54.
24. Silverstone SM (1973) Radiation therapy of glomus jugulare tumors. *Arch Otolaryngol* **97**: 43-48.
25. Smith CJ, Kohut RI and Million RR (1973) Chemodectomas of the nasopharynx. *Laryngoscope* **83**: 330-335.
26. Spector GJ, Maisel RH and Ogura JH (1973) Glomus tumors in the middle ear. I. An analysis of 46 patients. *Laryngoscope* **83**: 1652-1672.
27. Brackmann DE, House WF, Terry R and Scanlan RL (1972) Glomus jugulare tumors: Effect of irradiation. *Trans Am Acad Opth & Otolaryngol* **76**: 1423-1431.
28. Coleman MJ, Tonkin J, Bleasel K and Lim GHK (1972) Glomus jugulare tumor: A case report. *Aust & NZ J Surg* **42**: 64-68.
29. Glover GW and Block J (1972) Glomus jugulare tumors - radiotherapy or surgery. *Br J Surg* **59**: 947-953.
30. Hatfield PM, James AE and Schultz MD (1972) Chemodectomas of the glomus jugulare. *Cancer* **30**: 1164-1168.
31. Hudgins PT (1972) Radiotherapy for extensive glomus jugulare tumors. *Radiology* **103**: 427-429.
32. Maruyama Y (1972) Radiotherapy of tympano jugular chemodectomas. *Radiology* **103**: 659-663.
33. Westbrook KC, Guillamondegui OM, Medellin H and Jesse RH (1972) Chemodectomas of the neck. Selective management. *Am J Surg* **124**: 760-766.
34. Guttman R (1971) Unusual radiation response in various inoperable radioresistant tumors. *Am J Roent* **111**: 350-354.
35. Maruyama Y, Gold LHA and Kieffer SA (1971) Radioactive cobalt treatment of glomus jugulare tumors. *Acta Radiol* **10**: 239-247.
36. Myers EN, Newman JP, Kaseff L and Black FO (1971) Glomus jugulare tumor - a radiographic-histologic correlation. *Laryngoscope* **81**: 1838-1851.
37. Spitzer R, Borrison R and Castellino RA (1971) Functioning non-chromaffin paraganglioma (chemodectoma) of the urinary bladder. *Radiology* **98**: 577-578.
38. Ahmed A, Doge OG and Kirk RS (1969) Chemodectoma of the orbit. *J Clin Path* **22**: 584-588.
39. Diepeveen J, Hentzer E and Rovsing H (1969) Non-chromaffin paragangliomas. *Acta of Laryngologica* **68**: 142-155.
40. McNeil R and Bras G (1969) Tumors of the chemoreceptor system. *West Ind Med J* **18**: 46-52.
41. House WF and Glasscock ME (1968) Glomus tympanicum tumors. *Arch Otolaryngol* **87**: 550-554.
42. Oberman HA, Holtz F, Sheffer LA and Magielski JE (1968) Chemodectomas (non-chromaffin paragangliomas) of the head and neck. *Cancer* **21**: 838-851.
43. Parisier SC and Sinclair GM (1968) Glomus tumors of the nasal cavity. *Laryngoscope* **78**: 2013-2023.
44. Simonton KM (1968) Paraganglioma (chemodectoma) of the middle ear and mastoid. *JAMA* **206**: 1531-1534.
45. Brown JS (1967) Glomus jugulare tumors. Methods and difficulties of diagnosis and surgical treatment. *Laryngoscope* **77**: 26-67.
46. Fuller AM, Brown HA, Harrison EG and Siekert RG (1967) Chemodectomas of the glomus jugulare tumors. *Laryngoscope* **77**: 218-238.
47. Schermer KL, Pontius EE, Dziabis MD and McQuiston RJ (1966) Tumors of the glomus jugulare and glomus tympanicum. *Cancer* **19**: 1273-1280.
48. Grubb WB and Lampe I (1965) The role of radiation therapy in the treatment of chemodectomas of the glomus jugulare. *Laryngoscope* **75**: 1861-1871.
49. Shapiro MJ and Neues DK (1964) Technique for removal of glomus jugulare tumors. *Arch Otolaryngol* **79**: 219-224.
50. Miller JD (1962) Results of treatment in glomus jugulare tumors with emphasis on radiotherapy. *Radiology* **79**: 430-434.
51. Bradshaw JD (1961) Radiotherapy in glomus jugulare tumors. *Clin Radiol* **12**: 227-228.

Chordoma

Management of chordomas is difficult. Surgical excision alone is inadequate because of location, thus leading to the recommendation of radiation therapy in the majority of patients. Local recurrences are frequent, and the best results have been with radical surgical procedures followed by high doses of radiation. However, this conventional treatment has yielded disappointing long-term survival rates, and new innovative approaches have been sought. Preliminary data using particle therapy suggest improved local control rates. Patients with chordomas should be treated in regional centers on protocols designed to improve therapy over historical experience. Eighty-four percent of radiation oncologists in the national survey would treat chordoma.

Chordoma

Author, Year	Total # Pts.	Site Age	Treatment	Results	Notes
Amendola et al, 1986	21	Clivus - 11 Sacrum - 3 Thoracic Spine - 1 Cervical Spine - 3 Lumbar Spine - 3 Age 7-82 years, mean age 50 years.	Surgery followed by radiotherapy in 17 patients (18%). Doses ranged from 50-66 Gy in 5-6 1/2 weeks.	Irradiation produced significant tumor control with remission of symptoms 1-6 years. Five year actuarial survival was 50%; ten year survival was 20%.	Larger tumor control was achieved with planned post-operative radiation, rather than radiation for recurrent disease. Chordomas of clivus fared better than those of spine.
Belza and Urich, 1986	1	Cervical	Subtotal resection followed by 5500r	During next six years, the patient underwent four subsequent surgical procedures for recurrent disease, demonstrating progressive transformation to malignant fibrous histiocytomas.	The cause of the transformation remains obscure.
Duncan et al, 1986	1	Sacrum	Neutron irradiation, 13.8-18.3 Gy.	Partial response. Patient died at nine months with recurrent local disease.	
Lybeert and Meerwaldt, 1986	18	Sacrococcygeal - 14 Basisphenoid - 3 Lumbar - 1 Age 35-76, mean 61 years.	Radiation only four. Surgery only four. Surgery and post-operative radiation only ten.	The ten patients receiving post-operative radiation fared the best. High doses of radiation (60-65 Gy) gave the longest recurrence-free survival.	Two of 14 irradiated patients developed marginal recurrences suggesting the importance of accurate tumor volume assignment.
Saunders et al, 1986	8	Sacral Age 39-69 years, mean 60 years.	Helium and neon ion beam therapy. 70-80.5 GyE (gray equivalent).	Seven of eight have local control of their tumor.	Follow-up 33 months is too short to assess long-term tumor control rate. No significant complications.
Austin-Seymour et al, 1985	67	Base of skull or cervical spine, chordoma or low-grade chondrosarcoma. Age 7-65 years, mean 40 years.	Subtotal resection followed by proton radiation, 160 MeV protons. Dose - 69 cGE (cobalt gray equivalent).	Actuarial three year local control rate is 89% and five year local control rate is 79%. Four treated failures and two marginal recurrences.	Median follow-up 27 months. Four patients have had severe complications.

Historical Data: Chordoma

Author, Year	Total # Pts.	Site Age	Treatment	Results	Notes
Bernstein and Gutin, 1985	5	Recurrent clivus chordomas.	I^{125} interstitial therapy. Estimated peripheral tumor doses of 5000–15000 rad.	Of five recurrent patients: 2 recurred 19 and 28 months after treatment, 2 died of other causes with stable tumor, and 1 died of progressive tumor outside the irradiated volume.	
Raffel et al, 1985	26	Cranial chordomas. Mean age 39.6 years.	Surgery and radiation therapy including external beam therapy, heavy charged particles and interstitial implants 3600–8000 rad.	Mean follow up was 5.6 years. 14 of 26 patients (54%) survive.	All patients with the chordroid variant of chordoma survive.
Rich et al, 1985	48	Base of skull – 14 Vertebrae – 15 Sacral – 18 Ages 10–79 years.	Surgery alone – 14 Surgical excision and radiation – 17 Biopsy and radiation – 15 Pre-op radiation – 2	Of 48 patients, 14 are alive with no disease, 6 are alive with disease, and 22 patients had local failure. 5 year actuarial survival rate for irradiated patients – 50%.	Higher radiation doses achieved longer responses.
Saunders et al, 1985	19	Base of skull or spinal chordoma – 10 Chordosarcoma – 5 Meningioma – 4.	Helium ion therapy 60–80 GyE (gray equivalent). Mean – 69.	Of 19 patients, 13 alive with no evidence of disease, 2 alive with recurrence, 2 dead with recurrence and 2 stable.	Mean follow up 22 months, too short to assess value.
Chetiyawardana, 1984	69	Sarcrococcygeal – 37 Clivus – 17 Spine – 13 Petrous Bone – 2 Ages 1–86 years, mean age 51 years.	48 patients treated with radiotherapy.	Of 65 evaluable patients, 5 year actuarial survival is 45%, 10 year actuarial survival rate is 23%.	Patients who received radical surgery and radical XRT fared best. 16% developed metastases.
Halpern et al, 1984	1	Sacrum Age 68 years.	7000 rad, 5 years later patient received another 4000r for recurrence.	Two years after second course of radiotherapy patient had biopsy proven sacral malignant fibrous histocytoma with pulmonary metastases.	At autopsy, there was no evidence of chordoma.
Cummings et al, 1983	24	Base of skull – 10 Sacrococcygeal – 12 Spine – 3 Ages 2–77 years, median age 53 years.	All patients had postoperative radiotherapy 3000–6000 cGy.	5 year survival – 62%, 10 year survival – 28%, most patients had residual tumor at death or last follow up.	Some patients received multiple daily fractions.
Reddy et al, 1981	10	Cranial – 5 Lumbar – 1 Sacrococcygeal – 4 Ages 14–73 years, median age 40 years.	Surgery followed by radiation therapy in 8 of the 10. Dose: 4200–8000 rad.	6 or 10 patients recurred. 3 of 10 are alive and disease free.	
Saxton, 1981	19	Basisphenoid – 6 Lumbar – 2 Sacrococcygeal – 11	Surgery followed by radiation in 9, 6 radiation alone, 3 surgery alone.	Radiation – palliates large inoperable tumors. Excision followed by radiation produces best local control	

References

1. Amendola BE, Amendola MA, Oliver E and McClatchey KD (1986) Chordoma: Role of radiation therapy. *Radiology* **158**: 839–843.
2. Belza MG and Urich H (1986) Chordoma and malignant fibrous histiocytoma. Evidence for transformation. *Cancer* **58**: 1082–1087.
3. Duncan W, Arnott SJ and Jack WJL (1986) The Edinburgh experience of treating sarcomas of soft tissues and bone with neutron irradiation. *Clin Radiol* **37**: 317–320.
4. Lybeert ML and Meerwaldt JH (1986) Chordoma. Report on treatment results in eighteen cases. *Acta Radiol [Oncol]* **25**: 41–43.
5. Saunders WM, Castro JR, Chen GTY, Gutin PH, Collier JM, Zink Sr, Phillips TL and Ganger GE (1986) Early results of ion beam radiation therapy for sacral chordoma. *J Neurosurg* **64**: 243–247.
6. Austin-Seymour M, Munzenrider JE, Goitein M, Gentry R, Gragoudas E, Koehler AM, McNulty P, Osborne E, Ryugo DK, Seddon JH, Urie M, Verhey L and Suit HD (1985) Progress in low-LET heavy particle therapy: Intracranial and paracranial tumors and uveal melanomas. *Radiat Res [Suppl]* **5**: 219–226.
7. Bernstein M and Gutin PH (1985) Interstitial irradiation of skull base tumors. *Can J Neurol Sc* **12**: 366–370.
8. Saunders WM, Chan GT, Austin-Seymour M, Castro JR, Collier JM, Gauger G, Gutin P, Phillips TL, Pitluck S, Walton RE and Zink SR (1985) Precision high dose radiotherapy. II. Helium ion treatment of tumors adjacent to critical central nervous system structures. *Int J Radiat Oncol Biol Phys* **11**: 1339–1347.
9. Raffel C. Wright DC, Butin PH and Wilson CB (1985) Cranial chordomas: Clinical presentation and results of operative and radiation therapy in twenty-six patients. *Neurosurgery* **17**: 703–710.
10. Rich TA, Schiller A, Suit HD and Mankin HJ (1985) Clinical and pathologic review of 48 cases of chordoma. *Cancer* **56**: 182–187.
11. Chetiyawardana AD (1984) Chordoma: Results of treatment. *Clin Radiol* **35**: 159–161.
12. Guthrie W (1984) Dundee chordomas. *Scott Med J* **29**: 227–233.
13. Halpern J, Kopolovic J and Catane R (1984) Malignant fibrous histiocytoma developing in irradiated sacral chordoma. *Cancer* **53**: 2661–2662.
14. Cummings BJ, Hodson DI and Bush RS (1983) Chordoma: The results of megavoltage radiation therapy. *Int J Radiat Oncol Biol Phys* **9**: 633–642.
15. Reddy EK, Mansfield CM and Hartman GV (1981) Chordoma. *Int J Radiat Oncol Biol Phys* **7**: 1709–1711.
16. Saxton JP (1981) Chordoma. *Int J Radiat Oncol Biol Phys* **7**: 913–915.

Choroid Plexus Papilloma

Papillomas of the choroid plexus are friable vascular lesions which have a predilection for children. Complete surgical excision is the recommended therapy. Controversies exist regarding the need for post-operative radiation when there is incomplete removal or biopsy only. Certainly some patients who have received post-operative radiotherapy following incomplete surgical excision have been long term survivors. Some of these lesions are large, invasive and non-resectable at the time of presentation. Radiation has been shown to shrink these vascular lesions, allowing complete resection at a later date. As many of these patients are youngsters, attention to late complications such as brain necrosis, and later social or intellectual changes is mandatory. Seventy-three percent of radiation oncologists in the national survey would not treat choroid plexus papilloma.

Choroid Plexus Papilloma

Author, Year	Total # Pts.	Site Age	Treatment	Results	Notes
Aristizabal and Runyon, 1981	1	4th ventricle, 20 mos.	Biopsy, 4500r in 30 fractions in 43 elapsed days.	No neurologic deficits at 3 year follow-up. Continued decrease in size on follow-up CT scans	Surgically unresectable.
Naguib et al, 1981	1	Left cerebellopontine angle with bone involvement. 29 years	Subtotal excision, 4950r in 32 fractions in 33 days.	At 16 months follow-up, regression of tumor size.	

Choroid Plexus Papilloma (Continued)

Author, Year	Total # Pts.	Site Age	Treatment	Results	Notes
Hawkins, 1980	17	Lateral ventricle - 3. 4th ventricle - 4. 4 mos - 8yrs.	Surgical excision. Post-operative radiation therapy for those incompletely resected, and those malignant histologically; 3000-4000r given.	Five children underwent radiation, with persistence of neurologic deficits.	Pre-operative radiation. Shrunk tumor allowing for total removal, in 1 case.
Carrea and Polak, 1977	2	4th ventricle, 13 mos, 7 yrs.	3000r pre-operative radiation followed by radical surgery.	Radiation shrunk the vascular stroma, makeup definitive surgery possible.	

References

1. Aristizabal SA and Runyon TD (1981) Radiotherapy of unusual benign disease. *Int J Radiat Oncol Biol Phys* **7**: 1437-1440.
2. Naguib MG, Chou SN and Mastri A (1981) Radiation therapy of a choroid plexus papilloma of the cerebellopontine angle with bone involvement. *J Neurosurg* **54**: 245-247.
3. Hawkins JC (1980) Treatment of choroid plexus papillomas in children: A brief analysis of twenty years' experience. *Neurosurgery* **6**: 380-384.
4. Carrea R and Polak M (1977) Preoperative radiotherapy in the management of posterior fossa choroid plexus papillomas. *Child's Brain* **3**: 12-24.

Craniopharyngioma

This embryonal rest of Rathke's pouch proves more than troublesome. There is general agreement that surgical excision and radiation therapy are appropriate for treatment, but the degree of surgical excision is worthy of review in the articles cited. Following surgical excision and radiation, it is reasonable to anticipate a 70% five-year and 60% ten-year survival in this disorder, dependent in part on the degree of extension of the tumor at the time of presentation. Radiotherapists should consider the potential sequelae of radiation treatment plans that require 5500 to 6500 rad when determining the risk vs. benefit ratio for these patients. Parameters are reviewed in the reports of Kramer and Thompson and Calvo; standard texts and references should be consulted. In treating the cystic form of the tumor, where drainage has not been possible, isotope instillation has been carried out with some success. Ninety-five percent of the radiation oncologists responding to the national survey would treat craniopharyngioma.

References

1. Fischer EJ, Welch K, Belli JA, Wallman J, Shullite JJ, Winston KR and Cassady JR (1985) Treatment of craniopharyngioma in children 1972-1981. *J Neurosurg* **45**: 496-501.
2. Hoogenhout J, Otten BJ, Kazem I, Stoelinga GBA and Walder AHD (1984) Surgery and radiation therapy in the management of craniopharyngioma. *Int J Rad Oncol Biol Phys* **10**: 2293-2297.
3. Calvo FA, Horendo J, Arellano A, Sachetti A, DelaTorre A, Aragon G and Otero J (1983) Radiation therapy in craniopharyngiomas. *Int J Rad Oncol Biol Phys* **9**: 493-496
4. Kramer S (1983) Childhood craniopharyngioma survival, local control. Endocrine and neurologic function following radiotherapy. *Int J Rad Oncol Biol Phys* **9**: 171-175.
5. Strauss L, Strum V, George P, Schelgl W, Ostertag H, Clorias JH and VanKarck G (1982) Radioisotope therapy of cystic craniopharyngiomas. *Int J Rad Oncol Biol Phys* **8**: 1581-1585.
6. Shapiro K, Till K and Grant DN (1979) Craniopharyngiomas of childhood: A rational approach to treatment. *J Neurosurg* **50**: 617-623.
7. Thompson IL, Griffin TW, Parker RG and Blasko JC (1978) Craniopharyngioma: the role of radiation therapy. *Int J Rad Oncol Biol Phys* **4**: 1059-1063.
8. Urdaneta N, Chessin H and Fischer JJ (1976) Pituitary adenomas and craniopharyngiomas: analysis of 99 cases treated with radiation therapy. *Int J Rad Oncol Biol Phys* **1**: 895-902.

Cushing's Disease

The inhibition of secondary sequelae from pituitary derived Cushing's disease is reported to be effective in 50-75% of the patients treated with radiation. Improvement in pre-treatment assessment, methods of radiation delivery and treatment planning should continue to yield high response rates. Standard texts and references should be reviewed.

References

1. Jennings AS, Liddle GW and Ortho DN (1970) Results of treating childhood Cushing's disease with pituitary irradiation. *New Eng J Med* **297**: 957.
2. Edmonds MW, Simpton WJK and Meaking JW (1972) External irradiation of hypophysis for Cushing's disease. *Calif Med Assoc J* **107**: 860.
3. Dohan FC, Raventos A and Boncot N (1957) Roentgen therapy in Cushing's syndrome without adrenocortical tumor. *J Clin* Endocrinol Metab **17**: 8.

Cystic Hygroma, Lymphangioma

Lymphangiomas are benign neoplasms of the lymphatic system considered to be developmental lymphatic malformations. The accepted appropriate therapy is surgical excision. When they are incompletely excised, recurrence is common. Occasionally repeated surgical procedures are unsuccessful at controlling these lesions. In rare circumstances for tumors in unusual locations, and in refractory symptomatic patients, radiation therapy may be indicated. Low doses in the range of 15-20 Gy appear to be effective in preventing continual chylous effusion and in reducing the tumors.

On the other hand, cystic hygroma is a lesion composed of lymphatic tissue presenting in the neck and treated with surgical excision. The majority of these lesions present in infants and youngsters and are best managed surgically. Considering the risks of radiation in the pediatric age group, it would require very special circumstances to allow the use of radiation for cystic hygroma.

In the national survey 68% of radiation oncologists would not treat lymphangioma and 85% would not treat cystic hygroma.

Cystic Hygroma Radiotherapy and/or Surgery

Author, Year	Total # Patients	Treatment	Results	Notes
Ninh and Ninh, 1974	7	Radiotherapy (no details).	No improvement. All were subsequently operated on.	Lymphangitis and lymphedema.
	126	Excision (4 subtotal excisions).	4 deaths (3.1%) 2 cases of spontaneous regression.	Partial facial paralysis.
Barrand and Freeman, 1973	2	Radiotherapy.	Caused an increase in size which necessitated urgent surgery.	
	2	Aspiration.	Ineffective.	Massive infiltrating cystic hygroma of the neck in infancy.
	8	Surgical excision (these include those cases listed above in which other methods of treatment failed).	Tumor could not be completely removed in any case. 5/8 important structures were damaged. 4/8 died.	Authors recommended that surgery be deferred until after the age of 1 year, if the child is thriving.

Historical Data: Cystic Hygroma Radiotherapy and/or Surgery

Author, Year	Total # Patients	Treatment	Results	Notes
Galofre et al, 1962	57	Radiotherapy (x-irradiation, radium or radon seeds).	17/35(58%) good results.	Authors emphasized that the "good" results in the nonsurgical group were not as good as the correspondingly labeled ones in the surgical category. Such things as atrophy of the face, problems in dental development, and actinodermatitis were common complications in the nonsurgical series.
	69	Excision.	40/69(58%) good results.	
Perzik, 1960	1	External and interstitial irradiation and injections of sclerosing solution. Surgical excision.	Continued enlargement after treatment with irradiation and sclerosing agents. Several episodes of recurrent infection post-op. Subsequent satisfactory regression.	Age 3 1/2 months. Cervical cystic hygroma.
Martin, 1954	9	Radium applicator therapy (usually 700mg hrs. repeated 2–3 times) and/or radiotherapy (900–2400r/5–9 days, 200–220Kv). Prior partial surgical excision in one case.	7/9 satisfactory response (but three of these required plastic surgical repair after treatment to remove redundant skin folds).	Retarded development of right shoulder girdle and breast in one patient receiving radiotherapy to the axilla and supraclavicular area.
Pfahler and Perlman, 1950	1	2400r(air)8F/5 months. Additional intermittent treatments in the next 2 years to bring the total surface dose to 4000r. Technical Factors: 180Kv, 15ma, 0.5mm Cu plus 1mm Al filtration, FSD, 50cm. Three portals: anterior neck & chest, posterior neck & chest, and right axilla.	Progressive reduction of the mass.	Mass involved neck and mediastinum.
Portmann, 1945	1	600r/6F/6 wks to each side of the neck and mediastinum. Field size: 10 x 10cm. Technical Factors: 200Kv, HVL, 0.9mm Cu, FSD, 50cm.	Cervical masses began to diminish in size but surgery was attempted elsewhere. Child died during 2nd operation.	Age 10 months. Mass involved neck and mediastinum.
	1	Fourteen radon seeds (each 1.4mc, filter 0.3mm gold) were inserted into substernal mass extending posterior to the trachea and downward into the mediastinum.	Mass regressed. No recurrence at 9 year follow up.	Age 2 years. Mass involved neck and mediastinum.
	1	1,200r in 100r increments over a 2 year period. Field Size: 10 x 10cm. Technical Factors: 200Kv, HVL, 0.9mm Cu, FSD, 50cm.	Progressive reduction of the mass.	Age 5 weeks. Mass involved neck and mediastinum.
Hodges et al, 1939	7	50–150r(125–135Kv) at 1–2 month intervals to a total dose of 600–900r.	4/7 excellent results.	Ages 11 weeks to 11 years.

Historical Data: Cystic Hygroma Surgery Only

Author, Year	Total # Patients	Treatment	Results	Notes
Chait et al, 1974	26	Surgical excision (preceded by incision and drainage in one pt. until child's condition improved).	24/25 cured.	3 patients have recurrence but were cured after second excision.
	1	Sclerosing agents.	No regression.	
Miller and Taboada, 1974	1	Surgical excision.	Healed uneventfully. No recurrence at one year follow up.	Age 63 years. Mass in shoulder.
Brooks, 1973	3	Surgical excision.	No recurrences at 20 months, 3 years or 14 year follow up.	Ages 5 weeks to 19 years. Cystic hygroma of the neck.
Feutz et al, 1973	3	Surgical excision.	Complete excision. Post-op course was uneventful. Only partial excision because of involvement with superior vena cava and right innominate vein. Second excision 2 years later. Again only partial excision was accomplished.	Ages 30-55 years. Intrathoracic cystic hygroma.
Mills and Grusfield, 1973	4	Surgical excision.	No recurrences at 4 months, two years, or 4 year follow up.	Ages 4-23 months. Cervicomediastinal masses.
Seeler et al, 1971	1	Surgical excision.	Difficulty with skin closure and slow wound healing.	Age 5 weeks. Cystic hygroma at the flank.
Bratu et al, 1970	1	Surgical excision.	No recurrence at 1 year follow up.	Age 5 months. Cystic hygroma at the flank.
Noone and Brown, 1970	2	Surgical excision.	No recurrences at 15 and 16 month follow ups.	Ages 7 weeks and 5 years. Cystic hygroma of the parotid gland.
Ward et al, 1970	15	Surgical excision.	One death. Four cases required multiple excisions. No recurrences at follow up of 6 months to 10 1/2 years.	Ages 3 weeks to 19 years at surgery. Cystic hygroma of the neck.
Yacoub and Lise, 1969	3	Surgical excision (only partial excision in one case).	No recurrences at follow ups of 5 and 9 years.	Ages 33-65 years. Intrathoracic cystic hygroma.
Nanson, 1968	3	Surgical excision.	No recurrences.	Ages 14 months-2 years. Cystic hygroma at the mediastinum.
Woodring, 1968	1	Surgical excision.	All vital structures were intact at the conclusion of surgery.	Age 57 years. Cyst was beneath sternocleidomastoid muscle.
Barnhart and Brown, 1967	1	Partial surgical excision (approximately 40% of mass removed). Cauterization at base of tongue 6 days later. Further excision 2 months later.	No further follow up data.	Age 2 days. Cystic hygroma of the neck.

Historical Data: Cystic Hygroma Surgery Only (Continued)

Author, Year	Total # Patients	Treatment	Results	Notes
Feldman and Cotton, 1966	1	Surgical excision.	No recurrences.	Age 19 years. Hygroma of the scrotum.
Kirschner, 1966	1	Surgical excision.	Steady recovery.	Age 2 months. Cervicomediastinal mass.
Bill and Summer, 1965	61	Surgical excision (radiotherapy was used briefly for a lymphangioma of the tongue with no benefical results).	3 deaths.	35/61 were less than 1 year old. 29/61(48%) post-op edema of neighboring tissues with lymph accumulation and lymphatic drainage.

Historical Data: Lymphangioma and Cystic Hygroma

Author, Year	Total # Pts.	Site Age	Treatment	Results	Notes
Johnson et al, 1986	1	Posterior mediastinum, 11 years.	Unsuccessful surgical management, followed by 2000cGy/10 fractions mediastinal radiotherapy.	Prompt and permanent resolution of the chylothorax. No recurrence with two years follow up.	
O'Cathail et al, 1985	1	Lateral chest wall, 50 years.			Multiple surgical procedures from age 11; each with multiple recurrences prior to radiotherapy.
Aristizabal and Runyon, 1981	1	Peritoneum, 27 years.	2600r whole abdomen followed by 1400r whole pelvis.	No evidence of disease at 6 year follow up.	Three previously unsuccessful surgical attempts prior to radiotherapy.
Stromberg et al, 1976	3		Radiation therapy.	No response when used as initial therapy or subsequent therapy.	
Saijo et al, 1975	1	Lip and cheek, age 3.	Radon seeds	No visible swelling or facial asymmetry, no bone abnormality at age 41, 38 years of follow up.	

References

1. Johnson DW, Klazynski PT, Gordon WH and Russell DA (1986) Mediastinal lymphangioma and chylothax: The role of radiotherapy. *Am Thorac Surg* **41**: 325–328.
2. O'Cathail S, Rostom AY and Johnson ML (1985) Successful control of lymphangioma circumscription by superficial x-rays. *Br J Dermatol* **113**: 611–615.
3. Aristizabal SA and Runyon TD (1981) Radiotherapy of unusual benign disease. *Int J Radiat Oncol Biol Phys* **7**: 1437–1440.
4. Aristizabal SA, Galindo JH, David JR and Boone M (1977) Lymphangiomas involving the ovary: Report of a case and review of the literature. *Lymphology* **10**: 219–223.
5. Stromberg BV, Weeks PM and Wray RC (1976) Treatment of cystic hygroma. *South Med J* **69**: 1333–1335.
6. Saijo M, Munro IR and Mancer K (1975) Lymphangioma: A long-term follow-up study. *Plast Reconstr Surg* **56**: 642–651.
7. Chait D, Yonkers AJ, Beddoe GM and Yarington CT (1974) Management of cystic hygromas. *Surg Gynec Obstet* **139**: 55–58.
8. Miller JM and Taboada JC (1974) Cystic hygroma colli in an adult. *Johns Hopkins Med J* **134**: 233–236.
9. Ninh TN and Ninh TX (1974) Cystic hygroma in children: A report of 126 cases. *J Pediactr Surg* **9**: 191–195.
10. Barrand KG and Freeman NV (1973) Massive infiltrating cystic hygroma of the neck in infancy. *Arch Dis Child* **48**: 523–531.

11. Brooks JE (1973) Cystic hygroma of the neck. *Laryngoscope* **83**: 117–128.
12. Feutz EP, Yune HY, Mandelbaum I and Brashear RE (1973) Intrathoracic cystic hygroma. *Radiology* **108**: 61–66.
13. Mills NL and Grusfield JL (1973) One-stage operation for cervicomediastinal cystic hygroma in infancy. *J Thorac Cardiovasc Surg* **65**: 608–611.
14. Seeler RA, Lal SJ and Laxminarayana MS (1971) Cystic hygroma in the flank of a newborn. *Clin Pediat* **10**: 354–356.
15. Bratu M, Brown M, Carter M and Lawson JP (1970) Cystic hygroma of the mediastinum in children. *Am J Dis Child* **119**: 348–351.
16. Noone RB and Brown HJ (1970) Cystic hygroma of the parotid gland. *Am J Surg* **120**: 404–407.
17. Ward PH, Harris PF and Downey W (1970) Surgical approach to cystic hygroma of the neck. *Arch Otolaryngol* **91**: 508–514.
18. Yacoub MH and Lise M (1969) Intrathoracic cystic hygromas. *Br J Dis Chest* **63**: 107–111.
19. Nanson EM (1968) Lymphangioma (cystic hygroma) of the mediastinum. *J Cardiovasc Surg* **9**: 447–452.
20. Woodring AJ (1968) Cervical cystic hygroma: A review of the literature and report of an unusual case. *Ann Otol Rhinol Laryngol* **77**: 978–983.
21. Barnhart RA and Brown AK (1967) Cystic hygroma of the neck. *Arch Otolaryngol* **86**: 74–78.
22. Feldman MA and Cotton RE (1966) Hygroma of the scrotum. *Br J Surg* **53**: 642–645.
23. Kirschner PA (1966) Cervicomediastinal cystic hygroma: One-stage excision in an eight-week-old infant. *Surgery* **60**: 1104–1107.
24. Bill AH and Summer DS (1965) A unified concept of lymphangiomas and cystic hygroma. *Surg Gynec Obstet* **120**: 79–86.
25. Galofre M, Judd ES, Perez PE and Harrison EG (1962) Results of surgical treatment of cystic hygroma. *Surg Gynec Obstet* **115**: 319–326.
26. Perzik SL (1960) Early management in extensive cervical cystic hygroma and macroglossa. *Arch Surg* **80**: 460–463.
27. Martin JA (1954) Treatment of cystic hygroma. *Texas State J Med* **50**: 217–222.
28. Pfahler GE and Perlman HH (1950) Cystic hygroma of the neck and mediastinum successfully treated by roentgen rays. *Am J Roent Rad Ther Nucl Med* **63**: 539–544.
29. Portmann UV (1945) Cystic hygroma. *Cleveland Clin Qrtly* **12**: 98–104.
30. Hodges FM, Snead LO and Berger RA (1939) Roentgen therapy of cystic hygroma of the neck in children. *Am J Roent Rad Ther Nucl Med* **42**: 551–555.
31. Goetsch E (1938) Hygroma colli cysticum and hygroma axillar; pathologic and clinical study. *Arch Surg* **36**: 394–479.
32. Figi FA (1929) Radium in treatment of multilocular lymph cysts of the neck in children. *Am J Roent Rad Ther Nucl Med* **21**: 473–480.

Desmoid-Aggressive Fibromatosis

Following surgical excision alone, local recurrences occur in 27–57 percent of cases of desmoid – aggressive fibromatosis. Radiation therapy in doses of 5000–6000 rad decreases local recurrence rates. Normal tissue tolerance may be limiting for the total dose of external beam radiation; therefore either post-operative brachytherapy or brachytherapy following external beam may be used. Regression rates may occur from eight months to two years following treatment. Desmoid – aggressive fibromatosis may occur in association with Gardner's syndrome and pregnancy. A seventy percent local control rate has been reported with external radiation. In the national survey eighty-two percent of radiation oncologists would treat desmoid – aggressive fibromatosis.

Desmoid-Aggressive Fibromatosis Radiotherapy and/or Surgery

Author, Year	Total # Patients	Treatment	Results	Notes
Assad et al, 1986	14 Median age – 31 years 11 Females and 3 Males	Surgery and brachytherapy plus external beam boost of 3000–5000r.	92% (11/12) local control rate with minimum two year follow up.	Three of fourteen had wound healing problems after brachytherapy; it should be initiated no longer than 72 hours after therapy.
Khorsand and Karakousis, 1985	19 Median age – 39 years 10 Females and 9 Males	Varied according to three groups: with Gardner's syndrome, recurrent and initial therapy.	Disease-free survivors in initial therapy group was 9/9 (100%) from 1–13 years.	Doses of XRT not provided.

Historical Data: Desmoid-Aggressive Fibromatosis Radiotherapy and/or Surgery

Author, Year	Total # Patients	Treatment	Results	Notes
Leibel et al, 1982	19 Median age – 27 years 11 Females and 8 Males	Radiation 5000–5500r	72% relapse-free survival 5–11 year follow up. 4 of 6 had recurrences at margin of field 1 had in-field recurrence.	Median follow up eight years. Local control not related to amount of disease. VAC chemotherapy used for radiation salvage.
Greenberger et al, 1981	9	Radiation 3000–6800r	8 of 9 controlled	Follow up 2–8 years.
Abadir, 1976	1	6000r/31F/45 days (Co^{60}) to tumor. 3900r/13F/40 days (10 Mev) to right upper anterior abdominal wall.	Tumor completely disappeared. Recurred one year later coincident with cystosarcoma phylloides of the breast.	The desmoid tumor was located in the upper anterior abdominal wall. The two tumors eventually became confluent and the patient expired.
Suit and Russell, 1975	6	7500r/54F/78 days. (Details of one case only).	All patients are alive and free from disease after 2–8 years.	Authors recommend: 6000r/ 7–8 weeks. All were extra-abdominal desmoids.
Hill, Newman and Phillips, 1973	4	5100–6100r/30–34F/42–53 days (Co^{60}), 4 Mev or 6 Mev.	Three patients are free from disease at 2 year follow up. Tumor has regressed to 20% of its original size in the fourth patient.	Extra-abdominal tumor (3) Abdominal tumor (1).
Gaches and Burke, 1971	1	2900r (superficial x-rays)/ 5 weeks. Second course of 2300r.	Tumor regressed noticeably after first treatment but had grown considerably 2 1/2 years later. Mass did not regress after second course.	Both were abdominal wall desmoids.
	1	Excision only	Free from disease at 8 month follow up.	
Cole and Guiss, 1969	2	Wide surgical excision. Recurrences treated by radiotherapy.	One half complete regression of recurrence following radiotherapy (patient is clinically free of disease at 3 year follow up).	All were extra-abdominal desmoids.
	2	Surgical excision. Recurrences treated by further excision and in one case, forequarter amputation.	Patients are clinically free of disease at 4 years and 12 years later.	
Rosen and Kimball, 1966	1	1800r/2 weeks.	Tumor contained for two years. Large mediastinal mass (from untreated intrathoracic portion of original tumor) was noted.	Both were extra-abdominal desmoids.
	1	Surgical excision. Recurrence treated with wide en block resection.	Second recurrence treated with forequarter amputation.	
Masson and Soule, 1966		Surgery alone (22 patients)	No recurrence in 5/18	4 lost to follow up. All were extra-abdominal tumors.
	34	Surgery plus irradiation (8 pts). Radium interstitially, 250Kv x-ray or Co^{60}.	No recurrences in 3/8	All were extra-abdominal tumors.
		Irradiation alone (4 pts).	No recurrence in 1/4.	All were extra-abdominal tumors.

Historical Data: Desmoid-Aggressive Fibromatosis Radiotherapy and/or Surgery (Continued)

Author, Year	Total # Patients	Treatment	Results	Notes
Benninghoff and Robbins, 1964	4	Excision followed by 2000-4000r/3-4 weeks. (In one case recurrence after radiotherapy was followed by two weeks of prednisone therapy.)	Regression of the tumor in all cases. No recurrences 2-7 years later.	Abdominal tumor (1) Extra-abdominal tumor (3)
Soule and Scanlon, 1962	1	560r(air) 1 week: Four weeks later, 610r/4 days to the same fields. Three weeks later, 660r to the same fields. (130-200 Kv, HVL 1.18-3.5cm). This was followed in three months by 600r/6 days to the same area plus 600r (single dose) to two new portals. (200 Kv, HVL 1.18mm Cu).	Six and one half years following the last x-ray treatment an undifferentiated fibrosarcoma was found in the center of the recurrent desmoid.	Extra-abdominal desmoid.
Gonatas, 1961	1	2600r through various portals.	Regression of tumor. At twelve year follow up, tumor was no larger than before.	All were extra-abdominal desmoids.
	5	Surgical excision.	Recurrence in 1/5.	
Musgrove and McDonald, 1948	7	Radium and/or x-rays (no details given).	No recurrence in 5/7.	All were extra-abdominal desmoids.
Pack and Ehrlich, 1944	17	Excision.	4/17 recurrences. All recurrences responded to radiation therapy except two. In one of these, the patient did not appear for follow up until the tumor had progressed considerably.	All were abdominal wall tumors. Three cases of malignant transformation.
	3	High voltage roentgen or radium element pack therapy. All were inoperable cases.	Tumor was satisfactorily controlled.	
		Recurrences of the above cases treated by surgery and/or radiation.	Surgery alone (for last recurrent tumor): six patients have had no further recurrences for 2-21 years. Radiation alone (for last recurrent tumor): five patients have had no further recurrences for 3-26 years. Surgery and radiation (for last recurrent tumor): One patient had no recurrence for 26 years.	

References

1. Assad WA, Nori D, Hilaris BS, Shiu MH and Hajdu SI (1986) Role or brachytherapy in the management of desmoid tumors. *Int J Radiation Oncology Biol Phys* **12**: 901-906.
2. Khorsand J and Karakousis CP (1985) Desmoid tumors and their management. *Am J Surg* **149**: 215-218.
3. Reitamo JJ (1983) The desmoid tumor IV. Choice of treatment results and complications. *Arch Surg* **118**: 1318-1322.
4. Leibel SA, Wara WM, Hill DR, Bovill EG, DeLorimer AA, Beckstead JH and Phillips TL (1982) Desmoid tumors: Local control and patterns of relapse following radiation therapy. *Int J Radiation Oncol Biol Phys* **9**: 1167-1171.
5. Greenberger HM, Goebel R, Weichselbaum RR, Greenberger JS, Chaffey JT and Cassady JR (1981) Radiation

therapy in treatment of aggressive fibromatosis. *Int J Radiation Oncol Biol Phys* **7**: 305–310.
6. Abadir R (1976) Desmoid tumor associated with cystosarcoma phylloides of the breast. *J Surg Oncol* **8**: 43–48.
7. Suit HD and Russell WO (1975) Radiation therapy of soft tissue sarcomas. *Cancer* **36**: 759–764.
8. Hill DR, Newman H and Phillips TL (1973) Radiation therapy of desmoid tumors. *Am J Roent Rad Ther Nucl Med* **117**: 84–89.
9. Gaches C and Burke J (1971) Desmoid tumor (fibroma of the abdominal wall) occurring in siblings. *Br J Surg* **58**: 495–498.
10. Brasfield RD and Das Gupta TK (1969) Desmoid tumors of the anterior abdominal wall. *Surgery* **65**: 241–246.
11. Cole NM and Guiss LW (1969) Extra-abdominal desmoid tumors. *Arch Surg* **98**: 530–533.
12. Enzinger FM and Shiraki M (1967) Musculo-aponeurotic fibromatosis of the shoulder girdle (extra-abdominal desmoid). *Cancer* **20**: 1131–1140.
13. Masson JK and Soule EH (1966) Desmoid tumors of the head and neck. *Am J Surg* **112**: 615–622.
14. Rosen RS and Kimball W (1966) Extra-abdominal desmoid tumor. *Radiology* **86**: 534–540.
15. Benninghoff D and Robbins R (1964) The nature and treatment of desmoid tumors. *Am J Roent Rad Ther Nucl Med* **91**: 132–137.
16. Dahn I, Jonsson N and Lundh G (1963) Desmoid tumors. *Acta Chir Scand* **126**: 305–314.
17. Soule EH and Scanlon PW (1962) Fibrosarcoma arising in an extra-abdominal desmoid tumor: Report of a case. *Staff Meetings of the Mayo Clinic* **37**: 443–451.
18. Gonatas NK (1961) Extra-abdominal desmoid tumors. *Arch Path* **71**: 214–221.
19. Hunt RT, Morgan HC and Ackerman LV (1960) Principles in the management of extra-abdominal tumors. *Cancer* **13**: 825–836.
20. Musgrove JE and McDonald JR (1948) Extra-abdominal desmoid tumors. *Arch Path* **45**: 513–540.
21. Pack GT and Ehrlich HE (1944) Neoplasms of the anterior abdominal wall with special consideration of desmoid tumors. *Int Abst Surg* **79**: 177–198.

Dupuytren's Contracture

There is general agreement that Dupuytren's contracture should be managed surgically if it is to be treated. No modern series could be located to indicate the use of radiation therapy. In the national survey 85% of radiation oncologists would not treat Dupuytren's contracture.

Historical Data: Dupuytren's Contracture Radiotherapy

Author, Year	Total Cases	Treatment	Results	Side Effects or Complications	Notes
Finney, 1955	43	X-ray applicator: Palmar mold covering the palmar fascia and adjacent tissues or grip cylinder. Surface dose of 300r in 7–8 days.	15/25 (60%) good functional results		
		Medium voltage x-ray therapy (140Kv, 5ma, HVL 5.7mm Al) 1500r in 3 fractions in 5 days.	8/18 (44.4%) good functional results		
Skoog, 1948	2	Deep x-ray therapy (no technical details given)	1 case-treatment given post-op lesion regressed. 1 case-radiation as primary treatment – deformity progressed.		
	69	Operative treatment- McIndoe's operation (aponeurosectomy)	57/69 (83%) good functional results		
Beatty, 1938	10	100Kv, 5ma, 1m-2mm Al filtration, HVL .11-.14mm Cu FSD 30cm. 100–200r (air) x 3–4 at weekly intervals.	7/10 improvement with loss of pain, reduction of palmar nodes, and relief of contracture.		

Historical Data: Dupuytren's Contracture Alternate Modes of Treatment

Author, Year	Total # Patients	Treatment	Results	Notes
Orlando et al, 1974	128	1. Radical fasciectomy (23 pts) 2. Partial fasciectomy (96 pts)	1. 69% good-very good results. 2. 72% good-very good results.	Average follow up of 2.3 years. Complications in 128 operations: Wound separation (8) Loss of flap (8) Haematoma (6) Primary infection (2)
Quetglas, 1972	80	Aponeurectomy both of the fibers of the palm as well as the fingers.	1/80 recurrence Total recovery usually at 3-6 months.	
Honner et al, 1971	138	Fasciectomy	66% good-excellent results. 25% fair results.	Classification of results: Excellent – Full flexion and extension of the fingers, full function, no recurrences. Good – Slight limitation of flexion or extension. Fair – Limitation of extension or flexion with joint stiffness. Authors also provided review of 11 previously reported operative series in the literature. Good-excellent results ranged from 61% to 100%.
McFarlaine et al, 1966	86	Limited fasciectomy, some radical.	70/86(80%) good results. 10/86(13%) fair results.	
Webb-Jones, 1965	40	Radical fasciectomy.	32/40(80%) clear of recurrence or extension at 3 year, 8 months.	Complications: Haematoma (1) Oedema (11) Digital nerve injury (3) Delayed wound healing (3)

References

1. Ketchum LD and Hixson FP (1987) Dermofasciectomy and full-thickness grafts in the treatment of Dupuytren's contracture. *J Hand Surg Am* **12**: 659–664.
2. Schneider LD, Hankin FM and Eisenberg T (1986) Surgery of Dupuytren's disease: A review of the open palm method. *J Hand Surg Am* **11**: 23–27.
3. Matton G and Beck F (1982) Our experience with 186 operated Dupuytren hands. Comparison of two techniques. *Acta Orthop Belg* **48**: 775–793.
4. Robbins TH (1981) Dupuytren's contracture: The deferred z-plasty. *Ann R Coll Surg Engl* **63**: 357–358.
5. Tubiana R, Fahrer M and McCullough CJ (1981) Recurrence and other complications in surgery of Dupuytren's contracture. *Clin Plast Surg* **8**: 45–50.
6. Orlando JC, Smith JW and Goulian D (1974) Dupuytren's contracture: A review of 100 patients. *Br J Plast Surg* **27**: 211–217.
7. Viganto JA (1973) Dupuytren's contracture: A review. *Semin Arthritis-Rheum* **3**: 155–176.
8. Quetglas J (1972) Dupuytren's disease. Comments on 80 cases operated on. *Acta Chir Plast* **14**: 244–254.
9. Honner R, Lamb DW and James JIP (1971) Dupuytren's contracture. Long term results after fasciectomy. *J Bone & Joint Surg Am* **53**: 240–246.
10. McFarlane RM and Jamieson WG (1966) Dupuytren's contracture. The management of one hundred patients. *J Bone & Joint Surg Am* **48**: 1095–1125.
11. Webb-Jones A (1965) Dupuytren's contracture. The results of radical fasciectomy. *Br J Plast Surg* **18**: 377–384.
12. Finney R (1955) Dupuytren's contracture. *Br J Rad* **28**: 610–614.
13. Finney R (1953) Dupuytren's contracture. *Lancet* **2**: 1064–1066.
14. Skoog TS (1948) Dupuytren's contracture with special reference to etiology and improved surgical treatment; its occurence in epileptics; note on knuckle-pads. *Acta Scand* **96**: 1–190.
15. Beatty SR (1938) Roentgen therapy of Dupuytren's contracture. *Rad* **30**: 610–612.

Epithelial Hemangioendothelioma

There is considerable variation in the histologic classification and biology of the vascular endothelial tumors of bone. Some tumors called hemangioendothelioma of bone by one pathologist, are termed angiosarcoma by another. Some of the tumors appear benign, while some clearly have a malignant course. Surgical excision is the primary therapy. For non-resectable lesions, however, and for those with microscopic residual disease, radiotherapy may be employed. Doses of 4000-5500 rad have been associated with long term local control. In the national survey seventy percent of radiation oncologists would not treat epithelial hemangioma of the bone.

Epithelial Hemangioendothelioma

Author, Year	Total # Pts.	Site Age	Treatment	Results	Notes
Friendly et al, 1982	1	Frontal bone, age 5.	Surgical excision. Eight months later a recurrence was re-excised, and the patient received 5000r.	Three years post radiotherapy, she had a negative surgical exploration and five years later there was no clinical evidence of disease or deformity.	
Finsterbush et al, 1981	1	Multifocal, involving bones of the hand, age 17.	4000r/8 weeks.	Doing well four years after treatment.	
Joachims and Cohen, 1974	1	Mastoid bone and ear, age 19.	Partial resection followed by 6000r cobalt therapy in 45 days.	Three years after treatment, there are no local recurrences or distant metastases.	Hearing is stable.
Deutsch et al, 1973	1	Penis, age 17.	Excision followed by post-operative radiotherapy, 3600r/18 fractions dose. One month later patient had thoracic spine lesions thought to be metastases and received palliative radiotherapy to spine and two courses of chemotherapy.	Patient had prompt response to his treatment and did well for six years when he developed extradural disease and preliminary metastases.	Biology of the disease suggested it to be very slow growing.
Pearlman, 1972	3	Leg, age 36. Arm, age 54. Foot, age 68.	Surgery, post-operative radiotherapy. Radiation doses: 4500r/23 days, 5000r/24 days, 6500r/38 days.	One patient had rapid progression of systemic metastases and died. One patient did well with no evidence of disease three years after treatment. One patient required an amputation for persistent local tumor six months after radiotherapy.	All three patients had hemangioendothelial sarcomas of bone.
Garcia-Moral, 1972	2	Dorsal spine, age 56. Proximal humerus, age 44.	Surgery and post-operative radiotherapy. Doses: 2600-4250r and 6000r.	One patient had no evidence of disease 19 months after treatment, while the other patient developed metastases, but was controlled locally four years after treatment.	

Historical Data: Epithelial Hemangioendothelioma

Author, Year	Total # Pts.	Site Age	Treatment	Results	Notes
Unni et al, 1971	22	Ages 7-78 years. 6 of 22 were multicentric. Multiple sites	Resection and/or radiation, depending upon location.	Eleven patients died, 1-18 months after diagnosis. Four patients were alive five years after diagnosis and two at least ten years after diagnosis.	
Morgenstern and Westing, 1969	1	Clavicle and scapula, age 40.	5000r to clavicle and scapula.	Prompt response. No evidence of disease at 14 year follow up.	

References

1. Friendly DS, Font RL and Milhorat TH (1982) Hemangioendothelioma of frontal bone. *Am J Ophthalmol* **93**: 482-490.
2. Finsterbush A, Husseini N and Rousso M (1981) Multifocal hemangioendothelioma of bones in the hand: A case report. *J Hand Surg (Am)* **6**: 353-356.
3. Joachims HZ and Cohen Y (1974) Hemangioendothelioma of the mastoid bone. *Laryngoscope* **84**: 454-458.
4. Deutsch M, Leen RLS and Mercado R (1973) Hemangioendothelioma of the penis with late appearing metastases: Report of a case with review of the literature. *J Surg Oncol* **5**: 27-34.
5. Garcia-Moral CA (1972) Malignant hemangioendothelioma of bone. Review of world literature and report of two cases. *Clin Orthop* **82**: 70-79.
6. Pearlman AW (1972) Hemangioendothelial sarcoma of bone: The role of irradiation and tumor growth studies. *Bull Hosp Joint Dis* **33**: 135-149.
7. Unni KK, Ivins JC, Beabout JW and Dahlin DC (1971) Hemangioma, hemangiopericytoma, and hemangioendothelioma (angiosarcoma) of bone. *Cancer* **27**: 1403-1414.
8. Morgenstern P and Westing SW (1969) Malignant hemangioendothelioma of bone. Fourteen-year follow-up in a case treated with radiation alone. *Cancer* **23**: 221-224.

Erythroplasia of Queyrat

Erythroplasia of Queyrat (Bowen's disease of the penis) represents intra-epithelial carcinoma. Ten to thirty percent of these lesions, if untreated, will convert to squamous cell carcinoma. There are multiple methods of treatment including external radiation or radium molds. Therapy should be directed toward not only irradiation, but should focus upon maintenance of sexual function, sensation, and maintenance of urinary function. Seventy-one percent of radiation oncologists in the national survey would not treat erythroplasia of Queyrat.

Erythroplasia of Queyrat Survey: Five Centers (1976)

Kv	Time and Dose	Field Size	Organ at Risk
Co^{60}	5000-6000r 6-7 weeks	As needed.	
100 Kv	5000r (6-15F) 3 weeks	Small margin	Skin
Co^{60}	175-6000r	5 x 5	
120 Kv	200r x 5	To cover lesion.	Penis
200 Kv	4500r/9F 2 weeks	6 x 8	

Erythroplasia of Queyrat

Author, Year	Total # Patients	Treatment	Results	Notes
Blank and Schnyder, 1985	4	Soft x-rays, 3200-4600 roentgens.	1 recurred.	
Goette et al, 1975	3	Topical fluorouracil (1%).	Lesions cleared completely in all three patients. Disease free follow up period of 20-60 months thus far.	Authors include review of five cases in the literature also treated with fluorouracil. Recurrence free period of nine months to sixteen years in four of these cases (one patient lost to follow up).
Graham and Helwig, 1973		Primary Treatment: 1. Surgical excision (74). 2. Desiccation, curettage and/or excision plus radiotherapy (6). 3. Radiotherapy. 4. Light desiccation and curettage (7) plus excision (8). 5. Topical treatment. Secondary treatment for recurrences. 6. Surgical excision (15). 7. Excision, desiccation and curettage (5). 8. Radiotherapy (1). 9. Excision plus radiotherapy (1).	Recurrences: 1. 10/74(13.5%) 2. 3/6 3. 3/4(75%) 4. 7/7(100%) without excision. 2/8 with excision. 5. 1/1(100%) 6. 5/15(33%) 7. 2/5(40%) 8. 1/1 9. 0/1	
Kaplan and Katch, 1973	1	Radium mold. Surface dose to shaft: 6900 gamma-Y^{90} Dose to glans: 6600 gamma-Y^{90}.	Shaft completely healed two months after treatment.	Authors suggest that the designation of erythroplasia of Queyrat be restricted to cases of Bowen's disease or intra-epithelial carcinoma of the glans penis in order to exclude the benign erythroplasias of the penis. In the case reported, biopsy was interpreted as erythroplasia of Queyrat with intra-epithelial carcinoma and areas of probable microinvasion.
Lewis and Bendle, 1971	1	Topical fluorouracil (1%).	Successful clearing of the lesion.	
Hueser and Pugh, 1969	1	Topical 5-fluorouracil (2%).	Lesion cleared.	
Mantell and Morgan, 1969	1	Y^{90} irradiation. Surface dose of 1500r/10 min.	Lesion cleared. No recurrence at three years.	
Andersson et al, 1967	2	Excision.	No recurrences at three years and five years.	Authors suggest that excision be used only if the disease is confined to the mucosa. Amputation or radiotherapy should be employed if deeper structures are involved.
Jansen, 1967	2	Topical 5-fluorouracil (5%).	Both lesions cleared but required reapplication to small areas after 6-9 months. Lesions cleared again.	

Erythroplasia of Queyrat (Continued)

Author, Year	Total # Patients	Treatment	Results	Notes
Brown, 1966	1	Radiotherapy, 3000r. Three years later a course of topical steroids was administered. Eight years after onset of disease excision was performed.	Temporary relief of irritability but no change in size or appearance of the lesion. Steroids provided only temporary relief of irritability. Complete symptomatic relief following excision.	
Shapiro et al, 1962	1	Excision biopsy followed by radiotherapy, 4950r (skin dose) 40F. HVL, 1.5mm Cu. Treatment to entire dorsum of the glans penis.	Patient clinically free of disease at 27 month follow up.	
McAninch and Moore, 1949	3	Surgical excision.	No recurrences at eight months to one year in the two cases where follow up data were available.	Excellent cosmetic and functional results were obtained in all three cases.
McDaniel and Mason, 1949				Authors provide a review of cases reported in the American literature. Of five cases treated with x-rays none benefited.

References

1. Blank AA and Schnyder VW (1985) Soft x-ray therapy in Bowen's disease and erythroplasia of Queyrat. *Dermatologica* **17**: 89–94.
2. Goette DK, Elgart M and Devillez RL (1975) Erythroplasia of Queyrat. Treatment with topically applied fluorouracil. *Southern Med J* **60**: 185–188.
3. Graham JH and Helwig EB (1973) Erythroplasia of Queyrat. A clinicopathologic and histochemical study. *Cancer* **32**: 1396–1414.
4. Kaplan C and Katch A (1973) Erythroplasia of Queyrat (Bowen's disease of the glans penis). *J Surg Onc* **5**: 281–290.
5. Lewis RJ and Bendle BJ (1971) Erythroplasia of Queyrat: Report of a patient successfully treated with topical 5-fluorouracil. *Candian Med Assoc J* **104**: 148–149.
6. McAninch JW and Moore CA (1970) Precancerous penile lesions in young men. *J Urol* **104**: 287–290.
7. Hueser JN and Pugh RP (1969) Erythoplasia of Queyrat treated with topical 5-fluorouracil. *J Urol* **102**: 595–597.
8. Mantell BS and Morgan WY (1969) Queyrat's erythroplasia of the penis treated by beta particle irradiation. *Br J Radiol* **42**: 855–857.
9. Andersson L, Jonsson G and Brehmer-Andersson E (1967) Erythroplasia of Queyrat-carcinoma in situ. *Scand J Urol Nephrol* **1**: 303–306.
10. Janson GT, Dillaha CJ and Honeycutt WM (1967) Bowenoid conditions of the skin: Treatment with topical 5-fluorouracil. *Southern Med J* **60**: 185–188.
11. Brown PB (1966) Erythroplasia of Queyrat. *Br J Plastic Surg* **19**: 378–382.
12. Shapiro L, Boyarsky S and Roberts TW (1962) Carcinoma developing in Queyrat's erythroplasia. *NY State J Med* **62**: 2999–3001.
13. McDaniel WE and Mason LM (1949) Malignant dyskeratosis, erythroplasia of Queyrat. *Arch of Derm* **60**: 419–424.

Extramammary Paget's Disease

New information regarding treatment with radiation for this disorder did not appear in our literature search of U.S. data, and past experience is too limited to draw a conclusion. Obviously, even if radiation is considered, it must be under circumstances where the conventional therapies have failed. Eighty-two percent of radiation oncologists in the national survey would not treat this disorder.

Extramammary Paget's Disease

Author, Year	Total # Patients	Treatment	Results	Notes
Williams et al, 1976		<u>Patients without underlying carcinoma</u>: 1. Wide local excision (2). <u>Patients with underlying carcinoma</u>: 2. Wide excision and/or radiotherapy plus chemotherapy (3). 3. Multiple wide excision (1) or abdominal perineal resection (1).	1. Both patients had recurrences which were eventually controlled by multiple excision. No evidence of disease at 12 and 17 years. 2. Radiation therapy was of short term value. Chemotherapy had no effect. All three died of disease at six months, twelve months and seventeen months. 3. Both patients alive with no evidence of disease at twenty-three months and seventeen years.	
Creasman et al, 1975		<u>Patients without invasion</u>: 1. Biopsy only (3). 2. Excision (6). 3. External irradiation (1). Patients with associated adenocarcinoma: 4. Radical vulvectomy (2) plus hysterectomy and vaginectomy (1). 5. 3000r to pelvis (palliation for pain). 6. Refused treatment.	Without invasion: 1. 2/3 dead at 49 months and 9 years. 1/3 alive 5 years. 2. 5/6 no evidence of disease at 6 months-5 1/2 years. 1/6 dead at 3 months. 3. No evidence of disease at 10 years. <u>With invasion</u>: 4. 2/3 no evidence of disease at 1-2 years. 1/2 recurrences (died 11 years after first treatment from metastatic adenocarcinoma and melanoma). 5. Little objective response of the metastatic lesions to irradiation. Patient died eight months later. 6. Died at one month.	All were cases of Paget's disease of the vulva.
Parmley et al, 1975	7	Primary treatment was vulvectomy with or without lymph node dissection. This was followed by radiotherapy to recurrences (2), to lymph nodes (2), or to the pelvis and para-aortic regions (1). Radiotherapy: 250 Kv or Co^{60}, 2700-4500r.	2/2 no response to 250 Kv x-rays, death in less than two years. 2/2 temporary response to Co^{60} therapy, death in 2.5 years or less. 1/1 treated with vulvectomy. 2/2 alive with no evidence of disease 1.5 years and 13 years after radical vulvectomy and lymph node dissection in both plus Co^{60} radiotherapy in one.	All patients had invasive vulvar Paget's disease.
Sharkey et al, 1975	1	Surgical excision.	No evidence of recurrence at five years.	Both were cases of perianal Paget's disease.

Historical Data: Extramammary Paget's Disease

Author, Year	Total # Patients	Treatment	Results	Notes
Taylor et al, 1975	18	Initial treatment: 1. Radiation therapy (2, one had a coexisting infiltrating carcinoma). 2. Surgery plus radiotherapy (4, two had coexisting carcinoma). 3. Surgical excision (15).	1. 2/2 local recurrence. 2. 3/4 local recurrence, two with infiltrating carcinoma died of disease. 1/4 no recurrence at 42 months. 3. Complete excision (uninvolved margins) 6/6 no recurrences. Involved margins: 7/9 recurrences.	All were cases of Paget's disease of the vulva. There was no underlying carcinoma in most of the cases.
Fethston and Friedrich, 1972	5	Surgical excision.	3/5 alive with no evidence of recurrence. One patient died at six years with no evidence of disease. One patient had three local recurrences treated by surgical excision followed by topical 5-FU therapy for an asymptomatic recurrence. At present there is complete regression of the lesion.	All were cases of vulvar Paget's disease.
Fenn et al, 1971	7	Surgical excision.	Follow up of 5 months - 8.5 years. 3/7 alive with no recurrence. 2/7 alive with no recurrence following a second surgical procedure. One patient died of disseminated carcinoma. One patient died of other causes.	All were cases of vulvar Paget's disease.
Kawatsu and Miki, 1971	1	Excision of bilateral axillary regions. Topical chemotherapy with 5% fluorouracil cream to the genital lesion. This was followed by 3400r (1000 Kv) ten months later.	No recurrences of axillary lesions at one year. Erosion of the genital lesion following fluorouracil therapy. Repeated biopsies showed new atrophic dermis with or without Paget's cells in the basal cell layer. The genital lesion cleared after irradiation.	A case of triple extramammary Paget's disease - bilateral axillary lesions and a genital lesion.
Vogel and Ayers, 1970	13	Simple vulvectomy.	One patient died at sixteen months from other causes. There was no evidence of Paget's disease. The other patient has had no recurrences at three years following treatment.	Both were cases of vulvar Paget's disease.
Hambrick et al, 1968	1	Various local remedies used without benefit. Radiotherapy: 1650r in three months (80 Kv, no filtration).	Partial resolution.	Extramammary Paget's disease of the groin.
Koss et al, 1968	7	Surgical excision.	4/7 no evidence of disease at 4-17 years. 2/7 recurrences treated by re-excision. 1/7 died in O.R.	Most patients had received prior therapy, including irradiation in three cases.

Historical Data: Extramammary Paget's Disease (Continued)

Author, Year	Total # Patients	Treatment	Results	Notes
Abell, 1965	2	Vulvectomies without lymph node dissection.	One patient died six months after treatment. The second is alive and free of disease six months after treatment.	Both were cases of vulvar Paget's disease.
Helwig and Graham, 1963	34	1. Radiotherapy (5). 2. Excision, radium and x-rays (1). 3. Excision, desiccation, and curettement (1). 4. Surgical excision (27).	1. 5/5 recurred or were unaltered by therapy. 2. Recurred. 3. Recurred. 4. 6/27(22%) recurred.	All were cases of anogenital Paget's disease.
Murrell and McMullan, 1962	1	Surgical excision.	No recurrence at 1.5 year follow up.	Paget's disease in the groin.
	1	Radiotherapy: 225r/3F/3 weeks. Second course of radiotherapy ten years after first treatment: 3000r to penis, scrotum and superpubic areas. 3000r to left inguinal region Co^{60}. Third series: 4290r to lower left abdominal region. Co^{60}.	Some improvement after radiotherapy. But six years later the lesion was still present and inguinal lymph nodes were palpable. Patient refused further treatment until four years later. After second course the inguinal nodes became non-palpable and the cutaneous lesions disappeared. But there was persistent edema of the left leg. This was treated with irradiation with no relief. Patient died eleven years after first treatment.	Authors state that although radiotherapy to the genital lesion produced clinically satisfactory results, tissue sections from the scrotal area revealed tumor cells in the skin lymphatics. They concluded that the radiation had good effect on the inguinal lymph nodes but was ineffective within the abdominal cavity.

References

1. Williams SL, Rogers LW and Quan SH (1976) Perianal Paget's disease. Report of seven cases. *Dis Colon & Rectum* **19**: 30–40.
2. Creasman WT, Gallager HS and Rutledge F (1975) Paget's disease of the vulva. *Gyn Onc* **3**: 133–148.
3. Parmley TH, Woodruff JD and Julian CG (175) Invasive vulvar Paget's disease. *Obst & Gyn* **46**: 341–346.
4. Sharkey FE, Clarke RL and Gray GF (1975) Perianal Paget's disease: Report of two cases. *Dis Colon & Rectum* **18**: 245–248.
5. Taylor PT, Stenwig JT and Kausen H (1975) Paget's disease of the vulva. A report of 18 cases. *Gyn Onc* **3**: 46–60.
6. Fethston WC and Friedrich EG (1972) The origin and significance of vulvar Paget's disease. *Obst & Gyn* **39**: 735–744.
7. Fenn ME, Morley GW and Abell MR (1971) Paget's disease of vulva. *Obst & Gyn* **38**: 660–670.
8. Kawatsu T and Miki Y (1971) Triple extramammary Paget's disease. *Arch Derm* **104**: 316–319.
9. Vogel EH and Ayers MA (1970) Primary epidermal Paget's disease of the vulva. *Obst & Gyn* **36**: 284–286.
10. Hambrick GW Jr, Whelan ST and Wood MG (1968) Extramammary Paget's disease. *Arch Derm* **97**: 598–599.
11. Koss LG, Ladinsky S and Brockunier A Jr (1968) Paget's disease of the vulva. Report of 10 cases. *Obst & Gyn* **31**: 513–525.
12. Abell MR (1965) Intraepithelial carcinomas of epidermis and squamous mucosa of vulva and perineum. *Surg Clin N Am* **45**: 1179–1198.
13. Helwig EB and Graham JH (1963) Anogenital extramammary Paget's disease. *Cancer* **16**: 387–403.
14. Murrell TW Jr, and McMullan FH (1962) Extramammary Paget's disease. *Arch Derm* **85**: 600–613.

Fibrosclerosis

Sclerosing cervicitis is similar to sclerosing retroperitonitis and sclerosing mediastinitis. It also is similar to idiopathic retroperitoneal fibrosis and idiopathic fibrous mediastinitis. The etiology is unknown. High-dose radiation has been used successfully in some cases to cause regressions in symptomatic patients with lesions located in critical areas. Cases are anecdotal and response rates irregular. In the national survey 97% of radiation oncologists would not treat fibrosclerosis.

Fibrosclerosis (see also Aggressive Fibromatosis, Desmoid)

Author, Year	Total # Patients	Treatment	Results	Notes
Rice et al, 1975	1	Cervical area, age 46. Biopsy, 5000 rad Cobalt therapy	Improvement at 11 months follow up.	Similar lesion to sclerosing retroperitonitis, and sclerosing mediastinitis.
Nelson et al, 1968	1	Retroperitoneum, age 68. Biopsy, 1688 rad Cobalt therapy	No improvement and at 9 months follow up required surgical removal.	

References

1. Rice DH, Batsakis JG and Gulthard SW (1975) Sclerosing cervicitis. Homologue of sclerosing retroperitonitis and mediastinitis. *Arch Surg* **110**: 120–122.
2. Nelson RM, Jenson CB, Horsley BL and Ershler I (1968) Idiopathic retroperitoneal fibrosis producing distal esophageal obstruction. *J Thorac Cardiovasc Surg* **55**: 216–224.

Fungal Infections

Past use of radiation has proven effective in inhibiting fungal infections. In tinea capitis where radiation treatment was given, the risk versus benefit was not understood. Radiotherapeutic considerations of dose distribution to normal tissue was neither applied nor was it considered. Statements such as "a procedure which has proven safe in thousands of cases" appeared in the literature. Thus, reports as late as 1951 reviewed as many as 1,004 patients treated for tinea capitis.

It is interesting to note that by 1959 the need for gonadal shielding was appreciated, and the recommendation to carry it out stimulated publication by two sets of authors. The now well established skin cancers, thyroid, head and neck, and central nervous system tumors that result from such radiation demonstrate the need for evaluating or projecting the long term sequelae in any young patient receiving external radiation for benign disorders.

In a series of 2,200 children followed for up to 40 years, there was a 20% incidence of skin cancers; the minimal latency period seemed to be 20 years. The skin cancer incidence occurred in Caucasian patients rather than in black patients, suggesting an obvious interaction with ultraviolet light exposure. A similar number of patients, some untreated and some exposed to 300–600 rad x-rays, was followed for 26 years and showed a 10-fold increase in skin cancer for the treated patients. Of 10,842 patients whose thyroids were irradiated, a 3-fold increase in abnormalities and malignancies was observed compared to unirradiated controls. With the availability of modern antifungal agents, we consider it inappropriate to treat fungal infections with radiation. Ninety-four percent of radiation oncologists responding to the national survey would not treat fungal infections with radiation.

References

1. Shore RE, Albert RE, Reed M, Harley N and Pasternack BS (1984) Skin cancer incidence among children irradiated for ringworm of the scalp. *Rad Res* **100**: 192–204.
2. Ron E and Modan B (1980) Benign and malignant thyroid neoplasms after childhood irradiation for tinea capitis. *JNCI* **65**: 7–11.

3. Pousti A (1979) Malignant tumors of the scalp resulting from x-ray treatment of tinea capitis. *Br J Plastic Surg* **32**: 52-54.
4. Spallone A, Gagbardi FM and Vagnozzi R (1979) Intracranial meningiomas related to external cranial irradiation. *Surg Neurol* **12**: 153-159.
5. Shore RE, Albert RE and Pasternack BD (1976) Follow up study of patients treated by x-ray epilation for tinea capitis I: Resurvey of post-treatment illness and mortality. *Arch Environ Hlth* **31**: 21-28.
6. Andrews GC and Domonkos AN (1959) The reduction of gonadal dose in dermatological radiotherapy. *AMA Arch Dermatol* **79**: 449-454.
7. Cepollaro AC, Kullos A and Ruppe JP (1959) Measurement of gonadal radiations during treatment for tinea capitis. *New York J Med* **39**: 3033-3040.
8. Beare JM and Cheeseman EA (1951) Tinea capitis: review of 1004 cases. *Br J Dermatol* **63**: 165-186.

Giant Cell Tumor

Although sometimes described as a benign tumor, malignant tranformation occurs independent of radiation. This tumor is often treated because of major bone destruction which could be devastating.

Eighty-three percent of radiation oncologists in the national survey would treat giant cell tumors if they are threatening.

Giant Cell Tumor

Author, Year	Total # Patients	Treatment	Results	Notes
Larsson et al, 1975	5	Radiotherapy only (2). Surgery plus radiotherapy (1). Surgery only (2). Details of radiotherapy: Total dose of 3100-5000r.	Follow up of 6-16 years. No recurrences.	All were cases of giant cell tumors of the spine. Authors emphasize that radiotherapy should not be used for tumors in other regions, but that it seems justified for tumors of the spine.
Larsson et al, 1975	43	Primary treatment: 1. Curettage alone. 2. Curettage plus grafting. 3. Radiotherapy alone. 4. Radiotherapy plus curettage. 5. Resection. 6. Amputation.	1. 5/8(28%) remissions. 2. 9/12(75%) remissions. 3. 4/10(40%) remissions. 4. 2/4(50%) remissions. 5. 1/7(14%) remissions. 6. 1/2 remissions.	Giant cell tumor of bone. There were six deaths (11.3%) due to a malignant course of the tumor. The patient had received radiotherapy.
DePalma et al, 1974	10	Complete en bloc excision followed by fusion of joint or bone grafting.	Follow up of 2-12 years. No recurrences.	All were cases of giant cell tumor of bone. 8/10 were located in the femur.
Martins and Dean, 1974	1	Radiotherapy: 5000r/40 days, Co^{60} 6.5x6.5cm opposing sellar ports.	Patient became asymptomatic for 2.5 years. From that time on the patient experienced progressive deterioration and death due to a poorly differentiated spindle cell sarcoma of the sphenoid sinus.	Case of giant cell tumor of the sphenoid bone.
Marcove et al, 1973	25	Curettage followed by cryosurgery.	2/25 obvious clinical recurrence. 6/25 residual foci as demonstrated by "second look" biopsy procedure.	Five of these eight tumors were controlled with repeat cryotherapy.

Giant Cell Tumor (Continued)

Author, Year	Total # Patients	Treatment	Results	Notes
McGrath, 1972	52	Primary treatment: 1. Curettage plus graft (20). 2. Curettage plus radiotherapy (5). 3. Curettage plus graft plus radiotherapy (2). 4. Local excision (1). 5. Local excision plus radiotherapy (1). 6. Resection (7). 7. Resection plus radiotherapy (1). 8. Radiotherapy alone (12). 9. Amputation (3). Radiotherapy dose: 3000–9500r/1–3 courses/up to 18 months.	Recurrences: 1. 9/20(45%). 2. 1/5(20%) malignant change of previously typical tumor. 3. 1/2(50%). 4. 0/1(0%). 5. 0/1(0%). 6. 0/7(0%). 7. 0/1(0%). 8. 6/12(50%) malignant change in four. 9. 0/3(0%).	Giant cell tumor of bone. There was no relationship between the dose and course of radiotherapy and the incidence of typical or malignant recurrences.
Shifrin, 1972	24	Includes both primary and secondary treatment. 1. Curettage (10). 2. Resections (5) or amputation (2). 3. Radiotherapy (7).	Recurrences: 1. 4/10. 2. 0/7. 3. 2/7.	All were cases of giant cell tumor of bone. Subsequent developments: Metastasis (1). Osteogenic sarcoma (1). Fibrosarcoma (1). Both had been treated by irradiation. Osteonecrosis and pathologic fracture (1).
Emley, 1971	1	Biopsy followed by radiotherapy, 4186r/1 month, Co^{60}.	Well and free of symptoms at 20 month follow up.	Giant cell tumor of the sphenoid bone.
Emley, 1971	14	1. Biopsy plus irradiation (6). 2. Excision only (3). 3. Excision and irradiation (5).	Includes thirteen previously reported cases plus the case reported by the author. 1. 4/6 favorable results (cured or improved). 2. 1/3 favorable result. 3. 1/5 favorable result.	Review of the literature of reported cases of giant cell tumors of the sphenoid bone.
Dahlin et al, 1970	195	Without radiation: 1. Curettage plus cautery and/or bone graft in some cases (41). 2. Excision (6). 3. En bloc resection (11). 4. Amputation (10). With radiation: 5. Curettage plus cautery and/or bone grafting in some cases (23). 6. Excision (13). 7. Radiation alone (7).	Minimum follow up of three years: Recurrences: 1. 16/41(39%) 2. 4/6(67%) 42.6% 3. 0/10 Amputation for non-union was subsequently performed in one patient. 4. 0/10. 5. 11/23(48%) 6/13(46%) 47.2% 6. 4/7 dead of disease within 2 years. 2/7 subsequently required amputation. 1/7 clinically well at 2 years.	All were giant cell tumors of bone. Seventy-seven percent were located at or near the end of a major tubular bone of the extremities. Seventeen patients (8.7%) had malignant giant cell tumors. In two patients the sarcomas were found in recurrent tumors. These patients had not been treated by irradiation at any time. In eleven patients, the sarcomas developed on an interval of 3.7 to 38 years. After therapy that included irradiation administered before supervoltage equipment was available.

Giant Cell Tumor (Continued)

Author, Year	Total # Patients	Treatment	Results	Notes
Goldenberg et al, 1970	218	1. Curettage (45). 2. Curettage plus graft (91). 3. Resection (44). 4. Resection plus graft (22). 5. Amputation (10). 6. Irradiation (10) Radiotherapy: Radium application, radon seeds, roentgen therapy, or Co^{60}. Dose range: 1120–5320r.	Recurrences and complications: 1. 37/45(82%). 2. 55/91(60%). 3. 28/44(64%). 4. 17/22(77%). 5. 0/10(0%). 6. 7/10(70%). Radiotherapy was used in conjunction with other therapy in forty-six cases. Results: 8/46 healing without complications and minimum follow up of three years. 29/46 recurrence, metastases or death.	All were cases of giant cell tumor of bone. Complications include recurrences or seeding, metastasis, nonunion of graft, fracture of graft, infection, foot drop, irradiation sarcoma and death. These cases were compiled from a variety of sources. Five had been previously reported. The patients with post irradiation sarcoma died 9–31 years after diagnosis.
Johnson and Riley, 1969	24	Initial treatment: 1. Curettage (16). 2. Irradiation (3). 3. Local resection (3) or amputation (2).	Recurrences: 1. 8/12 four lost to follow up. 2. 2/2 one lost to follow up. 3. 0/2 three lost to follow up.	All were cases of giant cell tumor of bone. Both patients in this series who died with malignant giant cell tumor had received irradiation at a time when the tumor was histologically benign in one case and clinically benign in the other case.
Friedman and Pearlman, 1968	58	Radiotherapy: GCT of the jaw (13): 1850r/22 day to 3000r/60 day GCT of the long bones (19): 2000r/21 days to 6264r/33 day (doses smaller than 3000r/21 days were unsuccessful). GCT of membranous bones (13): 2300r/34 days to 5700r/6 months (2 courses). GCT of spinal column (12): 980r/17 days to 6000r/120 days (successful tumor dose ranged from 2200r/21 days to 5100r/34 days).	Recurrences: GCT of jaw: 0/13. GCT, long bones: 9/20. GCT, membranous bones: 2/13. GCT, spinal column: 4/12. Death from radiation myelitis occurred in one patient who received 6000r/120 days.	All were giant cell tumors of bone. Eleven cases treated by the author, forty-six from the literature.
Riley et al, 1967	2	Case #1: Radiotherapy to GCT of left innominate bone followed by total excision (which necessitated resection of part of the vaginal wall). Case #2: Excision followed by radiotherapy 2125r/13F/2 weeks to head of 9th rib. Recurrence was treated by excision and radiotherapy 4000r.	Case #1: Submucosal nodules removed from the vaginal wall at the site of previous resection at seven months, seventeen months, and thirty-two months post-op. They were benign giant cell tumors similar histologically to the previously resected lesion.	Soft tissue recurrence of GCT of bone after irradiation and excision.

Giant Cell Tumor (Continued)

Author, Year	Total # Patients	Treatment	Results	Notes
			Case #2: First recurrence treated by excision and radiotherapy. Tumor involving the eight and ninth thoracic vertebrae was found two years after treatment for recurrence. There was also a nodule in the scar of the old incision which proved to be malignant GCT. Patient died fifteen months later from extensive disseminated tumor.	
Berman, 1964	5	Radiotherapy: 2500r/40 days to 5100r/34 days. One patient received 600r in two courses over a period of approximately six months.	2/5 alive and well for 4-12 years. 1/5 alive for 17 years with total disability. 2/5 dead, one with malignant transformation, one with complications due to the natural progression of the disease.	All were giant cell tumors of the vertebrae.
Mnaymneh et al, 1964	67	Primary: 1. Curettage (31). 2. Curettage plus irradiation (4). 3. Radiation (6). 4. Partial excision and post-op radiotherapy (3). 5. Partial excision only (2). 6. Total excision (21).	Recurrences: 1. 13/23, primary recurrence. 6/8, second recurrence. One with malignant change. 2. 4/4, one recurred as a fibrosarcoma. 3. 2/3, primary recurrences. 3/3, secondary recurrences. 4. 2/2, primary recurrences. 1/1, secondary recurrences. 5. One half tumor progressed as a fibrosarcoma. 6. No recurrences.	Giant cell tumor of bone. Of the nine tumors treated by radiation alone or radiation combined with curettage or partial excision, eight recurred. Malignant transformation in 4/67, who had received radiation therapy.

References

1. Larsson S, Lorentzon R and Boquist L (1975) Giant cell tumor of bone. A demographic clinical and histopathological study of all cases recorded in the Swedish cancer registry for the years 1958 through 1968. *J Bone & Joint Surg Am* **57**: 167-173.
2. Larsson S, Lorentzon R and Boquist L (1975) Giant cell tumors of the spine and sacrum causing neurological symptoms. *Clin Orth* **111**: 201-211.
3. Vistnes LM and Vermuellen WJ (1975) The natural history of a giant cell tumor. Case report. *J Bone & Joint Surg Am* **51**: 865-867.
4. DePalma AF, Ahmad I and Flannery G (1974) Treatment of giant cell tumors in bone. *Clin Orth* **110**: 232-237.
5. Martins AN and Dean DF (1974) Giant cell tumor of sphenoid bone: Malignant transformation following radiotherapy. *Surg Neurol* **2**: 105-107.
6. Marcove RC, Lyden JP, Huvos AG and Bullough PB (1973) Giant cell tumors treated by cryosurgery. A report of twenty five cases. *J Bone & Joint Surg Am* **55**: 1633-1644.
7. Barnes R (1972) Editorial. Giant-cell tumor of bone. *J Bone & Joint Surg Br* **54**: 213-215.
8. McGrath PJ (1972) Giant cell tumor of bone. An analysis of fifty-two cases. *J Bone & Joint Surg Br* **54**: 216-229.
9. Shifrin LZ (1972) Giant cell tumor of bone. *Clin Orth* **82**: 59-66.
10. Emley WE (1971) Giant cell tumor of the sphenoid bone. *Arch Otol* **94**: 369-374.
11. Dahlin DC, Cupps RE and Johnson EW (1970) Giant-cell tumor: A study of 195 cases. *Cancer* **25**: 1061-1070.
12. Goldenberg RR, Campbell CJ and Bonfiglio M (1970) Giant-cell tumor of bone. An analysis of two hundred and eighteen cases. *J Bone & Joint Surg Am* **52**: 619-664.
13. Johnson KA and Riley LH (1969) Giant cell tumor of bone. An evaluation of 24 cases treated at the Johns Hopkins Hospital between 1925 and 1955. *Clin Orth* **62**: 187-192.
14. Friedman M and Pearlman AW (1968) Benign giant-cell tumor of bone: Radiation dosage for each type. *Radiology* **91**: 1151-1158.
15. Riley LH, Hartman WH and Robinson RA (1967) Soft tissue recurrence of giant cell tumor of bone after irradiation and incision. *J Bone & Joint Surg Am* **49**: 365-368.
16. Berman HL (1964) The treatment of benign giant cell tumors of the vertebrae by irradiation. *Radiology* **83**: 202-207.
17. Mnaymneh WA, Dudley HR and Mnaymneh LG (1964) Giant cell tumor of bone. *J Bone & Joint Surg Am* **46**: 63-75.
18. Hutter RVP, Foote FW Jr, Frazell EL and Francis KC (1963) Giant cell tumors complicating Paget's disease of bone. *Cancer* **16**: 1044-1056.
19. Hutter RVP, Worcester JN Jr, Francis KC, Foote FW Jr

Gynecomastia (Prostate Cancer Managed with DES)

We consider pre-irradiation of the breasts an acceptable treatment to prevent gynecomastia in males planned to receive DES or feminizing hormones for the treatment of prostatic cancer. In the national survey 74% of radiation oncologists would treat to prevent gynecomastia.

Gynecomastia

Author, Year	Total # Patients	Treatment	Results
Fass, Steinfeld, Brown and Tessler, 1986	87 patients pre- and post-hormone status	1200–1500r 3 fractions 4Mev or Co-60	67/87 no gynecomastia 72/87 no mammalgia
Corvalan et al, 1969	20 patients	900r each breast single dose 100Kv	18/20 improved, avoided significant sequelae, 1 patient skin change
Malis, Cooper and Wolever, 1969	20 patients pre-hormone 11 patients on hormone	900r/3 fxs 140Kv	Pre-hormone: 11/18 no gynecomastia 7/8 mild hypertrophy 1 pt pain, tenderness Post-hormone: 10/11 gynecomastia 10/11 pain, 3 of these had later reduced symptoms
Gangai et al, 1967	13 patients 10 prior to hormone, 3 after hormone	900r in air 3 fractions	3/10 pre-hormone breast hypertrophy 0/10 pain nipple sensitivity, skin changes 1/3 post hormonal-improved in pain, sensitivity 3/3 breast size unchanged
Alfthan and Kettunen, 1965	25 patients	1425–2375r single dose both breasts prior to hormone	On hormone, pain and soreness relieved, but not gynecomastia, pre-hormone gynecomastia prevented.
Larsson and Sundbom, 1962	6 patients 1 breast treated	1000–1500r 1 treatment	Successful results

References

1. Fass D, Steinfeld A, Brown J and Tessler A (1986) Radiotherapeutic prophylaxis of estrogen-induced gynecomastia: a study of late sequelae. *Int J Radiat Oncol Biol Phys* **12**: 407–408.
2. Corvalan JF, Gill WM, Egleston TA, and Rodriguez-Antunez A (1969) Irradiation of the male breast to prevent hormone produced gynecomastia. *Am J Roentgenol Radium Ther Nucl Med* **106**: 839–840.
3. Malis I, Cooper JF and Wolever THS (1969) Breast radiation with carcinoma of the prostate. *J Urol* **102**: 336–337.
4. Gangai MP, Shown TE, Sieber PE and Moore CA (1967) External irradiation: a successful modality in preventing hormonally induced gynecomastia. *J Urol* **97**: 338–339.
5. Alfthan O and Kettunen K (1965) The effect of roentgen ray treatment of gynecomastia in patients with prostatic carcinoma treated with estrogenic hormones: a preliminary communication. *J Urol* **94**: 604–606.
6. Larsson LG and Sundbom CM (1962) Roentgen irradiation of the male breast. *Acta Radiologica* **58**: 253–256.

Hemangioma

These benign vascular tumors may lead to disastrous occurrences in the spinal cord subglottis region, brain, liver, larynx and orbit with platetet consumption. Treatment in these situations is acceptable, although in the pediatric age group medical management should be attempted first if possible. Complications from the use of steroids can be serious in this population. If hemangiomas are not treated soon enough in critical locations, they may be fatal. Seventy-five percent of the radiation oncologists in the national survey will treat hemangiomas.

Subglottic Hemangiomas

Author, Year	Total # Pts.	Site and Age of Patients	Treatment	Results	Notes
Holbrow and Mott, 1973	1	Subglottic Age 6 months.	Two gold grains (Au 198), 4mCi, implanted in the lesion. (One grain was coughed out two days later). Tracheostomy tube had also been inserted.	Airway had improved greatly in two months.	Gold grains were encased in platinum.
Bourne and Taylor, 1972	1	Laryngeal Age, 5 months.	Nasotracheal intubation and prednisone therapy followed by 500r (surface dose) with beta-ray applicator. A second dose of 500r was given eight months later.	Infant had improved by the next day and nasotracheal intubation was no longer necessary.	
Calcaterra, 1968	1	Subglottic. Age, 1 month.	Tracheostomy: 950r/5F/8 days (Co^{60}) through opposing lateral ports. Supravoltage irradiation.	No significant regression.	
Tefft, 1966	28	Subglottic Age, 3 weeks to 2 years at diagnosis	Tracheostomy: Initial dose of 100–300r. Final dose: 125r/2 days to 900r/12 days. Average final dose: 450r/3 days. Technical factors: 200Kv, 15ma, HVL, 2.6mm Cu.	Twenty-seven patients responded to irradiation but average time for complete regression and relief of respiratory symptoms was nine months.	Ten cases were irradiated without prior insertion of tracheostomy tube. Authors recommend a dose of only approximately 25r in such cases.
Ferguson and Flake, 1961	17	Subglottic. Age 1–11 months.	200–500r/1–6 days (250–350r may be given at one time if the infact has a tracheostomy). Technical factors: 200 Kv, 15ma, 0.4mm Tn plus 0.25mm Cu plus 1mm Al filtration, HVL 2.7mm Cu, FSD 50cm. Opposing or oblique fields. One patient received radium therapy.	Sixteen lesions regressed promptly (6–8 weeks).	Tracheostomy was done in six patients.

Historical Data: Subglottic Hemangiomas

Author, Year	Total # Pts.	Site and Age of Patients	Treatment	Results	Notes
Holbrow, 1958	1	Subglottic. Age, 6 months.	250r(deep x-ray) to subglottic region. One month later a second treatment to 200r was given. Digoxin, antibiotics and a third course of irradiation was given.	Considerable tracheal obstruction and respiratory distress following the first treatment. Tracheostomy tube was removed after second treatment but had to be replaced two days later. No adverse reactions following the third treatment and the patient progressed satisfactorily.	
	1	Subglottic Age, 1.5 months.	450r/2F/2 weeks.	No reaction. Stridor ceased two days following second treatment.	
Baker and Pennington, 1956	5	Larynx Age, 1-4 months.	400r/9 days. Repeated at intervals of 3 months to a total of 1200r.	Response difficult to evaluate. One patient died. One patient also had extensive involvement of the mediastinum which was not controlled.	
Kasabach and Donlan, 1945	1	Subglottic Age, 3 months.	Tracheostomy: 1050r/7F/7 days to each side of larynx. (200 Kv, .5mm Cu plus 1.25mm Al filtration, FSD, 50cm).	Regression of lesion.	
	1	Subglottic, lip anterior chest and nape of neck. Age 5.5 months.	Tracheostomy: 1000r/10F/7 days to each side of larynx. (200 Kv, 25ma, .5mm Cu plus 1.25mm Al filter, FSD 50cm). 1500r/5F/5 days to lip and to anterior chest. (130 Kv, 4ma, 1mm Al filter, FSD 25cm). Radium needles in nape of neck.	Regression of subglottic lesions. Regression of lip and chest lesions. Regression of neck lesion.	

Hemangiomas of Bone

Author, Year	Total # Pts.	Site and Age of Patients	Treatment	Results	Notes
McAllister et al, 1975	8	Vertebral Ages, 25–75 years.	1. Surgical removal (2). 2. Surgical removal followed by radiotherapy (1). 3. Decompression followed by post-op radiotherapy (2). 4. Ligation of feeding arteries followed by radiotherapy (4400r/ 3 weeks) (patient had a posterior spinal fusion). 5. Radiotherapy alone (2).	1. One died post-op. One good recovery. 2. Good results. 3. Considerable clinical improvement in both cases. 4. Lesion was found to be filling in with new bone at five months post-op. Patient was symptom free at twelve months. 5. Good recovery in both cases.	
Gomez-Aravjo et al, 1974	1	Maxilla Age, 19 years.	1000r/5F/6 months. Subsequent resection.	Some reduction in tumor size but not complete resolution following radiotherapy. Free of tumor four years post-op.	
	1	Mandible Age, 8 years.	Steroids – no results. Modified hemimandibulectomy and tracheostomy.	Free from tumor at four months follow up.	
Periman et al, 1974	1	Maxilla (central cavernous hemangioma). Age, 12 years.	4000r/1 month. Injection of a sclerosing agent (sodium morrhuate) six months later.	No regression following radiotherapy. Lesion repsonded to the sclerosing agent.	
	1	Mandible (central cavernous hemangioma). Age, 12 years.	1200r/4 days (6 Mev).	Good response to radiotherapy. Evidence of bone deposition in previously radiolucent areas at three month follow up.	
Hekster et al, 1972	1	Vertebral with spinal cord compression (patient was paraplegic). Age, 61 years.	Percutaneous catheter embolization followed by radiotherapy (3000r/12F/4 weeks, Co^{60}).	Patient was in excellent condition at seven month follow up.	
Macanash and Owen, 1972	1	Mandible Age, 12 years.	Short course of radiotherapy (dose not stated).	Lesion began filling with bone. Teeth became firmer.	
	1	Mandible Age, 13 years.	Profuse bleeding during preparation for operation to ligate the external carotid artery (mandibular right second molar had been extracted).	Patient died in O. R.	
Unni et al, 1971	56	Bone – most were located in the skull or vertebra. Ages, 4 1/2 to 70 years.	Curettage, total excision or resection of as much of the tumor as possible followed by radiotherapy in eleven cases, of which seven were vertebral lesions.	Vertebral lesions: 6/7 good results with decompression followed by radiotherapy.	

Historical Data: Hemangiomas of Bone

Author, Year	Total # Pts.	Site and Age of Patients	Treatment	Results	Notes
Loring, 1967	1	Mandible Age, 42 years.	1600r(skin dose)/4 days (250 Kv, HVL 0.5mm Cu, 1mm Al, FSD 50cm).	Swelling flattened, new bone formed.	
Abramson, 1965	1	Mandible Age, 38 years.	2700r/1 month (intra-oral cone technique).	Regeneration of bone exhibited at six month follow up.	
Topazian, 1964	1	Mandible Age, 16 years.	3000r(tumor dose)15F/3 weeks. (Co^{60}).	No increase in size at three months. (Parent's report). Subsequently lost to follow up.	
Bergstrand et al, 1963	13	Vertebral with spinal cord compression. Ages, 16-68 years.	Surgery - Laminectomy followed by removal. (One patient received prior to x-ray therapy but with poor results).	8/13 completely cured. 4/13 markedly improved. 1/13 no improvement.	
Rohan, 1960	1	Mandible Age, 15 years.	Ligation of left external carotid artery. Uncontrollable bleeding upon extraction of loose molar and premolar teeth. Three weeks later 2000r/2 weeks to the mandible was given.	Pulsation and bleeding in the buccal tumor ceased following ligation. Patient was free from recurrences at eight months following radiotherapy.	
Smith, 1959	1	Mandible Age, 25 year.	2464r/29 days.	At eight month follow up the facial asymmetry had disappeared and there was filling in of the active zone of destruction with new bone.	
Lindquist, 1951	1	Vertebral Age, 18 years.	Radiotherapy to five fields (three dorsal, two ventral). Tumor dose of 2100r. Four series of treatments in ten months were given.	The patient had clinical symptoms of compression of the spinal cord when first observed. After last series of treatment the only symptoms remaining were some numbness of the feet and some insecurity of balance. At nine year follow up mobility and sensibility were normal.	
Feber and Lampe, 1942	1	Vertebral - associated with spinal cord compression. Age, 52 years.	200r(air) day to a total of 2400r. Second course (2000r) given eight months later. Technical Factors: 200 Kv, 0.5mm Cu plus 1 mm Al filtration, HVL 0.9mm Cu, FSD 50cm, 13x15cm field.	Steady improvement. At eight month follow up (after second treatment) patient was normal except for areas of minimal hypalgesia in the lower extremities and mildly hyperactive deep tendon reflexes.	Authors report twelve cases in the literature similarly treated and also with excellent results.

Liver Hemangiomas

Author, Year	Total # Pts.	Site and Age of Patients	Treatment	Results	Notes
Slovis et al, 1975	3	Liver Ages, 1 day and 5 weeks.	150-600r (plus prednisone in two cases).	Tumors regressed but role of radiotherapy is difficult to evaluate.	Two of these patients also had congestive heart failure.
	1	Liver Age, 1 day.	Right lobectomy.	Patient well at seven year follow up.	
Ein and Stephens, 1974	8	Liver - hemangiomas (5). Hemangioendotheliomas (3). Newborn - 12 years of age.	Radiotherapy (4) followed by surgery in some cases.	Radiotherapy: 1/4 benefited. Surgery: 3/6 died in O.R. or post-op.	
McLean et al, 1972	1	Liver - multinodular hemangiomatosis. Age, 4 months.	2000r (6 Mev). Prednisone instituted when total irradiation had reached 1050r.	Little response to irradiation. Dramatic improvement following institution of steroids.	Capillary hemangioma difficulty involving the liver.
Kagan et al, 1971	1	Liver Age, 46 years.	5022r(mid tumor dose)/2 months (daily tumor dose was increased from 30r by increments of 10-114r daily, 5 days a week).	Marked improvement.	
Adam et al, 1970	6	Liver - diffuse involvement in four. Ages, 4 months - 60 years.	1500-2500r following laparotomy.	Progression of the disease was halted in all six but three were not completely relieved of symptoms. Tumor decreased in size of two.	Five of the patients were 48 years of age or over. Four of the patients had diffuse involvement of both lobes.
	10	Liver Ages, 26-72 years.	Resection (4 lobectomies, 6 wedge resections).	Two deaths, both following emergency resections. Post-op course uncomplicated in the other cases except for one who required drainage of bile in the subhepatic space.	
Park and Phillips, 1970	5	Liver Ages, 4 months - 67 years.	1300-2500r(tumor dose/2-4 weeks) 250 Kv, 1 Mev, or Co^{60}.	Improvement in 4/5.	All patients had undergone prior lobotomy and the tumors had been found to be nonresectable. Four of the patients were 48 years of age or over.
Issa, 1968	2	Liver Ages, 27-55 years.	2500r(tissue dose)/ 2 weeks or 2500r(tissue dose)/5 weeks.	Improvement in both cases.	
Shockman et al, 1963	1	Liver Age, 35 years.	1620r(air)/30 days to each of two portals for a calculated mid plane dose of 2000r. (250 Kv, 15ma, Th. II filter HVL 2.3mm Cu, FSD 70cm).	Size of liver decreased. At three years follow up patient was well and leading a normal life.	Cavernous hemangioma in both lobes in widespread distribution.

Liver Hemangiomas (Continued)

Author, Year	Total # Pts.	Site and Age of Patients	Treatment	Results	Notes
Wilson and Tyson, 1952	1	Liver Age, 53 years.	700r/2 weeks (HVL 0.95mm Cu) through two anterior-posterior ports Three months later 2700r/24 days (HVL 2.25mm Cu) was given.	Some decrease in the size of the liver. Jaundice diminished slightly.	Diffuse cavernous hemangioma involving the entire liver.
	2	Liver Ages, 39-44 years.	Resection.	Uneventful recovery.	

Subglottic or Cutaneous Hemangiomas Alternate Modes of Therapy

Author, Year	Total # Pts.	Site and Age of Patients	Treatment	Results	Notes
Donaldson et al, 1979	99	Multiple sites, one-28 months	90 Yttrium needles 900-2500r	Seventy-two percent complete resmission. Ninety-four percent good or average cosmesis.	Long term follow up no malignancies.
Lasser and Stein, 1973	1	Multiple, also had a variety of types.	Steroid therapy (prednisone). Was begun at five weeks of age and Continued until two years of age.	Growth of the hemangiomas was arrested within days. Resolution of laryngeal and pharyngeal hemangiomas occurred. But the patient still has hemangiomas and still developed some cosmetic effects.	Satisfactory response occurred in the capillary cavernous types of hemangiomas. There was no response in the port wine type.
Overcash and Putney, 1973	2	Subglottic Ages, 8 months and 3 months.	Prednisone.	Definite regression in both cases.	
Cohen and Wang, 1972	10	Subglottic (4) Tongue and floor of mouth (2) Parotid gland (1) External auditory canal (1) Face and chin (2) Most were infants less than nine months of age. Subglottic, ages 6.5-10 weeks.	Prednisone.	Marked regression in 8/10.	In several cases withdrawal of steroid therapy resulted in regrowth of the tumor.
Fost and Esterly, 1968	6	Face, tongue, neck, chest and trunk. Some had multiple hemangiomas. All were infants.	Prednisone.	Marked regression in 5/6.	Regression was noted within two weeks after beginning therapy. Three patients had regrowth when therapy was reduced or discontinued.

For a review of cases of hemangioma treated with corticosteroids reported prior to 1968 see Fost and Esterly and Katz and Askin.

Cutaneous Hemangiomas Radiotherapy

Author, Year	Total # Pts.	Site and Age of Patients	Treatment	Results	Notes
Hoehn et al, 1970	52	Head and neck. Includes both children and adults.	Surgery	17/29(59%) cured. 8/20(27%) controlled.	Total of 30 significant complications including: Radiation atrophy (4) Radiation actinodermatitis (2) Hemorrhage (post-op mortality) (1) Facial nerve paralysis, temporary (7) Facial nerve paralysis, permanent (2) Delay of wound healing (4) Cosmetic defect (10)
			Radiation (high voltage or radon seeds).	1/4(25%) cured. 2/4(50%) controlled.	
			Surgery and radiation.	8/19(42%) cured. 4/19(21%) controlled.	
Corby et al, 1969	1	Cheek Age, 3 months.	Prednisone - no response. 1200r/4F.	Platelet count rose to normal following radiotherapy. Hemangioma had completely regressed one year later.	Associated thrombocytopenia.
Pyesmany et al, 1969	1	Left side of neck (cavernous). Age, 4 1/2 months.	800r(300 Kv, 20ma, HVL 2mm Cu) through opposed AP ports.	Following irradiation patient was asymptomatic except for persistent petechiae. Patient completely asymptomatic at 22 weeks follow up.	Associated with intravascular coagulation.
Zaidi, 1966	1	Left temple Age, 7 weeks.	Prednisone, no improvement. 1500r/8F/31 days (140 Kv, 0.25mm Cu, 1mm Al filter).	Platelet count rose following radiotherapy. Tumor had regressed at two weeks.	Associated thrombocytopenia.
Duncan and Halnan, 1964	1	Shoulder Age, 3 months.	300r(skin dose) single dose (250 Kv, HVL, 1.6mm Cu, FSD, 40cm).	Lesion responded and platelet count rose.	Associated thrombocytopenia.
	1	Chest Age, not given.	375r(tumor dose) single dose (300 Kv, HVL 2.5mm Cu) followed by betamethasone two months later. Second course of radiotherapy of 1500r/8F/10 days was given.	Platelet count fell. No response to betamethasone, some improvement following second course radiotherapy but platelet remained low.	

Historical Data: Cutaneous Hemangiomas Radiotherapy

Author, Year	Total # Pts.	Site and Age of Patients	Treatment	Results	Notes
Nordberg and Sundberg, 1963	1087	Cavernous hemangiomas of the skin Ages, not given.	Contact therapy (for minor superficial hemangiomas): 50 Kv, 0.5mm Al filtration, FSD 20mm. The hemangiomas were compressed during treatment and the quality of the rays modified somewhat (an additional 0.5mm Al filtration added). The surface dose was 1000r for the first treatment and 600–800r for subsequent treatments. Radium treatment: 900–1000r surface dose (700–800r at 3mm depth) for the first treatment. 500–700r (3mm depth) for subsequent treatments.	Receiving one treatment: Radium: < 900r(surface dose) (56), 47% disappeared. > 900r(surface dose) (99), 61% disappeared. Contact therapy: < 900r(surface dose) (46), 68% disappeared. > 900r(surface dose) (262), 75% disappeared. Receiving two treatments: Radium: < 900r(surface dose, first treatment) (66), 32% disappeared. > 900r(surface dose, first treatment) (97), 36% disappeared. Contact therapy: 900r(surface dose, first treatment) (34), 40% disappeared. 900r(surface dose, first treatment) (147), 31% disappeared. Radium & contact therapy: 900r(surface dose, first treatment) (87), 30% disappeared. 900r(surface dose, first treatment) (58), 37% disappeared.	The results are at one year follow up.
Sutherland and Clark, 1962	1	Right submandibular and anterior cervical. Age, 3 months.	ACTH and prednisone. 675r(air)/7F/3 weeks.	Platelet count rose. Hemangioma had regressed markedly at one month follow up.	Associated thrombocytopenia.

For a review of hemangiomas associated with thrombocytopenia, see Duncan & Halnan, Sutherland & Clark and Shim.

Hemangioma of the G. I. Tract

Author, Year	Total # Pts.	Site and Age of Patients	Treatment	Results	Notes
Allred and Spencer, 1974	40	Colon, rectum, and anus. Average age, 45.7 years.	Treatment: Local removal Radical hemorrhoidectomy Resection Radiation Oral iron Transfusion	Failures: 1/13 0/2 0/4 0/2 1/6 0/2	If complete removal of the hemangioma is not feasible, treatment is directed at relieving the symptoms.
Abrahamson and Shandling, 1973	8	Bowel	Radium therapy Excision	2/3 cured. 5/5 cured.	

Hemangioma of the G. I. Tract (Continued)

Author, Year	Total # Pts.	Site and Age of Patients	Treatment	Results	Notes
Oppenheim and O'Brien, 1950	2	Rectum	Radium pack to the anterior pelvis and sacrum (1). 200r (skin dose) daily to total of 2552r tumor dose. (200 Kv, HVL, .9mm Cu, FSD 80cm, 20x20cm field).	Good results in both cases. No recurrence of gastro-intestinal complaints or bleeding.	

Hemangioma of the Urinary Tract

Author, Year	Total # Pts.	Site and Age of Patients	Treatment	Results	Notes
Liang, 1958	2	Bladder Ages, 52 and 64 years.	250r(air)/10F through an anterior port.	Good results in both cases.	

Hemangioma of the Joint

Author, Year	Total # Pts.	Site and Age of Patients	Treatment	Results	Notes
Moon, 1973	133	Knee joint	1. Radiotherapy (10). 2. Synovectomy (11). 3. Partial synovectomy (19). 4. Mass excised (86). 5. Partial excision (7).	1. 8 recovered. 1 functional limitation. 1 residual tumor. 2. 8 recovered. 2 recurrences. 3. 13(76%) recovered. 3 functional limitation. 1 recurrence. 4. 56(73%) recovered. 19 functional limitation. 2 residual tumor. 5. 2(29%) recovered. 4 residual tumor. 1 gangrene - amputation later performed.	The cases listed consist of two cases reported by Moon plus cases provided in a review of the literature reported in Moon's paper.

Skeletal Muscle Hemangiomas: Surgical excision is the treatment of choice. See Chavhan & Baird, Jones, and Scott.

Intracranial Angiomas

Author, Year	Total # Pts.	Site and Age of Patients	Treatment	Results	Notes
Zeller and Chuterian, 1975	1	Pons Age, 18 years.	3000r/4 weeks to the pons.	Patient died 2 months later.	
Amacher et al, 1972	50	Cerebral	Surgical removal.	One post-op death. Three cases of fatal re-bleeding.	64% subarachnoid hemorrhage and intracerebral hematoma. 22% subarachnoid hemorrhage only. 8% seizures. 60% intracerebral "steal" phenomenon.

Intracranial Angiomas (Continued)

Author, Year	Total # Pts.	Site and Age of Patients	Treatment	Results	Notes
Svien and McRae, 1965	68	Intracranial	No treatment.	16% died. 10% invalids.	
Paterson and McKissock, 1956	108	Intracranial	1. Total excision (36). 2. Ligation of the cortical vessels alone (15). 3. Ligation of the common carotid artery alone (4). 4. Radiotherapy alone (6) or following surgery (5). 5. No treatment (42).	1. 1 post-op death. 2 late deaths from intracerebral hemorrhage, 3 are incapacitated. 29 alive and doing full-time work. 1 lost to follow up. 2. 11 working full-time. 3 incapacitated. 1 too recent to assess results. 1 lost to follow up. 3. 2 no effect. 1 transient relief of headaches, symptoms worse at 1 year follow up. 1 died 24 hours post-op (was in deep coma pre-op). 4. No benefit in any case. 5. 3 deaths just after diagnosis. 5 hemorrhages. 1 death at seven years. 14 well at the end of follow up with no serious disabilities. 1 remained hemiplegic. All others lost to follow up.	
Potter, 1955	45	Cerebral	Treatment: Symptomatic Radiotherapy Radical excision	Survival after Rx (yrs) 0–5 5–10 10–20 28 7 3 – 2 1 3 4 6 1 – –	
Bergman, 1950	1	Pons Age, 4 years.	Total of 1750r(air) over a period of five years given in courses of approximately 750–1800r to each of three or four portals.	Recurrent attacks of bulbar palsy responded to radiotherapy. Patient died approximately five years after first treatment.	

References

1. Donaldson SS, Chassagne D, Sancho-Garnier H, Beyer HL (1979) Hemangiomas of infancy: Results of ^{90}Y interstitial therapy: A retrospective study. *Int J Rad Oncology Biol Phys* **5**: 1–11.
2. McAllister VL, Kendall BE and Bull JWD (1975) Symptomatic vertebral hemangiomas. *Brain* **98**: 71–80.
3. Slovis TL, Berdon WE, Haller JD, Casarella WJ and Baker DH (1975) Hemangiomas of the liver in infants. *Am J Roent Rad Ther & Nucl Med* **123**: 791–801.
4. Zeller RS and Chutorian AM (1975) Vascular malformations of the pons in children. *Neurology* **25**: 776–780.
5. Allred HW and Spencer RJ (1974) Hemangiomas of the colon, rectum, and anus. *Mayo Clin Proc* **49**: 739–741.
6. Bland KI, Abney HT, MacGregor AMC and Hawkins IF

(1974) Hemangiomatosis of the colon and anorectum. *Am Surg* **40**: 626–635.
7. Ein SH and Stephens CA (1974) Benign liver tumors and cysts in childhood. *J Pediatr Surg* **9**: 847–851.
8. Gomez-Aravjo JJ, Toth BB and Luna MA (1974) Central hemangioma of the mandible and maxilla: Review of a vascular lesion. *Oral Surg Oral Med & Oral Path* **37**: 230–238.
9. Li FP, Cassady JR and Barnett E (1974) Cancer mortality following irradiation in infancy for hemangioma. *Radiology* **113**: 177–178.
10. McNeill TW and Ray RD (1974) Hemangioma of the extremities: Review of 35 cases. *Clin Orthop* **101**: 154–166.
11. Perriman A, Uthman A and Kuzair KY (1974) Central hemangiomas of the jaws. *Oral Surg Oral Med and Oral Path* **37**: 502–508.
12. Abrahamson F and Shandling B (1973) Intestinal hemangiomata in childhood and a syndrome for diagnosis: A collective review. *J Pediatr Surg* **8**: 487–495.
13. Bucknill T, Jackson JW, Kemp HBS and Kendall BE (1973) Hemangioma of a vertebral body treated by ligation of the segmental arteries. *J Bone & Joint Surg* **55-B**: 534–539.
14. Chavhan ND and Baird D St C (1973) Skeletal muscle hemangiomas. An unusual case and a short review of the literature. *J Irish Med Assoc* **66**: 291–293.
15. Holbrow CA and Mott JJ (1973) Subglottic hemangioma in infancy. *J Laryngol & Otol* **87**: 1013–1017.
16. Lasser AE and Stein AE (1973) Steroid treatment of hemangiomas in children. *Arch Derm* **108**: 565–567.
17. Moon NF (1973) Synovial hemangioma of the knee joint. *Clin Ortho* **90**: 183–190.
18. Overcash KE and Putney FJ (1973) Subglottic hemangioma of the larynx treated with steroid therapy. *Laryngoscope* **83**: 679–682.
19. Amacher AL, Allcock JM and Drake CG (1972) Cerebral angiomas: The sequelae of surgical treatment. *J Neurosurg* **37**: 571–575.
20. Bourne RG and Taylor RGS (1972) Treatment of a juvenile laryngeal angioma with a beta-ray therapy applicator. *Radiology* **103**: 423–426.
21. Cohen SR and Wang C-I (1972) Steroid treatment of hemangioma of the head and neck in children. *Ann Otol Rhinol Laryngol* **81**: 584–590.
22. Hekster REM, Luyedijk W and Tan TI (1972) Spinal-cord compression caused by vertebral haemangioma relieved by percutaneous catheter embolisation. *Neuroradiology* **3**: 160–164.
23. Macanash JD and Owen MD (1972) Central cavernous hemangioma of the mandible: Report of cases. *J Oral Surg* **30**: 293–296.
24. McLean RH, Moller JH, Warwick WJ, Satran L and Lucas Jr RV (1972) Multinodular hemangiomatosis of the liver in infancy. *Pediatrics* **49**: 563–573.
25. Skalkeas G, Gogas J and Pavlatos F (1972) Mammary hypoplasia following irradiation to an infant breast. *Acta Chir Plast* **14**: 240–243.
26. Kagan AR, Jaffe HL and Kennamer R (1971) Hemangioma of the liver treated by irradiation. *J Nuclear Med* **12**: 835–837.
27. Unni KK, Ivins JC, Beabout JW and Dahlin DC (1971) Hemangioma hemangiopericytoma and hemangioendothelioma (angiosarcoma) of bone. *Cancer* **27**: 1403–1414.
28. Adam YG, Huvos AG and Fortner JG (1970) Giant hemangiomas of the liver. *Ann Surg* **172**: 239–245.
29. Hoehn JG, Farrow GM, Devine KD and Masson JK (1970) Invasive hemangioma of the head and neck. *Am J Surg* **120**: 495–500.
30. Park WC and Phillips R (1970) The role of radiation therapy in the management of hemangiomas of the liver. *JAMA* **212**: 1496–1498.
31. Touloukian RJ (1970) Hepatic hemangioendothelioma during infancy: Pathology, diagnosis and treatment with prednisone. *Pediatrics* **45**: 71–76.
32. Corby DC, Oquendo-Cobrera A and Louru JM (1969) Thrombocytopenia in a patient with a relatively small facial hemangioma. *Clin Pediatr* **8**: 728–731.
33. Pyesmany A, Ekert H, Williams K and Hittle R (1969) Intravascular coagulation secondary to cavernous hemangioma in infancy: Response to radiotherapy. *Canad Med Assn J* **100**: 1053–1055.
34. Williams HE, Phelan PD, Stocks JG and Wood H (1969) Hemangioma of the larynx in infants: Diagnosis, respiratory mechanics and management. *Aust Pedia J* **5**: 149–154.
35. Calcaterra TC (1968) An evaluation of the treatment of subglottic hemangioma. *Laryngoscope* **78**: 1956–1964.
36. Fost NC and Esterly NB (1968) Successful treatment of juvenile hemangiomas with prednisone. *J Pediatr* **72**: 351–357.
37. Issa P (1968) Cavernous hemangioma of the liver: The role of radiotherapy. *Br J Radiol* **41**: 26–32.
38. Katz HP and Askin J (1968) Multiple hemangiomata with thrombopenia. *Am J Dis Child* **115**: 351–357.
39. Shim WKT (1968) Hemangiomas of infancy complicated by thrombocytopenia. *Am J Surg* **116**: 896–906.
40. Kolar J, Bek V and Vrabec R (1967) Hypoplasia of the growing breast. *Arch Derm* **96**: 427–430.
41. Loring MF (1967) Hemangioma of the mandible. *Arch Otolaryng* **85**: 648–652.
42. Maier HC (1967) Hemangiomas of the subglottic region trachea and mediastinum in infancy and childhood. *Ann Thoracic Surg* **3**: 514–525.
43. Tefft M (1966) The radiotherapeutic management of subglottic hemangioma in children. *Radiology* **86**: 207–214.
44. Weldman AI, Zimany A and Kopf AW (1966) Underdevelopment of the human breast after radiotherapy. *Arch Derm* **93**: 708–710.
45. Zaidi ZH (1966) Hemangioma with thrombocytopenia. *Proc Roy Soc Med* **59**: 851–853.
46. Abramson BS (1965) Central hemangioma of the mandible: Report of a case. *J Oral Surg* **23**: 66–70.
47. Svien HJ and McRae JA (1965) Arteriovenous anomalies of the brain. Fate of patients not having definitive surgery. *J Neurosurg* **23**: 23–28.
48. Duncan W and Halnan KE (1964) Giant hemangioma with thrombocytopenia. *Clin Radiol* **15**: 224–231.
49. Topazian RG (1964) Central hemangioma of the mandible. *Oral Surg Oral Med & Oral Path* **18**: 1–6.
50. Bergstrand A, Hook U and Lidvall H (1963) Vertebral hemangiomas compressing the spinal cord. *Acta Neuro Scand* **39**: 59–66.
51. Nordberg UB and Sundberg J (1963) Indications and methods for radiotherapy of cavernous hemangiomas. *Acta Radiol [Ther]* **1**: 257–274.
52. Shockman AT, Wenger JA and Kohn NN (1963) Hemangioma of the liver. *Gastroent* **45**: 425–428.
53. Sutherland DA and Clark H (1962) Hemangioma associated with thrombocytopenia. *Am J Med* **33**: 150–157.
54. Ferguson CF and Flake CG (1961) Subglottic hemangioma as a cause of respiratory obstruction in infants. *Trans Am Bronchoesoph Assoc* **41**: 27–47.

55. Rohan RF (1960) Hemangioma of the mandible presenting as epistaxis. *J Laryngol & Otol* **74**: 178-181.
56. Lampe I and Latourette HB (1959) Management of hemangiomas in infants. *Pediatr Clinics of North Am* **6**: 511-528.
57. Smith HW (1959) Hemangioma of the jaws. *Arch Otolaryng* **70**: 579-587.
58. Doermann P, Lunseth J and Segnitz R (1958) Obstructing subglottic hemangioma of the larynx in infancy. *New England J Med* **258**: 68-71.
59. Holborow CA (1958) Subglottic hemangioma: Two infants with laryngeal stridor. *Arch Dis Child* **33**: 210-211.
60. Liang DS (1958) Hemangioma of the bladder. *J Urol* **79**: 956-960.
61. Scott JE (1957) Hemangiomata in skeletal muscle. *Br J Surg* **44**: 496-501.
62. Baker DC and Pennington CL (1956) Congenital hemangioma of the larynx. *Laryngoscope* **66**: 696-701.
63. Paterson HJ and McKissock W (1956) A clinical survey of intracranial angiomas with special reference to their mode of progression and surgical treatment: A report of 110 cases. *Brain* **79**: 233-266.
64. Potter JM (1955) Angiomatous malformations of the brain: Their nature and prognosis. *Ann Roy Coll Surg Eng* **16**: 227-243.
65. Jones KG (1953) Cavernous hemangioma of striated muscle. A review of the literature and a report of four cases. *J Bone & Joint Surg Am* **35**: 717-728.
66. Wilson H and Tyson WT (1952) Massive hemangiomas of the liver. *Ann Surg* **135**: 765-770.
67. Lindquist I (1951) Vertebral hemangioma with compression of the spinal cord. *Acta Radiol* **35**: 400-406.
68. Bergman PS (1950) Hemangioma of the pons. *J Mt Sinai Hosp* **17**: 119-131.
69. Oppenheim A and O'Brien JP (1950) Unusual anal, rectal and perirectal tumors palpable by rectal examination. *Am J Surg* **79**: 302-311.
70. Kasabach HH and Donlan CP (1945) Roentgen therapy of hemangioma of the larynx in infants. *J Pediatr* **26**: 374-378.
71. Feber L and Lampe I (1942) Hemangioma of vertebra associated with compression of the cord. Response to radiation therapy. *Arch Neurol & Psychiat* **47**: 19-29.

Herpes Zoster

Historically, irradiation of herpes zoster was said to be effective when the "bouquet" of lesions first formed over the sensory fibers. Careful scrutiny of the results of such treatments revealed no therapeutic benefit, viewed in light of the variability of the natural course of the disorder. Today acyclovir is indicated in clearly aggressive disease. Proper consultation and appreciation of the virulence of this disorder in immunosuppressed cancer patients, probably constitute the two most important means of controlling these lesions. Radiation treatment of herpes zoster is not indicated. Seventy-nine percent of radiation oncologists participating in the national survey would not treat herpes zoster with radiation.

Herpes Zoster Radiotherapy

Author, Year	Total # Patients	Treatment	Results	Notes
Rhys-Lewis, 1965	139	100r (skin dose) in 10 days to area overlying affect root-ganglion 1. Pts with slight symptoms 2. Pts with moderate symptoms 3. Pts with severe symptoms	Complete relief. 23/29 (1) 45/73 (2) 13/37 (3)	No clear evidence that radiation therapy is of any value.
	140	Controls - no treatment	Complete relief	
	26	Ophthalmic zoster only 1000r (skin dose) in 10 days to area overlying affected root-ganglion. 1. Pts with slight symptoms 2. Pts. with moderate symptoms 3. Pts with severe symptoms	Complete relief. 10/10 (1) 3/8 (2) 2/8 (3)	

Historical Data: Herpes Zoster Radiotherapy

Author, Year	Total # Patients	Treatment	Results	Notes
	36	1000r (skin dose) in 10 days to area over affected root-ganglion. 1. Pts with slight symptoms 2. Pts. with moderate symptoms 3. Pts with severe symptoms	Complete relief. 7/7 (1) 13/21 (2) 3/8 (3)	
	31	Ophthalmic zoster only (1, 2, 3) Same as directly above	Complete relief. 3/3 (1) 9/13 (2) 5/15 (3)	Treated prior to institution of controls
O'Brien, 1950	15	200 Kv, 0.5mm Cu plus 1mm Al filtration, FSD, 50cm. Field size: 15 x 10cm. 800r/4F/2 wks to the spinal nerve roots involved.	15/15 responded to irradiation	
Reeves and Waters, 1946	56	200 Kv, 0.5mm Cu plus 1mm Al filtration, FSD, 50cm. 800-1000r in 4-5 fractions over 4-5 days	38/56 cured	
McCombs, Tuggle and Guion, 1940	72	200 Kv, 1mm Cu plus 1mm Al filtration, FSD, 50cm. 6 x 15cm portal over spinal root ganglion of the nerves involved 1000-1200r in 5-6 fractions over 5-12 days	56/72 cured	46% cured within 8-14 days
	51	Controls (14 received injections of pituitrin)	51/51 cured	Only 16% cured within 8-14 days
Pillsbury and Fonde, 1936	50	100 Kv, no filter, FSD, 30cm. 260-325r in 4-5 fractions in 10-13 days	Effective in reducing the inflammatory recetion at the site of the lesion, but little effect on pain	
Keichline, 1934	62	Kv not given 3mm. Al filtration, FSD, 30cm. 148r to affected root ganglion - may be repeated if necessary	90% required single dose 8% give a second dose 2% given 3 doses at 10 day intervals	

Herpes Zoster Alternate Modes of Treatment

Author, Year	Total # Pts	Treatment	Results	Side Effects/ Complications	Notes
Simpson, 1975	50	Idoxuridine (5% or 40%) in dimethyl sulfoxide applied to the vesicles and on any prevesicular erythematous lesion 4 times a day for 4 days. (Did not paint the whole dermatome).	lesions healed more rapidly in 17/50 (34%) than would be expected without treatment Pain was relieved more rapidly in 26/47 (55%) than expected. No difference either in benefits or side effects between the two concentrations of IDU.	Transient stinging of the skin (29 pts)	

Historical Data: Herpes Zoster Alternate Modes of Treatment

Author, Year	Total # Pts	Treatment	Results	Side Effects/ Complications	Notes
Dawber, 1974	118	Idoxuridine (5%) in dimethyl sulfoxide applied every 4 hrs for 4 days. Idoxuridine (25%) in dimethyl sulfoxide applied every 2 hrs for four days. Only affected areas were painted.	Both concentrations shortened the period of vesiculation, healing time, and the duration of pain. No significant difference between the two concentrations.	Transient erythema (3) Urticarial oedema in 2 pts with dermatographia	
Juel-Jensen et al, 1970	20	Idoxuridine (5%) in dimethyl sulfoxide applied intermittently or Idoxuridine (40%) in dimethyl sulfoxide applied continuously for 4 days. Two control groups.	The group treated with Idoxuridine did much better than the two control groups. (Pain disappeared after a median of 3.5 days vs 14 days and 65 days for the control groups) Continuous 40% idoxuridine is superior to intermittent 5% idoxuridine (Pain disappeared after a median of 2.5 days vs 5 days)		
Faber and Burks, 1974	30	Chlorprothixene (orally or both orally and intramuscularly)	Relief of pain within 24 hrs: 11/30 (37%) Relief of pain within 72 hrs: 27/30 (90%)	Hallucinatory effects in one patient, took twice the prescribed dosage.	All patients had moderately severe to severe neuralgia.
Epstein, 1973	111	Triamcinolone injected subcutaneously beneath the visible lesions and in areas of burning, pain or pruritis.	Zoster: 52/58 (89%) excellent results. Post zoster neuralgia: 22/53 (41%) excellent results.	Sterile abscess (1) Series of abscesses (1) Cutaneous atrophy (3)	Of those patients with zoster, only 2 (3.5%) developed post zoster neuralgia.
Gailbraith, 1973	100	Amantadine hydrochloride (54 treated, 40 placebo)	The proportions of patients experiencing pain of long duration (longer than 28 days) was significantly reduced. No effect on the rate of healing or the appearance of new lesions.	Minimal side effects.	
Breen and Talukdar, 1965	50	Corticosteroids (27 treated, 23 controls)	Treated (27 cases): 4.1 days average duration of pain 0.8 days average duration of pyrexia. 4.5 days until onset of scabbing. Controls (23 cases): 15.5 days average duration of pain. 1.9 days average duration of pyrexia. 8.0 days until onset of scabbing.	No side effects on the short term regime used.	

Historical Data: Herpes Zoster Alternate Modes of Treatment (Continued)

Author, Year	Total # Pts	Treatment	Results	Side Effects/ Complications	Notes
Carter and Royds, 1957	20	Prednisone (systemic and local treatment to rash and to the eye) in ophthalmic zoster (10 treated, 10 controls)	Oedema was less, drying of rash was quicker and scarring was reduced in the prednisone group.		

References

1. Simpson JR (1975) Idoxuridine in the treatment of herpes zoster. *Practitioner* **215**: 226–229.
2. Dawber R (1974) Idoxuridine in herpes zoster: further evaluation of intermittent topical therapy. *Br Med J* **2**: 526–527.
3. Faber GA and Burks JW (1974) Chlorprothixene therapy for herpes zoster neuralgia. *South Med J* **67**: 808–812.
4. Epstein E (1973) Intralesional triamcinolone therapy in herpes zoster and post-zoster neuralgia. *EENT Monthly* **52**: 416–417.
5. Gailbraith AW (1973) Treatment of acute herpes zoster with amantadine hydrochloride (Symmetrel). *Br Med J* **4**: 693–695.
6. Juel-Jensen BE, MacCallum FO, and MacKenzie AMR (1970) Treatment of zoster with idoxuridine in dimethyl sulphoxide. Results of two double-blind controlled trials. *Br Med J* **4**: 776–780.
7. Breen GE and Talukdar PK (1965) Corticosteroids in acute infections. *Lancet* **1**: 158–160.
8. Rhys-Lewis RDS (1965) Radiotherapy in herpes zoster. *Lancet* **2**: 102–104.
9. Carter AB and Royds JE (1957) Further evaluation of intermittent topical therapy. *Br Med J* **2**: 526–527.
10. O'Brien FW (1950) Roentgen therapy and the relief of pain. *Am J Roent Rad Ther Nucl Med* **54**: 1–9.
11. Reeves RJ and Waters LB (1946) Herpes zoster. *Texas State J Med* **42**: 490–491.
12. McCombs P, Tuggle A and Guion CM (1940) Roentgen ray therapy in the treatment of herpes zoster. *Am J Med Sci* **200**: 803–808.
13. Pillsbury DM and Fonde GH (1936) The treatment of herpes zoster. *Med Clin North Am* **20**: 239–251.
14. Keichline JM (1934) Sixty-two cases of herpes zoster successfully treated with x-rays. *Radiology* **22**: 372–374.
15. Saral R, Ambinder RF, Burns WH, Angelopoulos CM, Griffin DE, Burke PJ and Lietman TS (1983) Acyclovir prophylactic against herpes simplex virus infections in leukemia patients: a randomized double blind placebo controlled study. *Ann Intl Med* **99**: 773–786.

Heterotopic Bone Formation

Radiation therapy to prevent the sequelae of heterotopic bone formation is indicated among patients known to be at high risk to develop this condition. Traditionally, 2000 rad in ten fractions has been employed, most effectively beginning within three to four days of surgery. Recent evidence indicates that lower doses of radiation may be effective and that tailoring treatment portals may reduce non-union. In the national survey, seventy percent of radiation oncologists would treat to prevent heterotopic bone formation.

Heterotopic Bone Formation

Author, Year	Total # Pts.	Sex/Age	Treatment	Results	Notes
MacLennan et al, 1984	58 (67 hips)	Average age 63 years. Ages 44–80 years. 18 Females and 40 Males.	Radiotherapy 2000 rad in 10 fractions.	Dramatic improvement in hip function.	Complications in fifteen. Treatment begins within five days of surgery.
Parkinson et al, 1982	51 (hips)	Mean 64 years. Ages 46–80 years. 17 Females and 34 Males.	Radiotherapy 2000 rad in 10 fractions.	Ninety-eight percent did not develop heterotopic bone formation.	Treatment should begin within first four days.

Historical Data: Heterotopic Bone Formation

Author, Year	Total # Pts.	Sex/Age	Treatment	Results	Notes
Schwartz and Kagan, 1979	1 (Zygomaticocaronoid ankylosis).	Male Age 51 years.	Excision followed by 2000 rad in 10 fractions.	Prevention of heterotopic bone formation.	Patient had trismus Nineteen month follow-up.

References

1. MacLennan I, Keys HM, Evarts CM and Rubin P (1984) Usefulness of post-operative hip irradiation in the prevention of heterotopic bone formation in a high risk group of patients. *Int J Radiat Oncol Biol Phys* **10**: 49–53.
2. Parkinson JR, Evarts CM and Hubbard LF (1982) Radiation therapy in the prevention of heterotopic ossification after total hip arthroplasty. *Hip, Proc, 10th Meeting*: 211–227.
3. Schwartz HC and Kagan AR (1979) Zygomatico-caronoid ankylosis secondary to heterotopic bone formation: Combined treatment by surgery and radiation therapy – a case report. *J Maxillofac Surg* **7**: 158–161.

Histiocytosis

Radiotherapy is useful in treating histiocytosis for relieving pain and preventing fracture in weight bearing bones. Local control is excellent (88–95%) in localized histiocytosis following low radiation doses, doses usually lower than 1000 rad. Radiation therapy has also proved useful in treating diabetes insipidus induced by histiocytosis. Results of the national survey indicate that 71% of radiation oncologists would treat histiocytosis.

Histiocytosis

Author, Year	Total Cases	Site and Age	Treatment	Results	Notes
Anonsen and Donaldson, 1987	24	Head and Neck 6mos to 36 years	Biopsy, radiation plus chemotherapy. Radiotherapy: 900–1600cGy in 200cGy fractions.	Local control in 14/16(88%) with mean. Follow up 5.7 years 2/16 – lost to follow up. 16/24(67%) disease-free with 6 year follow up.	Six of seven patients with diabetes insipidus were irradiated and all had easy control of their symptoms with vasopressin and radiotherapy. One had a complete response to radiation.
Sartoris and Parker, 1984	24	Seventy-one osseous lesions. 4 mos – 9.5 years	Chemotherapy, radiotherapy, combination or no treatment. Radiation therapy: 800–1500r	No difference in rates of healing by any specific therapy.	A radiologic study of resolution of osseous lesions.
Richter and D'Angio, 1981			Radiation therapy: 600–1000r sufficient for local control.	Biopsy and radiation is preferable to curettage alone for large lesions in weight-bearing bones. Radiation relieves pain associated with vertebrae body collapse.	Review article. No data presented, only the authors personal recommendations.

Histiocytosis (Continued)

Author, Year	Total Cases	Site and Age	Treatment	Results	Notes
Greenberger et al, 1979	127	Bone lesions and diabetes insipidus. Age: 1 mos-35years	Low radiation doses 100-2000r	95% local control from 100-2000r. 4/21 patients with diabetes insipidus had complete reversal of symptoms with radiotherapy.	
Griffin, 1977		Systemic advanced histiocytosis X. 4 mos of age	900r in 150r fractions hemi-body irradiation to upper half of body, with vincristine and prednisone.	Patient died 4 weeks after completion of radiation, from chemotherapy toxicity. Autopsy revealed no evidence of histiocytosis within the fields irradiated, but gross evidence of disease outside of the irradiation portals.	

Historical Data: Histiocytosis

Author, Year	# Cases	Treatment	Results	Notes
Ferris et al, 1974	1	Curettage and excision followed by radiotherapy 1500r/10 days.	Decrease in back pain and shrinkage of soft tissue mass over subsequent 2 month period. Possible additional focus of left parietal bone was noted.	Eosinophilic granuloma of the spine. Patient was 23 years of age.
Mehta et al, 1974	1	Removal of all accessible granulation tissue followed by radiotherapy, 100r/10F/10 days.	Uneventful recovery.	Eosinophilic granuloma of the temporal bone. Patient was 3 years of age.
West, 1973	1	Local radiation therapy, 300-330r, to lesions in a variety of locations (ribs, shoulders, long bones, spine, pelvis, hips, skull and mandible). After 14 years, radiotherapy was discontinued because of suspected skeletal resistance, fear of possible cerebral damage with further radiation, and diffuse skeletal involvement. Chlorambucil treatment begun. Velban therapy begun.	Patient responded well to local radiotherapy for 14 years. Marked progress of skull lesions. Chlorambucil was stopped. On Velban therapy, the left frontal lesion responded. No new lesions 1.5 years later. Patient felt well with no complaints when last seen after 85 months of Velban therapy.	Eosinophilic granuloma of bone. Patient was 15 years of age at start of treatment.
Schajowicz and Slullitel, 1973	106	Curettage (34) Curettage plus bone chips (8) Curettage plus radiotherapy (12) Radiotherapy (8) Radiotherapy and antibiotics (2)	The evolution was uniformly favorable in all unifocal bone lesions with any kind of conservative treatment. Results of treatment were variable with multiple and widely disseminated lesions, with and without Hand-	Eosinophilic granuloma of bone.

Historical Data: Histiocytosis (Continued)

Author, Year	# Cases	Treatment	Results	Notes
		Resection (13) and radiotherapy (1) Curettage, excision of gums and radiotherapy (1) Not known (2)	Schuller-Christian or Letterer-Siwe Syndrome.	
Synder et al, 1973	1	Biopsy plus 2000r to involved areas of mandible, 2000r to recurrence. Radiation, 1000r to second lesion which developed in left femur. Radiation, 2000r to third lesion in left iliac wing.	Mandibular lesion recurred 15 months later and was treated with radiotherapy. Two other lesions responded to radiotherapy. At present the patient is well without further evidence of recurrence.	Eosinophilic granuloma of bone. Patient was 28 years of age.
Johansen, 1973	1	Steroid therapy was discontinued after 16 months.	Patient is healthy and developing normally at 4 year follow up. No side effects of the corticosteriod therapy were observed.	Letterer-Siwe's disease. Patient was 9 months of age.
Kondl et al, 1972	1	Velban therapy.	Within 5 months, significant sclerosis and recalcification of all bony lesions had occurred. Maintenance therapy with Velban has produced a prolonged complete remission.	Diffuse eosinophilic granuloma of bone. Patient was 34 years of age.
Whitehead, 1972	1	Curettage and packing. Radiotherapy: 400r/single dose.	Granulation and epithelialization proceeded normally. Subsequent increase in size of lesion treated by radiotherapy. Patient was well and free of symptoms 6 months later.	Histiocytosis X.
	1	Radiotherapy to mandibular and skeletal lesions. Chlorambucil	White blood count has not been affected significantly. Patient is on chlorambucil to prevent further spread. No follow up data.	
Betts and McNeish, 1972	2	Vinblastine and prednisone.	Both patients had oral and dental manifestations. The gingiva appeared normal at 3 months follow up in one patient. The other patient deteriorated rapidly despite treatment and died 2 months after beginning treatment.	Letterer-Siwe disease. Age of patients 3–4 months.
El-Serafy and Reda, 1971	1	Surgical removal followed by radiotherapy plus prednisone.	No recurrence at 3 year follow up.	Eosinophilic granuloma of bone. Patient was 2 years of age.
	1	Radiotherapy plus prednisone. Radiotherapy was repeated twice in three years as new lesions occurred.	Some of the original lesions remain but there is definite evidence of good healing.	Eosinophilic granuloma of bone. Patient was 5 years of age.
	1	Curettage followed by radiotherapy and prednisone.	No signs of progression or recurrence during the last 7 months. Good radiologic evidence of healing of skull and vertebral lesions.	Eosinophilic granuloma of bone. Patient was 4 years of age.

Historical Data: Histiocytosis (Continued)

Author, Year	# Cases	Treatment	Results	Notes
	1	Radiotherapy plus prednisone.	Satisfactory healing.	Eosinophilic granuloma of bone. Patient was 2 1/2 years of age.
Rodrigues and Lewis, 1971	1	Curettage followed by radiotherapy, 1000r/16F/6 weeks.	Marked reduction in size of lesion with continuing gradual clinical improvement since discharge.	Eosinophilic granuloma of bone. Patient was 53 years of age.
Winkleman and Burgert, 1970	16	1. Radiotherapy alone (7) 2. Surgery (excision of curettage followed by radiotherapy (2) 3. Excision or curettage alone (5) 4. Biopsy alone (2)	1. 7/7 lesions healed at 2-5 year follow up 2. 2/2 lesions healed 3. 4/4 rapid healing of lesions. One patient lost to follow up 4. 2/2 subsequent spontaneous healing	Focal histiocytosis of bone.
	1	Radiotherapy.	Labial and palatal lesions had improved at 3-5 year follow up. But patient continued to lose her "floating" teeth because of involvement of gingiva.	Histiocytosis X of the skin (patient had granulomatous ulcers of the hard palate, upper gingiva, and labia minora). Patient was 23-60 years.
	10	Prednisone (8 patients) or triamcinolone (2 patients).	6/10 improved but complete clearing of the lung on roentgenogram was exhibited by only three patients.	Pulmonary histiocytosis X. Age range of patients was 23-60 years.
	11	1. Methotrexate and prednisone (3) 2. Prednisone alone (2) 3. Vinblastine (6)	1. 2/3 well at 3-6 year follow up 1/3 died, 1 month 2. 1/2 improved, off treatment 2 years 1/2 died, 3 months 3. 6/6 well or improving at follow up	Systemic histiocytosis X. Age range of patients was 1 month-9 years.
Burrow et al, 1970	6	Prednisone plus methotrexate in some cases.	5/6 died, in two there was obvious progression of the disease which appeared unresponsive to therapy. In the other three death occurred at a time when the disease appeared to be under control.	Letterer-Siwe disease patients were 2-14 months of age at onset of disease.
Fowles and Bobechko, 1970	40	Biopsy only (6) Biopsy plus radiotherapy (3) Biopsy plus curettage (2) Curettage only (19) Curettage plus bone graft or radiotherapy (10)	All of the patients improved regardless of the treatment.	Solitary eosinophilic granuloma of bone. Age range of 7 months to 14 years.
Davidson and Shillito, 1970	6	Biopsy, immobilization, and radiotherapy, 450-750r	6/6 cured	Eosinophilic granuloma of the cervical region. Patient was 11 years of age.
Lindenbaum and Getles, 1970	1	Curettage followed by radiotherapy, 1200r.	Gradual relief of symptoms; asymptomatic at 10 months.	Solitary eosinophilic granuloma of the cervical region. Patient was 11 years of age.

Historical Data: Histiocytosis (Continued)

Author, Year	# Cases	Treatment	Results	Notes
Bolton, 1970	1	Radiotherapy plus prednisolone	Lower anterior region responded well but lower molar and upper regions did not improve. Deterioration continued to take place necessitating extraction and curettage. Patient also developed a lesion in right femur and in pelvis. Radiotherapy to skull, jaw, femur. No recurrence of oral condition for 2 years. Subsequent prednisolone given to relieve headaches.	Hand-Schuller-Christian disease.
Nyholm, 1970	7	Radiotherapy: 50-950r in 6 patients. One patient received 2400r.	Remission of symptoms in all cases.	Solitary granulomas of bone.
	11	Locally applied radiotherapy 75-430r. Four patients had one or two osseous foci excised.	Focal response was usually prompt and local symptoms subsided. Healing was complete in most cases and there were no recurrences during 2-20 year follow up. Failure to respond to treatment in only one patient. Appearance of new lesion in 10 patients.	Multiple granulomas of bone.
Tos, 1969	1	Excision of granulomatous polyp followed by radiotherapy to the temporal bones (6000r/10 days to each side).	Function of the facial nerve improved to normal within one month.	Hand-Schuller-Christian disease with facial palsy. Patient was 4 years of age.
Esterly and Swick, 1969	1	Prednisone for 10 weeks followed by vinblastine sulfate. Cyclophosphamide for recurrence.	No response to prednisone. Striking response to vinblastine. Eight months later patient treated with cyclophosphamide for exacerbation of the eruption. Dramatic response: prompt clearing of the lesion. Treatment discontinued 6 months later with no further medication.	Cutaneous Letterer-Siwe disease. Patient was 8 months of age.
Gibson and Papa, 1968	1	1. Low fat, high carbohydrate diet and cytellin therapy. 2. Cholestyramine resin therapy, lowered carbohydrate intake and polyunsaturated fats.	Treatment 1. slight cholesterol drop and observable serum turbidity Treatment 2. dramatic lipid levels drop and clearing of skin lesions	Congenital acholangic biliary xanthomatosis. Patient also developed multiple yellowish papules on fingers and anterior surface of the elbow and knees. Patient was 13 years of age.
Roe, 1968	1	1. Cholestyramine therapy. 2. Clofibrate.	Treatment 1. ineffective in controlling the hyperlipemia; some reduction in skin lesion size. Treatment 2. reversion of serum lipid values to within the normal range; slow resolution of xanthomata.	Essential hyperlipemia with xanthomatosis. Patient was 44 years of age.

Historical Data: Histiocytosis (Continued)

Author, Year	# Cases	Treatment	Results	Notes
Hertz and Hambrick, 1968	1	Prednisone and vincristine sulfate.	Many of the old skin lesions cleared and very few new lesions appeared. Gradual attenuation and cessation of therapy. At 2 years of age physical examination was unremarkable without organomegaly or skin eruptions.	Congenital Letterer-Siwe disease.
Cornelius, 1967	2	Dietary therapy – carbohydrate restriction.	Rapid patient response. From start of dietary therapy, cutaneous lesions vanish within 2 months.	Eruptive xanthoma. Patients were 24 and 40 years of age.
Ito et al, 1967	1	Cholestyramine resin of several courses	Apparent success observed for first two courses of therapy: decreased itching and jaundice; softening and thinning of xanthomatosis lesions; and marked decrease of serum phospholipids. Serum cholesterol levels remained at more than 1000mg/100ml and fresh xanthomatous lesions appeared on post-op scar and the vermillion of the lips.	Atresia of the intrahepatic bile ducts with xanthomatosis.
Goldberg and Diamond, 1965		Corticosteroids (methylprednisone sodium succinate).	Striking therapeutic response and remission.	Letterer-Siwe disease.
Arcomano et al, 1961	1	Radiotherapy, 1200r to lesions of the right and left hemicranium. Details: 200Kv, 20ma, 0.5mm Cu plus 1mm Al filtration HVL 0.9mm Cu, FSD 50cm.	Patient improved, became asymptomatic.	Hand-Schuller-Christian disease. Patient was 6 years of age.
		Radiotherapy: 400r to skull 400r to thorax 400r to pelvis 400r to cervical spine 2nd course to spine and pelvis one year later.	Temporary subjective improvement. Two month temporary improvement following second course. Patient developed chicken pox and deteriorated rapidly. Patient eventually expired from a combination of causes.	Hand-Schuller-Christian disease. Patient was 3 1/2 years of age when first seen.
	1	Radiotherapy: 1000r/5 wks Details: 200Kv, 20ma, 0.5mm Cu plus 1mm Al filtration, HVL 0.9mm Cu, FSD 50cm.	Complete recovery	Lesion of the spine-eosinophilic granuloma. Patient was three years of age.
	1	No specific therapy other than bed rest and analgesics.	Patient asymptomatic within two months.	Eosinophilic granuloma. Patient was 2 1/2 years of age.

Historical Data: Histiocytosis (Continued)

Author, Year	# Cases	Treatment	Results	Notes
Arcomano et al, 1961 (Continued)	1	Curettage	Patient completely asymptomatic after treatment.	Eosinophilic granuloma. Patient was 2 1/2 years of age.
McGavran and Spady, 1960	28	1. Biopsy (2) 2. Biopsy followed by radiotherapy, 300-3500r (2). One patient received an additional 1800r to recurrence. 3. Curettage plus bone grafting in some cases (9) 4. Curettage plus radiotherapy 500-2420r (4). One patient also had bone grafting. 5. Excision (9 pts) 6. Excision plus radiotherapy, 1600r (1).	1. 2/2 alive and well at 3-5 year follow up. 2. 9/9 alive and well at 3-9 year follow up. 3. 4/4 alive and well at 4-9 year follow up. 4. 9/9 alive and well at 3-32 year follow up. 5. 1/1 alive and well at 3 year follow up.	Eosinophilic granuloma of bone.
Hedges, 1959	1	Radiotherapy: 400r (air)/10days Details: 100Kv, 15ma, HVL, 3.0mm Al, FSD, 24.5cm.	Granulomatous iris lesions disappeared in 3 days. Right eye normal at 3 months.	Neuroxanthoendothelioma of the eye. Patient was three months of age.
Childs and Kennedy, 1951	12	Radiotherapy: 150-200r(air) to each portal. Number of portals depending on site of the lesion.	9/12 responded well to treatment and the disease is considered to be arrested. 3/12 condition progressed rapidly and death ensued. (Little healing of the lesions, after several courses of treatment leukopenia, anemia, and thrombocytopenia developed. The patients failed rapidly and died.)	Reticuloendotheliosis of the Hand-Schuller-Christian disease.
Liebman et al, 1966	1	Radiotherapy: Dose ranging from 440-1980r of x-rays and Sr^{90} irradiation of 6000 rep/6 wks to ocular lesions. 200-400 roentgens to xanthomas on the anterior abdominal wall. This was combined with curettage and chemotherapy (used intermittently from the ages of 4-8 years).	Impossible to detect any definite suppression of the growths both ocular and cutaneous. New skin lesions stopped appearing and the old ones began to fade by the age of 4.5 yrs.	Corneal xanthomas. Presented the usual picture of xanthoma dissemination. Patient was 9 years of age.
Liebman et al, 1966 (Continued)	1	Sr^{90} irradiation, 6000 reps/2 months to lid lesion.	No observable change in treated lesion; appearance of two new lesions. Treated lesion smaller and paler 2 months after radiotherapy; untreated lesion was also reduced in size. At 4.5 years of age the cutaneous and mucosal xanthomas began to involute. Patient died of leukemia at age 5 years.	Typical features of juvenile xanthogranuloma associated with monomyelocytic leukemia and cafe au lait spots.

Historical Data: Histiocytosis (Continued)

Author, Year	# Cases	Treatment	Results	Notes
Webster et al, 1966	1	Biopsy followed by radiotherapy, 600r to heart and pericardium and 795r to skin lesion, 2000Kv, 1.5ma 5.0mm lead filter, HVL 7.0mm lead	Child was healthy but no change in skin lesions at follow up 13 months of age.	Juvenile xanthogranuloma with extracutaneous lesions.
Avioli et al, 1965	10	Oral prednisone	The clinical and laboratory manifestations of the disease were favorably altered in all cases. The cutaneous lesions responded favorably in all cases.	Histiocytosis X (Hand-Schuller-Christian disease).

References

1. Anonsen CK and Donaldson SS (1987) Langerhan's cell histiocytosis of the head and neck. *Laryngoscope* **5**: 537–542.
2. Sartoris DJ and Parker BR (1984) Histiocytosis X: rate and pattern of resolution of osseous lesions. *Radiology* **152**: 679–684.
3. Richter MP and D'Angio GJ (1981) The role of radiation therapy in the management of children with histiocytosis X. *Am J Pediat Hermatol Oncol* **3**: 161–163.
4. Greenberger JS, Cassady JR, Jaffe N, Vawter G and Crocker AC (1979) Radiation therapy in patients with histiocytosis: Management of diabetes insipidus and bone lesions. *Int J Radiat Oncol Biol Phys* **5**: 1749–1755.
5. Griffin TW (1977) The treatment of advanced histiocytosis X with sequential hemibody irradiation. *Cancer* **39**: 2435–2436.
6. Ferris RA, Pethrone FA, McKelvie AM, Twigg HL and Chun BK (1974) Eosinophilic granuloma of the spine. An unusual radiographic presentation. *Clin Orth* **99**: 57–63.
7. Gregg JA and Utz DC (1974) Eosinophilic cystitis associated with eosinophilic gastroenteritis. *Mayo Clin Proc* **49**: 185–187.
8. Mehta DN, Romani GV, Chatterjee AK and Subramanyam CSV (1974) Eosinophilic granuloma of the temporal bone. *J Laryn & Otol* **88**: 185–191.
9. Johansen AG (1973) A case of Letterer-Siwe disease. Successful result with long term steroid treatment. *Dermatologica* **146**: 297–302.
10. Schajowicz F and Slullitel (1973) Eosinophilic granuloma of bone and its relationship to Hand-Schuller-Christian and Letterer-Siwe syndromes. *J Bone & Joint Surg Br* **55**: 545–565.
11. Snyder SR, Merkow LP and White NS (1973) Eosinophilic granuloma of bone. Report of case. *Oral Surg* **31**: 712–715.
12. West WO (1973) Velban as treatment for diffuse eosinophilic granuloma of bone. Report of a case. *J Bone & Joint Surg Am* **55**: 1755–1759.
13. Betts PR and McNeish AS (1972) Oral manifestations of Letterer-Siwe disease. *Arch Dis in Child* **48**: 463–464.
14. Kondl ES, Deckers PJ, Gallitano AL and Khung CL (1972) Diffuse eosinophilic granuloma of bone. A dramatic response to Velban therapy. *Cancer* **30**: 1169–1173.
15. Vogel JM and Vogel P (1972) Idiopathic histiocytosis: A discussion of eosinophilic granuloma, the Hand-Schuller-Christian syndrome and the Letterer-Siwe syndrome. *Sem Hemat* **9**: 349–369.
16. Whitehead FIH (1972) Histiocytosis X. *Br J Oral Surg* **10**: 199–204.
17. El-Serafy F and Reda M (1971) Histiocytosis. *J Laryngol & Otol* **25**: 857–867.
18. Rodrigues RJ and Lewis HH (1971) Eosinophilic granuloma of bone. Review of literature and case presentation. *Clin Orth* **77**: 183–192.
19. Bolton R (1970) Hand-Schuller-Christian disease. Report of a case. *Br J Oral Surg* **7**: 116–123.
20. Burrow D, Kelly AMT, Bridges JM and Connolly JH (1970) Letterer-Siwe disease. Report of six cases. *Br J Derm* **83**: 135–142.
21. Davidson RE and Shillito J (1970) Eosinophilic granuloma of the cervical spine in children. *Ped* **45**: 746–752.
22. Fowles JV and Bobechko WP (1970) Solitary eosinophilic granuloma in bone. *J Bone & Joint Surg Br* **52**: 238–243.
23. Lindenbaum B and Getles NI (1970) Solitary eosinophilic granuloma of the cervical regions. A case report. *Clin Orth* **68**: 112–114.
24. Nyholm K (1970) Eosinophilic xanthomatous granulomatosis and Letterer-Siwe disease. *Acta Path & Micr Scand Suppl* **216**: 59–69.
25. Winkleman RK and Burgert EO (1970) Therapy of histiocytosis X. *Br J Derm* **82**: 169–175.
26. Esterly NB and Swick HM (1969) Cutaneous Letterer-Siwe disease. *Am J Dis Child* **117**: 236–238.
27. Tos M (1969) Facial palsy in Hand-Schuller-Christian disease. *Arch Otol* **90**: 563–567.
28. Gibson WB and Papa CM (1968) Congenital acholangic biliary xanthomatosis. *Arch Derm* **97**: 600–602.
29. Hertz CG and Hambrick GW (1968) Congenital Letterer-Siwe disease. A case treated with vincristine and corticosteroids. *Am J Dis Child* **116**: 553–556.
30. Roe DA (1968) Essential hyperlipemia with xanthomatosis. Effects of cholestyramine and clofibrate. *Arch Derm* **97**: 436–445.
31. Cornelius CE (1967) Disappearance of eruptive xanthoma following carbohydrate restriction. *Arch Derm* **96**: 45–50.
32. Ito J, Sugai T and Saito T (1967) Atresia of the intrahepatic bile ducts with xanthomatosis. *Arch Derm* **96**: 53–58.
33. Liebman SD, Crocker AC and Feiser CF (1966) Corneal xanthomas in childhood. *Arch Ophth* **76**: 221–228.

34. Webster SB, Reister HC and Harmon LE (1966) Juvenile xanthogranuloma with extracutaneous lesions. A case report and review of the literature. *Arch Derm* **93**: 71-76.
35. Avioli LV, Lasersohn JT and Lopresti JM (1965) Histiocytosis X (Schuller-Christian Disease): A clinopathological survey, review of ten patients and the results of prednisone therapy. *Med* **42**: 119-147.
36. Goldberg LC and Diamond A (1965) Letterer-Siwe Disease. *Arch Derm* **92**: 561-565.
37. Lichtenstein L (1964) Histiocytosis X (eosinophilic granuloma of bone, Letterer-Siwe disease, and Shuller-Christian disease). *J Bone & Joint Surg Am* **46**: 76-90.
38. Arcomano JP, Barnett JD and Wunderlich HO (1961) Histiocytosis X. *Am J Roent Rad Therp & Nuc Med* **85**: 663-679.
39. McGavran MH and Spady HA (1960) Eosinophilic granuloma of bone. A study of twenty-eight cases. *J Bone & Joint Surg Am* **42**: 979-992.
40. Hedges CC (1959) Neuroxanthoendothelioma of the eye treated with superficial x-ray therapy. *Am J Ophth* **47**: 683-684.
41. Childs DS and Kennedy RLJ (1951) Reticulo-endotheliosis of children: Treatment with roentgen rays. *Radiology* **57**: 653-658.

Hypersalivation in Amyotrophic Lateral Sclerosis

Hypersalivation in amyotrophic lateral sclerosis (ALS) is a secondary phenomenon associated with progressive difficulty in swallowing observed in this neurologic disorder. The patient's long term prognosis is dismal and palliative relief of frothing can be achieved rapidly with 2000 rad in five fractions to a port which encompasses the parotid, submaxillary and submandibular salivary glands, yet does not extend beyond the pre-vertebral fascia, thereby avoiding the spinal cord. Other fractionation schemes may be used to dry the mouth, but these involve more clinic visits for these pre-terminal patients. Dental care, which ordinarily would be a consideration, usually is not of concern due to shortened survival. There is no formal literature for this humane treatment. It is, however, usually easily agreed upon by neurologists, patients, family and radiation oncologists. In the national survey, 71% of radiation oncologists would not treat hypersalivation from amyotrophic lateral sclerosis.

Hypersplenism

Enlargement of the spleen may be painful and associated with hemolytic anemia, thrombocytopenia, granulocytopenia and, in some instances, extramedullary hematopoiesis. Lymphoma, leukemia, sickle cell anemia and myelosclerosis are all potential etiologic factors in hypersplenism. Irradiation to reduce splenomegaly and pain must be carried out cautiously, especially if the spleen is the source of extramedullary hematopoiesis. Very small incremental fractional doses in association with daily pre-treatment CBCs are needed to guide therapy. Significant palliative benefit may be achieved. In some instances, subsequent splenectomy after x-ray reduction is appropriate.

We prefer semi-log recording of WBC and platelets to evaluate not only absolute count, but also the rate of descent of the counts. Thus, a very high platelet count that falls, but to a still substantial absolute count, requires cessation of splenic radiation until the count stabilizes at some acceptable level. For example, if a platelet count falls from 200,000 to 125,000, treatment would be stopped, as more than likely the platelet count would continue to fall before recovering. Continued therapy would probably result in a life-threatening grade four thrombocytopenia. Yet a drop in platelet count in another patient from 110,000 to 100,000 represents an acceptable reduction allowing cautious continued therapy. In myelosclerosis, where the spleen is a site of extramedullary hematopoiesis, the goal is to reduce splenic size and discomfort without unduly risking life; WBC and platelets must be arduously followed. Seventy-six percent of radiation oncologists in the national survey would treat hypersplenism.

Hypersplenism Radiotherapy

Author, Year	Total # Pts.	Underlying Disease	Hematologic Manifestations of the Disease	Treatment	Results
Byhardt et al, 1975	14	Chronic lymphocytic leukemia	Progressive leukocytosis, lymphocytosis, thrombocytopenia and anemia.	Splenic midlplane dose, 200-1750r/3-14 days, Co-60. Field size: shaped to cover the palpable spleen and reduced as the spleen regressed. Fourteen pts received a total of 23 courses of irradiation.	14/18 relief of splenic pain. 8/23 splenomegaly was reduced by 5% or more. 12/23 splenomegaly was reduced by 25-50%. 11/23 peripheral WBC showed a 75% reduction or more. 12/23 peripheral absolute lymphocyte counts show a reduction of more than 75%. 14/23 platelet counts stable or increased to above 50,000/mm. 12/23 hemoglobin unchanged at 12-13mg/100ml one rose to this level. 3/7 reduction of lymphadenopathy of 50% or more.
Szur et al, 1973	3	Myelosclerosis	Anemia (2)	1000-2000r/14-26 days, Co-60, through a single anterior port usually over the lower part of the spleen. Field size: 15 x 15cm, 11 x 14cm or 12 x 12cm.	3/3 reduction of splenic size and abolishment of erythropoiesis (but not phagocytic activity in the spleen).
Sommer and Kontras, 1971	1	Sickle cell anemia	Anemia	1150r/7F, Co-60	Hemoglobin level and reticulocyte count rose. Reduction in splenic size.
Comas et al, 1968	8	Chronic lymphatic leukemia (3) Myeloproliferation (2) Lymphosarcoma (2) Liver cirrhosis (1)	Hemolytic anemia (7) Thrombocytopenia (6) Granulocytopenia (3)	700-2000r (mid plane dose)/8-17 days, Co-60, through opposing anterior and posterior fields which included all of the spleen.	No increase in granulocytes. No change in thombocytopenia. No change in hemolytic anemia. Some clinical improvement related to reduction in spleen size. Subsequent splenectomy in 6 pts. 5/6 obtained good relief of their hypersplenism.
Awwad et al, 1967	18	CML (8 pts) CLL (10 pts)		CML: 200r/4 wks to 400r/6 wks (skin dose per portal) CLL: 175r/3 wks to 374r/5 wks 250Kv, 15ma, HVL 1.5mm CU, FSD 50cm.	General reduction in splenic size, improvement in blood levels, and control of associated anemia.

Historical Data: Hypersplenism Radiotherapy

Author, Year	Total # Pts.	Underlying Disease	Hematologic Manifestations of the Disease	Treatment	Results
Djaldetti et al, 1962	8	Chronic lymphocytic leukemia.	Hemolytic anemia (8) All had failed to respond to drug therapy.	100r(air)/day for total of 200-700r (until WBC count dropped to 1/2 initial value) through two opposed fields, abdominal and dorsal. Technical factors: 100Kv, 0.5mm Cu filtration, FSD 50cm. Some pts also received steroid therapy.	5/8 remission anemia 5/8 reduction splenic size 8/8 decreased WBC count. Complications: GI bleeding (1)
Cook and Romano, 1962	117	Chronic lymphocytic leukemia		200r(air) at tri-weekly intervals. If lymphadenopathy is present, the enlarged lymph nodes are irradiated weekly and then at gradually spaced intervals with 150-200r in air.	At one year: 86/91 excellent response 3/91 good response 2/91 poor response excellent = relief of symptoms, blood picture returned to near normal, tumor fractions decreased markedly and pt able to return to a relatively normal life.
Hotchkis and Block, 1962	11	Chronic myelogenous leukemia	Anemia and leukocytosis in all patients.	950-3880r(air)/13-36 days localized to the spleen. Treatments were given in daily increments of 50-200r until the white cell count was reduced to 20,000-25,000. Technical factors: 250Kv, 30ma, Thoraeus II filter, FSD 40-50cm.	9/11 clinical remission (white cell count fell, hemoglobulin rose) which lasted from 1-9 months.
Szur and Smith, 1961	5	Myelosclerosis		Partial splenic irradiation.	All 5 patients benefited symptomatically.
Parsons et al, 1954	12	Chronic granulocytic leukemia	The validity of these studies has been questioned in that it is now believed that bone marrow smears do not accurately reflect the structure of the marrow	840-3240r/3-12F/3-12 days over 3-9 splenic fields. Technical factors: 130Kv, HVL 0.3mm Cu, FSD, 40.6cm. Field size: 50-75 sq cm	Results were assessed by sternal marrow counts. 8/12 significant decrease in the myeloid-erythroid layer. A fairly uniform decrease in all cells of the granulocytic series occurred.
Gunz, 1953	15	Chronic myeloid leukemia	The validity of these studies has been questioned in that it is now believed that bone marrow smears do not accurately reflect the structure of the marrow	600-2000r total dose. X-rays were in the 2-2.3 Mev range.	Results were assessed by sternal marrow counts: 6/8 either a few in the number of immature myeloid cells or a rise in the number of immature erythroid cells.

Historical Data: Hypersplenism Radiotherapy (Continued)

Author, Year	Total # Pts.	Underlying Disease	Hematologic Manifestations of the Disease	Treatment	Results
					6/12 a significant reduction of mitoses in immature myeloid cells 80 minutes after irradiation.
Hickling, 1953	7	Osteosclerosis or myelosclerosis.	Large increase in circulating leukocytes (5). Slight - moderate anemia (2).	X-ray treatment to the spleen alone or to the spleen and long bones.	5/7 benefited (decreased size of spleen and/or decrease in leukocytes and immature cells.) The two who received no benefit did not have increased leukocytes prior to treatment. Side effects/complications: Leukopenia (2), Anemia (1).
Stats et al, 1947	1	Giant follicular lymphoblastoma	Anemia	150r/3F to the 4 abdominal quadrants both anteriorly and posteriorly	No effect on the severity of the anemia. Spleen reduced greatly in size. Treatment halted due to fall in WBC count to 1650.

References

1. Byhardt RW, Brace KC and Wiernik PH (1975) The role of splenic irradiation in chronic lymphocytic leukemia. *Cancer* **35**: 1621–1625.
2. Jacobs HS (1974) Hypersplenism: mechanisms and management. *Br J Haematology* **27**: 1–5.
3. Szur L, Pettit JE, Lewis SM, Bruce-Tagoe AA and Short MD (1973) The effect of radiation on splenic function in myelosclerosis: studies with ^{52}Fe and ^{99}Tm. *Br J Radiology* **46**: 295–301.
4. Sommer A and Kontras SB (1971) Splenomegaly with hypersplenism in sickle cell anemia treated by radiation - case report. *Pediatrics* **48**: 457–458.
5. Comas FV, Andrews GA and Nelson B (1968) Spleen irradiation in secondary hypersplenism. *Am J Roent Rad Ther and Nucl Med* **104**: 668–673.
6. Awwad AK, Badeeb AO, Massoud GE and Salah M (1967) The effect of splenic x-irradiation on the ferrokinetics of chronic leukemia with a clinical study. *Blood* **29**: 242–256.
7. Cook JC and Romano W (1962) Chronic lymphocytic leukemia and radiation therapy. *Am J Roent Rad Ther and Nucl Med* **82**: 892–901.
8. Djaldetti M, de Vries A and Levie B (1962) Hemolytic anemia in lymphocytic leukemia. *Arch Int Med* **110**: 449–455.
9. Szur L and Smith MD (1961) Red-cell production and destruction in myelosclerosis. *Br J Haematology* **17**: 147–168.
10. Parsons WB, Watkins CH, Pease GL and Childs DS (1954) Changes in sternal marrow following roentgen ray therapy to the spleen in chronic granulocytic leukemia. *Cancer* **7**: 179–189.
11. Gunz FW (1953) Bone marrow changes in patients with chronic leukemia treated by splenic x-irradiation. *Blood* **8**: 687–692.
12. Hickling RA (1953) Treatment of patients with myelosclerosis. *Br Med J* **2**: 411–414.
13. Hotchkis DJ and Block MH (1952) Effect of splenic irradiation on systemic hematopoiesis. *Arch Int Med* **109**: 695–711.
14. Stats D, Rosenthal N and Wasserman LR (1947) Hemolytic anemia associated with malignant diseases. *Am J Clin Path* **17**: 585–613.

Hyperthyroidism

Classic treatment is by surgical and either medical or radioisotopic techniques.

Hyperthyroidism I 131 Therapy

Author, Year	Total # Patients	Treatment	Results	Notes
Thjodleifsson, 1975	174	1. I 131: Average initial dose 4.8mCi (37 patients). 2. Thyroidectomy (137).	1. 29/137(78.3%) euthyroid 7/37(18.9%) hypothyroid 2. 93/137(67.9%) euthyroid 11/137(8.1%) hypothyroid 33/137(24%) relapses	Graves' disease.
Wise et al, 1975	50	I 131: 10-12mCi for impalpable or small goiters, and 15mCi for larger goiters.	At six months: 46-50(92%) hypothyroid 4/50(8%) euthyroid.	All had diffuse goiters. Authors state that the rate of clinical improvement in 42(86%) early responders was such that antithyroid drugs were regarded as unnecessary.
Cevallos et al, 1974	102	I 131 Low dose: Mean thyroid dose of 5578r. High dose: Mean thyroid dose of 9986r.	Low dose: 56/102 euthyroid 19/102 hypothyroid 27/102 hyperthyroid High dose: 17/35 euthyroid 16/35 hypothyroid	Graves' disease.
Tunbridge et al, 1974	105	I 131 therapy: details not given.	Two year follow up: 85/105(81%) euthyroid 13/105(12%) hypothyroid	Author measured TSH levels, serum triiodothyronine levels, serum protein bound iodine and serum thyroxine. They concluded that raised serum TSH levels are not necessarily indicative of hypothyroidism.
Rapport et al, 1973	85	I 131 therapy: Retained dose of 50 uc/gm estimated to deliver 4130r to the thyroid. This was supplemented when necessary with antithyroid drugs.	At one year follow up: 33/85(38.8%) euthyroid 6/85(7.1%) hypothyroid 46/85(54.1%) hyperthyroid	All patients had diffuse toxic goiter (Graves' disease). Authors concluded that low dose sodium I 131 therapy has no short term advantage over anti-thyroid drugs alone due to the large number of patients that are still hyperthyroid at one year and to the fact that permanent hypothyroidism is not avoided.
Douglas, 1973	94	I 131: Mean dosage of 3-23mCi.	Cumulative incidence of hypothyroidism. 37.8% One year. 54.4% Five years. 81.3% Fifteen years.	Graves' disease.

Historical Data: Hyperthyroidism I 131 Therapy

Author, Year	Total # Patients	Treatment	Results	Notes
Blahd and Hayes, 1972	241	I 131 therapy: Dose: Calculated to give 5900–6000r to the thyroid (assuming 120r/1uc/gm). Estimated thyroid gland weight was obtained by empirical weight calculations. 132 patients received one dose. 72 patients received two doses. 36 patients received three or more doses.	Percentage hypothyroid (corrected for length of follow up): 10.4% at one year. 21.2% at five years. 39.5% at ten years. 70.8% at fifteen years.	All had Graves' disease. The entire patient population in this series was male. Percentage hypothyrodism increased by an increment of 2.7% per year in years 1 to 5, 3.7% per year in years 5 to 10, and 6.3% per year in years 10 to 15.
Glennon et al, 1972	55	I 131: Dose, mean dose of 2.7mCi.	3.7% hypothyroid at the end of one year. Annual incidence rate increase of 3.4% for 5–7 years. Total of 48% hypothyroid at 17 years.	There was a plateau in the incidence of hypothyroidism from the first to the fifth year.
McDougall and Greig, 1972	74	Combined carbamizone – I 131 treatment: Carbamizole given for five months stopped for two weeks when dose of I 131 was given, was restarted one week later and continued for five more months. (.1mg thyroxine daily was also given during this last phase). Two dose regimes: Standard dose (mean dose of 7.6mCi) low dose (mean dose of 3.8mCi). The two doses differ by a factor of two.	Standard dose group: 16/38(42.1%) euthyroid 14/38(36.8%) relapsed 8/38(21.1%) hypothyroid Low dose: 16/36(44.4%) euthyroid 17/36(47.2%) relapsed 3/36(8.4%) hypothyroid	
Sachs et al, 1972	603	I 131: Dose, majority received 3–6mc.	Using life table method. 12.3% hypothyroidism at the end of 1 year. 2.5% became hypothyroid in the second year. Decreasing incidence of hypothyroidism was found at eleven years, 40% hypothyroid, overall incidence of 23.6%.	
Jackson, 1971	131	The majority of patients received 1–4mc total dose of I 131.	One year follow up: 85/93(91.3%) euthyroid 5/93(5.3%) hypothyroid Two year follow up: 62/66(93.9%) euthyroid 4/66(6%) hypothyroid Total series results (minimum of three months follow up). 112/131(85%) euthyroid 15/131(11%) hypothyroid	20% required two or more treatments.

Historical Data: Hyperthyroidism I 131 Therapy (Continued)

Author, Year	Total # Patients	Treatment	Results	Notes
Jonckheer, 1971	40	I 131 therapy: Dose: 2-8mCi	65% initial drop in total serum thyroxine followed by a rebound into hyperthyroid levels. The dose was insufficient to produce euthyroid serum thyroxine levels in 85% of the patients.	Diagnosis: Graves' disease (28) Toxic nodular goiter (12) Authors recommend that complementary treatment be delayed for about four weeks in order to obtain full benefit from I 131 therapy.
Lewitus et al, 1971	99	1. Small dose I 125 (average 2.5mCi) (45 patients). 2. Intermediate dose I 125 (11 patients). 3. I 125 (average dose 3mCi) plus I 131 (average dose 3.8mCi) (43 patients).	1. 18/45 fair-good results. 3/45 permanent hypothyroidism. 2. 6/11 good results. 1/11 hypothyroidism. 3. 39/43 fair-good results. 3/43 hypothyroidism.	
Franco, 1970	18	I 131 and propranolol (a beta adrenergic blocking agent). Dose: 5mCi of I 131 10-40mg. q.i.d. propranolol. Propranolol was discontinued when there was no additional clinical need for symptomatic treatment.	Follow up of 2-16 months. Symptomatic improvement was immediate. No laboratory or clinical relapses to date. 5/18 developed clinical and/or laboratory signs of hypothyroidism and were put on replacement therapy.	Diagnosis: In all patients, diffuse thyroid hyperplasia with hyperthyroidism.
Kaipainen et al, 1970	243	I 131: 5.5mc	At one year: 22% hyperthyroid 7.4% hypothyroid At two years: 11% hyperthyroid 8.6% hypothyroid	
Viherkoski et al, 1970	387	Pretreatment with carbimazole in 55(14%). I 131 dose calculated to give 100-130uCi/gm in diffuse goiter and 140-160uCi/gm in nodular goiter. Post treatment with carbimazole in 186(43%).	Incidence of hypothyroidism at one year: 11.8% toxic nodular goitre 25.6% toxic diffuse goitre Yearly increment of 10,2%. 14% of the patients were pretreated with antithyroid drugs. In those not so treated severe post treatment reactions occurred in 4%. In addition the incidence of hypothyroidism was lower in the group of patients treated without carbimazole or with only post treatment carbimazole (21-22%).	
Burke and Silverstein, 1969	484	I 131: Mean therapeutic dose was 8.9 + 7.2mCi.	Incidence of hypothyroidism: 31% at one year. 44% at five years. 54% at eight years.	Graves' disease.
Goolden and Fraser, 1969	181	I 131 therapy: Dose, 150uCi/gm of thyroid tissue. 83 patients were given pretreatment with carbimazole for 2-4 months.	Follow up of one year. Carbimazole plus I 131: 63% euthyroid 14% hypothyroid 23% toxic	Pretreatment with carbimazole did not significantly alter subsequent response to I 131 therapy.

Historical Data: Hyperthyroidism I 131 Therapy (Continued)

Author, Year	Total # Patients	Treatment	Results	Notes
			I 131 only: 67% euthyroid 13% hypothyroid 20% toxic	
Reinwein et al, 1969	310	I 131 therapy: Fractionated therapy. Mean total dose of 5.4mCi in patients without a goiter and 7.1–12.9mCi in patients with a goiter. Mean number of doses was 1.7–2.7.	294/310(95%) euthyroid 7/310(2%) hypothyroid 9/310(3%) hyperthyroid	Follow up of 2–11 years. Four of the seven cases of hypothyroidism had subtotal thyroidectomy in addition to radioiodine therapy. Subtotal thyroidectomy in addition to radioiodine therapy was done in 27 cases. Some patients also received premedication or interim treatment with antithyroid drugs.

Skillman et al, 1969	70	I 131:
		1. 6mc (24 patients).
		2. 9mc (28 patients).
		3. 12mc (18 patients).
			At 2.5 years post treatment:
			1. 29% euthyroid
			   62% hypothyroid
			2. 36% euthyroid
			   50% hypothyroid
			3. 28% euthyroid
			   50% hypothyroid	

Feibush and Sherman, 1968	149	I 131 therapy: Dose, 2–4mc (first dose) up to a maximum of 15.2mc (total dose). 56.4% received only one dose.	12/149(8.6%) permanently hypothyroid.	Minimum follow up of three years. Nine of the twelve patients who became permanently hypothyroid did so within six months following therapy.
Hamburger and Pual, 1968	356	I 131: Large dose: initial or subsequent dose of 20mCi or greater.	Large dose (56): 36/56 euthyroid 19/56 hypothyroid Conventional doses (302) 82% euthyroid after a single dose. The remaining 18% required two or more doses.	
Hagen et al, 1967	116	Low dose: 80uc I 131/gm thyroid tissue followed by potassium iodide therapy in 97 patients.	90/116(77%) euthyroid after one dose. 7/116(6%) permanently hypothyroid.	Thirty-six patients were pretreated with a thiouracil derivative but there were no complications in this group as compared to those without treatment. Mean follow up period of 1.9 months.
	40	High dose: 160uc I 131/gm thyroid tissue.	16/40(40%) euthyroid after one dose. 13/40(33%) permanently hypothyroid.	Mean follow up period of eleven months. All patients in both groups had diffuse goiters.

Smith and Wilson, 1967	539	1. Conventional dose (271 patients) 5.0+2.0mCi.
		2. Half dose (268 patients) 2.8+1.6mCi
			At one year:
			1. 47.9% euthyroid
			   44.2% hyperthyroid
			   7.9% hypothyroid
			2. 30.8% euthyroid
			   65% hyperthyroid
			   4.3% hypothyroid	

Historical Data: Hyperthyroidism I 131 Therapy (Continued)

Author, Year	Total # Patients	Treatment	Results	Notes
Trezcan et al, 1967	120	I 131 therapy: Dose, 3-5mCi initial dose (total dose ranged from three to greater than 20mCi, but the majority of patients received less than 10mCi total dose).	Follow up of 12 years. Overall results: 100/120(83%) euthyroid 16/120(13.3%) hypothyroid 4/120 hyperthyroid Based on group at risk follow up: 11/120(9.2%) hypothyroid at one year. 9/33(27.3%) hypothyroid at five years.	Multinodular (17) Diffuse (98) Toxic nodule (5) The incidence of hypothyroidism was highest in the multinodular group (12.5%). It was only 6.7% in the diffuse group, and 0% in the toxic nodular group. 49/120 had prior drug or surgical treatment.
Donovan and Turtle, 1966	170	I 131 therapy: Dose, 5-12mCi initial dose ranged from 5-79mCi) 111(65%) were controlled with a single dose. 48(28%) required multiple doses.	Follow up of eleven years. 22/170(13%) hypothyroid 11/170(6.5%) were not controlled by I 131 and required other forms of treatment or additional I 131.	21/22 who developed hypothyroidism did so within the first two years following treatment.
Edsmyr and Einhorn, 1966	2035	I 131: Dose, calculated to give 5000-12000r.	First 796 cases, minimum follow up of two years. 7.5% hypothyroidism within one year. Annual increment of 3% to 27% hypothyroid at seven years.	No palpable goiter (541). Diffuse enlargement of the thyroid gland (811). Nodular goiter (683). Nine deaths within one month of therapy, three of these possibly due to an exacerbation after treatment.
Nofal et al, 1966	969	I 131 (848 patients) average dose of 10mc. 2/3rd of the patients received antithyroid medication prior to I 131 therapy or surgical treatment (121 patients).	I 131 treated: 44% hypothyroid at one year. Cumulative percentage of hypothyroidism increased 5.5%/month during the first 6 months, 1.3%/month during the second six month period and 2.8%/year thereafter. Surgically treated: 27% hypothyroid at one year. Cumulative percentage of hypothyroidism increased 3.7%/month during the first six months, 0.51%/month during the second six month period, and 1.7%/year thereafter.	Thyroid size at treatment: I 131: 13% normal 6.7% not palpable 53.9% diffusely enlarged 9.1% enlarged, solitary nodules 17.1% enlarged, multiple nodules Surgery: 2.5% normal 0% not palpable 68.6% diffusely enlarged 14.9% enlarged, solitary nodules 14% enlarged, multiple nodules
Saferborg and Einhorn, 1966	157	I 131 therapy: 1. Nonfractionated therapy (123). 2. Fractionated therapy (34).	1. Nonfractionated therapy: 38% cured by 1 treatment (none of these developed hypothyroidism). 76% cured by two treatments. 9/123(7.3%) hypothyroid 2. Fractionated therapy: 19/34 cured The remaining fifteen patients were given additional radioiodine and were ultimately cured. 4/34 hypothyroid.	All of the patients had large toxic nodular goiters with tracheal compression in some cases. All of the cases were unsuitable for surgery. Minimum follow up of one year. 1. Three deaths within 30 days. 2. No deaths within four months.

Historical Data: Hyperthyroidism I 131 Therapy (Continued)

Author, Year	Total # Patients	Treatment	Results	Notes
Neal, 1965	196	I 131 therapy: Standard calculated dose of 10000r to the gland.	74.0% euthyroid 13.8% hypothyroid 12.2% hyperthyroid	
	500	I 131 therapy: Calculated dose of 5000-8000r to the thyroid gland.	79.8% euthyroid 8.2% hyperthyroid 12% hypothyroid	
Dunn and Chapman, 1964	1452	I 131, 160uc/gm thyroid tissue, 1391 patients. I 130, 681uc/gm thyroid tissue, 61 patients.	I 131: 808/1391(58%) euthyroid 365/1391(26%) hypothyroid 96/1391(9%) probably hypothyroid I 130: 24/61(39%) euthyroid 27/61(44%) hypothyroid 6/61(10%) probably hypothyroid	In patients followed for ten years or more the incidence of hypothyroidism rose to 43%.
Beling and Einhorn, 1961	791	I 131: Dose calculated to give 6000-10000r to the gland.	At one year: 7.46% hypothyroid During subsequent observation approximately 3% developed hypothyroidism per year. At seven years: 26.5.% hypothyroid	Hyperthyroidism without demonstrable goiter (298 patients). Diffuse toxic goiter (218 patients). Toxic nodular goiter (167 patients).

Historical Data: Hyperthyroidism I 125 Therapy

Author, Year	Total # Patients	Treatment	Results	Notes
Siemsen et al, 1974	100	I 125: Dose - 200uCi/gm (60 patients) 100uCi/gm (40 patients)	High dose (minimum follow up of 12 months): 30/42(71%) euthyroid 10/42(24%) hyperthyroid 2/42(5%) hypothyroid Low dose (minimum follow up of 9 months): 12/28(43%) euthyroid 15/28(53%) hyperthyroid 1/28(4%) hypothyroid	
Weidinger et al, 1974	63	I 125 therapy: Dosage ranged from 0.5 to 3.5 times the dosage of I 131 used that would have been given.	Minimum follow up of four months: 37/63(60%) euthyroid 17/63(10%) hypothyroid 19/63(30%) hyperthyroid	All patients had Graves' disease (toxic diffuse goiter). 61/63 received propranolol either before or after I 125 therapy, and with or without antithyroid drugs.
Bremmer et al, 1973	297	I 125 therapy: 1000-6000r, or 300uCi/gm of thyroid.	Percentage hypothyroid at four year follow up: 39% (1000uCi dose) 34% (600uCi dose) 18% (300uCi dose)	Authors concluded that I 125 has no advantage over I 131, in the control of thyrotoxicosis.
Gimlette and Hoschl, 1973	31	I 125 therapy: Dose: 3-6mCi	Results after single dose: 9/31(29%) euthyroid 3/31(9.7%) hypothyroid 18/31(58.1%) thyrotoxic	Follow up of 23-36 months.

Historical Data: Hyperthyroidism I 125 Therapy (Continued)

Author, Year	Total # Patients	Treatment	Results	Notes
	421	I 131 therapy: Similar dosage schedule as that used for I 125.	Results after single dose: 218/421(51.8%) euthyroid 45/421(10.7%) hypothyroid 137/421(32.5%) thyrotoxic	Mean follow up of 26 months.
Werner et al, 1970	13	I 125: Series A: Dose of 8-10mCi (6 patients). Series B: Dose of 150-300uCi/gm (7 patients).	Series A: 5/16 hypothyroid 1/6 hyperthyroid Series B: 6/7 euthyroid 1/7 hyperthyroid	All patients had toxic diffuse goiters. Follow up to 54 months.

Historical Data: Hyperthyroidism Surgical and Medical Treatment

Author, Year	Total # Patients	Treatment	Results	Notes
Vaidya et al, 1974	75	Propylthiouracil	40% achieved remission with medical treatment alone. The average duration of medical treatment was 3.2 years. Thirty-two cases were treated surgically, thirteen because of non-compliance with drug treatment and thirteen because of recurrence following discontinuation of the drug.	All were cases of juvenile thyrotoxicosis.
Caswell and Maier, 1972	72	Subtotal thyroidectomy.	60/72(83%) euthyroid 7/72(10%) hypothyroid 5/72(7%) hyperthyroid	All of the patients in whom post-op hypothyroidism developed had diffuse toxic goiters.
Michie et al, 1972	278	Subtotal thyroidectomy.	151/278(51%) euthyroid 137/278(49%) hypothyroid	
Hedley et al, 1970	146	Subtotal thyroidectomy	80/146(54.8%) euthyroid 7/146(4.8%) equivocal 53/46(36.3%) hypothroidism 15/146(10.2%) hyperthyroidism	No evidence of a cumulative incidence of hypothyrodism after subtotal thyroidectomy. Authors also include a review of recent reported results of subtotal thyroidectomy. Percentage hypothyroid range from 3-28%. Percentage total morbidity range from 0-28%.
McNeil and Thomson, 1968	123	Thyroidectomy	100/123(81.3%) euthyroid 8/123(6.5%) hypothyroidism 15/123(12.2%) hyperthyroidism	Long term complications: Subjective voice disturbance (13). Unsightly scars (4). Hyperthyroidism (3).

Historical Data: Hyperthyroidism
Long Term Follow Up Studies on Patients Treated with I 131 for Hyperthyroidism

Author, Year	Total # Patients	Treatment	Results	Notes
Safa et al, 1975	87	I 131: Dose, 2.9–31mCi (mean 9.75 + 6.5)	Follow up of 5–24 years (mean 12.3 + 3.5). No deaths and no cancer or leukemia were observed in patients or their offspring. Reproductive history and health status of the progeny of I 131 treated patients were not different from those of the general population.	Patients were 3–18 years of age when treated. Major cause of goiter regrowth was Hashimoto's thyroiditis.
Hayek et al, 1970	30	I 131 (28 patients) I 130 (2 patients)	Average follow up of 9.2 years. No deaths and no evidence of cancer or leukemia. One female treated with I 130 has an abnormal reproductive history.	Patients were 8–18 years of age when treated. Authors also provide a review of reported cases of patients treated in childhood with radioiodine for thyrotoxicosis. Of 177 such cases benign nodules in 14 (8%).
Saenger et al, 1968	36,000	I 131 (22,000 patients) surgery or antithyroid drugs (14,000 patients) (Cooperative thyrotoxicosis study).	Incidence of leukemia in the two groups did not differ.	

References

1. Turner JG, Brownlie BEW and Rogers TGH (1976) Lithium as an adjunct to radioiodine therapy for thyrotoxicosis. *Lancet* **1**: 614–616.
2. Braverman LE (1975) Consequences of thyroid radiation in children. *New Eng J Med* **292**: 204–205.
3. Foster RS (1975) Thyroid irradiation and carcinogenesis. Review with assessment of clinical implications. *Am J Surg* **130**: 608–611.
4. Malone JF (1975) The radiation biology of the thyroid. *Curr Top Rad Res Quart* **10**: 263–368.
5. Safa AM, Schumacher OP and Rodriguez-Antunea A (1975) Long term follow up results in children and adolescents treated with radioactive iodine (I 131) for hyperthyroidism. *New Eng J Med* **292**: 167–170.
6. Sterling K (1975) Radioactive iodine therapy. *Med Clin N Am* **59**: 1217–1220.
7. Thjodleifsson B (1975) A study of Graves' disease in Iceland. *Acta Med Scand* **198**: 309–314.
8. Wise PH, Burnet RB, Ahmad A and Harding PE (1975) Intentional radioiodine ablation in Graves' disease. *Lancet* **2**: 1231–1232.
9. Barnes HV and Gann DS (1974) Choosing thyroidectomy in hyperthyroidism. *Surg Clin North Am* **54**: 289–307.
10. Cevallos JL, Hagen GA, Malouf F and Chapman EM (1974) Low dosage I 131 therapy of thyrotoxicosis (diffuse goiters): a five year follow up study. *New Eng J Med* **290**: 141–143.
11. Dobjns BM, Sheline GE, Workman JB, Thompkins EA, McCohahey WM and Becker DV (1974) Malignant and benign neoplasm of the thyroid in patients treated for hyperthyroidism: A report of the cooperative thyrotoxicosis therapy follow up study. *J Clin Endocr & Metab* **38**: 974–998.
12. McDougall IR (1974) Thyroid cancer after iodine 131 therapy. *JAMA* **227**: 438.
13. Siemsen JK, Wallack MS, Martin RB and Nicoloff JTR (1974) Early results of I 125 therapy of thyrotoxic Graves' disease. *J Nuc Med* **13**: 257–260.
14. Tunbridge WMG, Harsoulis P and Goolden AW (1974) Thyroid function in patients treated with radioactive iodine for thyrotoxicosis. *Br Med J* **31**: 89–92.
15. Vaidya VA, Bongiovanni AM, Parks JS, Tenore A and Kirkland RT (1974) Twenty-two years experience in the medical management of juvenile thyrotoxicosis. *Ped* **54**: 565–570.
16. Weidinger P, Johnson PM and Werner SC (1974) Five years experience with iodine 125 therapy of Graves' disease. *Lancet* **2**: 681–685.
17. Bremmer WR, McDougall IR, Greig WR (1973) Results of treating 297 thyrotoxic patients with I 125. *Lancet* **2**: 281–282.
18. Douglas JG (1973) The Vanderbuilt experience with I 131 treatment for Graves' disease. *Soc Med J* **66**: 92–97.
19. Gimlette TM and Hoschl R (1973) Treatment of thyrotoxicosis with iodine 125 in moderately low dosage. *Clin Rad* **24**: 263–266.
20. Rapport B, Caplan R and DeGroot LJ (1973) Low dose sodium iodine I 131 therapy in Graves' disease. *JAMA* **224**: 1610–1613.

21. Michie W (1973) Symposium on modern trends in the management of thyrotoxicosis. *Br J Surg* **60**: 757-769.
22. Blahd WH and Hayes MT (1972) Graves' disease in the male. *Arch Int Med* **129**: 33-40.
23. Caswell HT and Maier WP (1972) Results of surgical treatment for hyperthyroidism. *Surg Gyn & Obst* **134**: 218-220.
24. Glennon JA, Gordon ES and Swain CT (1972) Hypothyroidism after low dose I 131 treatment of hyperthyroidism. *Ann Int Med* **76**: 721-723.
25. Kendall-Taylor P (1972) Hyperthyroidism. *Br Med J* **2**: 337-341.
26. McDougall IR and Greig WR (1972) Combined carbimazole I 131 treatment for thyrotoxicosis. *Scot Med J* **17**: 57-61.
27. Michie W, Pegg CAS and Brewsher FD (1972) Prediction of hypothyroidism after partial thyroidectomy for thyrotoxicosis. *Br Med J* **1**: 13-17.
28. Sachs BA, Siegel E, Kass S and Dolman M (1972) Radioiodine therapy of thyrotoxicosis. *Am J Roent Rad Ther & Nuc Med* **115**: 698-705.
29. Becker DV and Hurley JR (1971) Complications of radioiodine treatment of hyperthyroidism. *Semin Nuc Med* **1**: 442-460.
30. Dworkin HJ (1971) Treatment of diffuse toxic goiter with I 131. *Sem Nuc Med* **1**: 339-410.
31. Jackson GL (1971) Radioiodine therapy of thyrotoxicosis. *Am J Roent Rad Therp & Nuc Med* **112**: 726-731.
32. Jonckheer MH (1971) Thyroid function after radioiodine. *Lancet* **1**: 1296-1297.
33. Lewitus A, Lubin E, Ben-Poarth M and Feige Y (1971) Treatment of thyrotoxicosis with I 125 and I 131. *Sem Nuc Med* **4**: 411-421.
34. McDougall IR, Greig WR and Gillespie FC (1971) Radioactive iodine (I 125) therapy for thyrotoxicosis. *New Eng J Med* **285**: 1099-1104.
35. Franco J (1970) Propranolol and I 131 in the treatment of diffuse hyperplasia with hyperthyroidism. *J Nuc Med* **11**: 219-220.
36. Surveyon I and Harris-Jones JN (1970) I 131 treatment for thyrotoxicosis. *Lancet* **2**: 1035-1036.
37. Hayek A, Chapman EM and Crawford JD (1970) Long term results of treatment of thyrotoxicosis in children and adolescents with radioactive iodine. *New Eng J Med* **283**: 949-943.
38. Hedley AJ, Fleming CJ, Chesters MI, Michie W and Crooks J (1970) Surgical treatment of thyrotoxicosis. *Br Med J* **1**: 519-523.
39. Kaipainen WJ, Vuopala U, Salokannel J, Rakkunen J and Timonen T (1970) Low dose radioactive iodine in the treatment of hyperthyroidism. A two year follow up study. *Ann Clin Res* **2**: 122-125.
40. Viherkoski M, Lamberg A, Hernberg CA and Niemi E (1970) Treatment of toxic nodular and diffuse goitre with radioactive iodine. *Acta Endocr* **64**: 159-170.
41. Werner SC, Johnson PM and Foodwin PN (1970) Long term results with iodine 125 treatment for toxic diffuse goitre. *Lancet* **2**: 681-685.
42. Burke G and Silverstein GE (1969) Hypothyroidism after treatment with sodium iodide I 131. *JAMA* **210**: 1051-1058.
43. Goolden AWG and Fraser TR (1969) Effect of pretreatment with carbimazole in patients with thyrotoxicosis subsequently treated with radioactive iodine. *Br Med J* **3**: 443-444.
44. Reinwein D, Miss H, Horster FA, Berger H, Klein E and Oberdisse K (1969) Late results of fractionated radioiodine therapy. *Germ Med Mth* **14**: 234-238.
45. Skillman TG, Mazzaterri EL and Gwinup G (1969) Random dosage of I 131 in the treatment of hyperthyroidism: Results of a prospective study. *Am J Med Sci* **257**: 382-386.
46. Starr P, Jaffe HL and Oettinger L Jr (1969) Later results of I 131 treatment in 73 children and adolescents: 1967 follow up. *J Nuc Med* **10**: 586-590.
47. Bhatig SK, Hadden DR, Montgomery AD and Weaver JD (1968) The management of thyrotoxicosis with therapeutic radioiodine. *I J Med Sci* **1**: 449-457.
48. Eipe J, Johnson SA, Kiamko RT and Bronsky D (1968) Hypoparathyroidism following I 131 therapy for hyperthyroidism. *Arch Int Med* **121**: 270-272.
49. Feibush JS and Sherman AA (1968) Low incidence of hypothyroidism following radioiodine therapy. *NY St J Med* **68**: 2158-2160.
50. Hamburger JI and Pual S (1968) When and how to use higher I 131 doses for hyperthyroidism. *New Eng J Med* **279**: 1361-1365.
51. McNeil AD and Thomson S (1968) Long term follow up of surgically treated thyrotoxic patients. *Br Med J* **3**: 643-646.
52. Philip JR, Harrison MT, Ridley EF and Crooks J (1968) Treatment of thyrotoxicosis with ionizing radiation. *Lancet* **2**: 1307-1310.
53. Saenger EL, Thoma GE and Thompkins EA (1968) Incidence of leukemia following treatment of hyperthyroidism. *JAMA* **205**: 855-862.
54. Zellman HE, Matiz H, Bartels EC and Bell GO (1968) Radioactive iodine in hyperthyroidism. *Lahey Clin Fd Bull* **17**: 137-143.
55. Block MA (1967) Surgery versus radioactive iodine for hyperthyroidism. *Surg Gyn & Obst* **125**: 1083-1084.
56. Einhorn J and Wickland H (1966) Hypothyroidism following I 131 treatment for hyperthyroidism. *J Clin Endocr & metab* **26**: 33-36.
57. Hagen GA, Quellette RP and Chapman EM (1967) Comparison of high and low dosage levels of I 131 in the treatment of thyrotoxicosis. *NEJM* **177**: 559-562.
58. Hamburger JI and Pual S (1968) When and how to use higher I 131 doses for hyperthyroidism. *New Eng J Med* **279**: 1361-1365.
59. Pennington, JS and Martin FIR (1967) Hypothyroidism following treatment of thyrotoxicosis with radioiodine. *Med J Austr* **2**: 641-642.
60. Smith RN and Wilson GM (1967) Clinical trial of different doses of I 131 in treatment of thyrotoxicosis. *Br Med J* **1**: 129-132.
61. Staffurth JS and Young J (1967) Delay in control of thyrotoxicosis after treatment with radioactive iodine. *J Clin Endocr & Metab* **27**: 1062-1064.
62. Trezcan UP, Frelick RW and MecKelnburg RL (1967) Low dose therapy of hyperthyroidism. *Del Med J* **39**: 142-146.
63. Caswell HT, Robbins RR and Rosemond GP (1966) Definitive treatment of 536 cases of hyperthyroidism with I 131 or surgery. *Ann Surg* **164**: 593-599.
64. Donovan JK and Turtle JR (1966) The results of radioiodine therapy in thyrotoxicosis. *Med J Aus* **2**: 271-272.
65. Edsmyr F and Einhorn J (1966) Complications in radioiodine treatment of hyperthyroidism. *Acta Rad (Therp)* **4**: 49-54.
66. Einhorn J and Wickland H (1966) Hypothyroidism fol-

lowing I 131 treatment for hyperthyroidism. *J Clin Endocr & Metab* **26**: 33–36.
67. Greig WR and Macgregor AG (1966) Clinical and radiobiological consequences of therapeutic thyroid irradiation (abridged). *Proc Roy Soc Med* **59**: 599–602.
68. Hershman JM (1966) The treatment of hyperthyroidism. *Ann Int Med* **64**: 1306–1314.
69. Nofal MN, Beierwaltes WH and Patro ME (1966) Treatment of hyperthyroidism with sodium iodide I 131. *JAMA* **197**: 87–92.
70. Saferborg NE and Einhorn J (1966) Fractionated I 131 therapy in large toxic goitres. *Acta Endoc* **51**: 7–14.
71. Buchanan WW, Koutras DA, Crooks J and Harden RM (1965) A comparison of pretreatment with potassium perchlorate and methylthiouracil on results of I 131 therapy. *Br J Rad* **38**: 536–540.
72. Neal FE (1965) Results of radioactive iodine treatment in thyrotoxicosis. *Nuc Med* **2**: 304–309.
73. Dunn JT and Chapman EM (1964) Rising incidence of hypothyroidism after radioactive iodine therapy in thyrotoxicosis. *New Engl J Med* **271**: 1037–1042.
74. Hadden DR, Montgomery DAD, Shaks RG and Weaver JA (1963) Propranolol and iodine 131 in the management of thyrotoxicosis. *Lancet* **2**: 852–854.
75. Beling U and Einhorn J (1961) Incidence of hypothyroidism and recurrences following I 131 treatment of hyperthyroidism. *Arch Rad* **56**: 275–288.

Hyperthyroid Ophthalmopathy

In well selected cases, external beam radiation to the retro-orbital muscles and tissues produces responses in soft tissue signs, ocular mobility, visual acuity and decrease in proptosis. Doses used commonly are 2000 cGy in 10 × 200 rad fractions. Treatment whether unilateral or bilateral requires simulation, treatment planning, dose calculation, and care in not exceeding tolerances. Precision in administration using beam shielding devices is essential. Cases should be selected with care, as all patients with ophthalmopathy are not candidates for radiotherapy. In the national survey 75% of radiation oncologists would treat ophthalmopathy resulting from Graves' disease.

Graves' Ophthalmopathy Radiotherapy

Author, Year	Total # Patients	Treatment	Results	Notes
Olivotto et al, 1985	28	2000 cGy/10 fractions over 12 days using 4 Mev linear accelerator to retrobulbar area. Half beam block technique to eliminate lens exposure.	26/28(93%) responded 19/28(68%) good to excellent response 14/28 have undergone post-XRT surgery 24/28(86%) spared long-term high dose corticosteroids.	No complications. Mean follow up 17 mos.
Hurbli et al, 1985	62	High dose prednisone (60–120 mg/d). Those with poor response underwent radiotherapy to orbit. 2000 cGy/10 fractions over 12–14 days. Beam angled 5° posteriorly to avoid contralateral lens.	34 of 46(74%) motility problems improved 12 of 28(53%) pts with symptoms greater than 6 mos. responded compared to 13 of 18(72%) whose problems were present far less than 6 mos (not significant) 10 of 14 with optic neuropathy improved, but 4 had recurrences.	No morbidity
Ouwerkerk et al, 1985	24	200cGy in 10 fractions of 200 cGy in 2 weeks using 4 Mev photons to orbit. Most patients also were given prednisone 30–60 mg/day	Decrease in proptosis. Increase in visual acuity. All patients could be tapered off prednisone.	Median duration of eye symptoms before irradiation – 12 months. Follow up 2–4.5 years.

Historical Data: Graves' Ophthalmopathy Radiotherapy

Author, Year	Total # Patients	Treatment	Results	Notes
Kinyoun et al, 1984	4	Intended: 2000 cGy in 10 200 cGy fractions to orbit. Actual: 4000 cGy in 10 400 cGy fractions	All 4 developed radiation retinopathy, decreased acuity, and 3/4 are blind.	Major dosimetric error occurred in which patients actually received 400 cGy to the midplane each day, rather than the prescribed 200 cGy. Thus, a total dose of 4000 cGy/10 fractions @ 400 cGy/fraction.
Brennan et al, 1983	14	2000cGy in 10 days to orbit	13 of 14 had reduced soft tissue inflammation. 12 of 14 had decreased proptosis 1-3 mm. Myopathy stabilized permitting subsequent strabismus surgery.	Follow up: 6 mos-3 years. No sequelae and no recurrences.
Yamamoto et al, 1983	6	Steroid therapy, super voltage orbital radiotherapy 2000 rad/10 days	Decrease in proptosis, decrease in muscle enlargement	Improvements noted 3-7 mos after therapy. Duration of response > 18 mos.
Yamamoto et al, 1982	9	Radiation therapy plus steroid therapy, plasmapheresis to orbit. Radiation: 2000 rad/10 days 10/200 rad fractions.	4 – good results 1 – fair results 4 – no response at 4 week evaluation.	No long-term follow up.
Teng et al, 1980	20	2000 rad/12 days in 200 rad fractions to orbit using 4.2 Mev linear accelerator	7/20(35%) showed response within 3 weeks; 4 pts (20%) minimal response; 9 pts (45%) unchanged.	Long-term follow up < 25 mos. Pts had long duration of eye symptoms prior to therapy.
Trobe et al, 1978	6	1500-2000 rad in 10 daily fractions using 4 Mev photon to orbit.	6 of 12 eyes were improved at 8 week evaluation	5 of the 6 responding eyes had rapid decline in vision just prior to XRT.
Covington et al, 1977	7	2000 rads/2 weeks using 6 Mev linear accelerator to orbit	5 of 7 improved within 3 mos of treatment	No complications
Ravin et al, 1975	37	Radiotherapy: 1500r (in air)/10F/10 days Lateral orbital fields 6 x 7cm lead shield to protect the lens	Class 3 patients (4): No significant decrease in exophthalmometer measurement. Class 4 patients (18): 2/18 progressed to class 5 disease after treatment. 1 pt with limitation of movement prior to treatment gained full range of motion. Class 5 patients (6): 5/6 visual acuity was good before and after treatment. 1/6 with severe exposure keratitis was not improved after treatment – subsequently underwent corneal transplantation. Class 6 patients (9): 9/9 visual acuity improved (within 2 wks. in most pts.) 7/8 optic nerve congestion improved within 4 months. 4/5 scotomas resolved in 1-6 months.	Classification of Ocular Changes of Graves' Disease: 0 – No signs or symptoms 1 – Only signs (upper lid retraction and stare, with or without eyelid lag and proptosis), no symptoms 2 – Soft tissue involvement (signs and symptoms) 3 – Proptosis 4 – Extra ocular muscle involvement 5 – Corneal involvement 6 – Sight loss (optic nerve involvement)

Historical Data: Graves' Ophthalmopathy Radiotherapy (Continued)

Author, Year	Total # Patients	Treatment	Results	Notes
Donaldson et al, 1973	23	Radiotherapy: 2000r (total orbital dose)/10F/2 wks. 4-6 MeV Fields: Left and right lateral roughly triangular in cross section to cover the muscular cone of the globe and nothing else. Fields were angled to avoid the contralateral lens.	Overall clinical assessment: 15/23(65%) good-excellent results 6/23(26%) fair results 2/23(9%) no response There was good agreement between the clinical assessment and the change in ophthalmopathy index.	All 23 pts. had previous treatment for thyrotoxicosis. 16 had received previous treatment for ophthalmopathy (14 of these had corticosteroids)
Blahut et al, 1963	18	1500r (air)/10F/10 days to each field. Technical details: 250Kv, 13ma, 0.44mm Sn, 0.25mm Cu plus 10mm Al filtration, HVL 2.7mm Cu, FSD 50cm Fields: Two opposing lateral fields, approx. 7 x 7 cm each to include both the pituitary, the lower part of the hypothalamus and the retrobulbar tissues.	13/18(72%) decrease in exophthalmometer readings of 2mm or more in at least one eye (6 in two eyes) during the course of therapy. 1/18 no decrease in exophthalmometer readings, but decrease in chemosis and subjective complaints. 1/18 decrease of 2mm exophthalmometer reading 2 months after therapy.	4/13(31%) who obtained a decrease of 2mm or more during treatment showed an increase in exophthalmous to pretreatment levels within 6 months after treatment.
Gedda and Lindgren, 1954	19	Pituitary and/or orbital radiotherapy. Orbital irradiation: 900r(skin dose)/6-9 F/6-9 days to each field followed after an interval of 4-5 wks by a second course of 100-900r. Technical details: 170Kv, 15ma, 0.5mm Cu plus 1mm Al filtration, HVL 0.9mm Cu, FSD 50cm, lateral fields, 10-15cm². Pituitary irradiation: 1500r(skin dose)/4-5F/4-5 days to each field followed in 5 weeks by a second course of 600-900r. Technical details: 170Kv, 15ma, 0.5mm Cu, FSD, 52-60cm, four temporal fields, 5 x 6cm.	Pituitary & orbital irradiation (16 pts) 10/16(63%) lacrimation, photophobia, and ophthalmoplegia disappeared. 6/7 eyelid edema disappeared. 2/2 chemosis disappeared 10/10 hyperthyroid patients became symptom free. Additional irradiation to the anterior part of the orbit was given to those six patients who did not respond. The results of this were: 4/5 disappearance of eye signs 5/6 eyelid edema disappeared. 2/2 chemosis disappeared. Orbital irradiation only (3 pts) 2/3 disappearance of eye signs 1/3 no response. 11/19 had previous thyroidectomy for hyperthyroidism.	
Beierwaltes, 1953	28	X-ray to the pituitary, 1550r/10F/10 days to each field, 200Kv, 25ma, 0.5mm Cu plus 1mm Al filtration, HVL, 1mm Cu, FSD, 50cm.	Follow up of 9 months - 12 yrs. 13/28(46%) decrease of 2mm or more in exophthalmometer measurements in at least one eye. Average of 19 months required for maximum recession. 10/12 decreased lid edema. 7/11 decrease or disappearance of bulbar conjunctival edema.	All patients treated presented two or more eye signs of malignant exophthalmos. Four patients exhibited no evidence of thyroid disease.

Historical Data: Graves' Ophthalmopathy Radiotherapy (Continued)

Author, Year	Total # Patients	Treatment	Results	Notes
Jones, 1951	29	Varied dosage schedules: 200r(skin dose)/56 days to 1000r/14 days. Technical details: 190-250Kv, 15ma, HVL 1.3-1.85mm Cu, FSD 25-60mm. Fields: anterior and lateral orbital. The anterior field extends from the supraorbital ridge to the molar region (8 x 6cm). The lateral field may be restricted to the bony orbit (4 x 6cm). Lead shield to protect the lens in mild cases.	Follow up of 9 months - 5 years True progressive exophthalmos (22 pts) 1. Malignant exophthalmos. 2/2 exophthalmos disappeared. 2. Chronic progressive exophthalmos. 9/19(47%) complete or moderate regression of exophthalmos. 7/19(37%) slight regression of exophthalmos. 3/19(15%) no regression. 20/20 edema greatly diminished or abated. 15/18 ocular movements normal or improved. Thyrotoxic exophthalmos (7 pts) 3/7 some decrease in exophthalmos and ophthalmoplegia. 2/7 substantial relief from conjunctivitis.	22 patients had progressive exophthalmos. 7 patients had thyrotoxic ophthalmopathy. Sequelae: Cataracts (1)

Historical Data: Exophthalmos Alternate Modes of Treatment

Author, Year	Total # Patients	Treatment	Results	Notes
Clarke, 1975	20	Lateral orbital decompression (bilateral in 14, unilateral in 20).	18/20 relieved of orbital discomfort, photophobia, and pain on eye movement. 8/12 disappearance of diplopia.	4 patients had no thyroid abnormality.
Gorman et al, 1974	18	Surgical decompression. Transantral procedure (10 pts) Transfrontal procedure (9pts) One patient was treated by both approaches.	Both procedures were successful in treating proptosis (mean recession of 4-6mm) and visual acuity. Neither procedure can be counted on to correct diplopia.	7 patients reported no history of thyrotoxicity. 14/18 had received oral therapy or retrobulbar steroid injections. Complications: Numbness of upper lip secondary to course of oral antrostomies(1). There was no surgical mortality.
Ogura and Lucente, 1974	120	Orbital decompression.	2mm-12mm decrease in exophthalmometer readings following surgery. 75% eyes balanced with 1mm. Complications: post-op sinusitis (2) aneurysm of the anterior cerebral artery (1) Two patients required revision for a more satisfactory result	3/120 had no history of hyperthyroidism. Indications for surgical decompression loss of visual acuity, changes in corneal epithelium, progressive loss of extraocular muscle function, conjunctival chemosis, and orbital edema.

Historical Data: Exophthalmos Alternate Modes of Treatment (Continued)

Author, Year	Total # Patients	Treatment	Results	Notes
Asregadoo, 1970	7	Guanethidine sulphate (5%) Double blind study.	3/7 significant ptosis was produced. 4/7 decreased intraocular pressure.	All patients had endocrine exophthalmos.
Burrow et al, 1970	5	Azathioprine (immunosuppressive therapy)	Despite evidence of immune suppression there was no objective evidence of significant improvement in eye changes. There was improvement in chemosis and conjunctival injection in one patient.	All patients had Graves' disease.
Cant, 1970	18	Triamcinolone acetonide injection. One orbit randomly selected was treated. The other was used as a control.	16/18 orbitonometer reading improved (mean improvement) 14/18 symptomatic improvement with reduction of pain on the treated side.	All patients had bilateral chronic lymphoid infiltration. All patients had been hyperthyroid.
MacCarty et al, 1970	46	Removal of roof, lateral walls and lateral sphenoid ridge. Forty patients had bilateral decompression. Six patients had unilateral decompression.	Visual acuity: 9/31(29%) normal 13/31(42%) improved 3/31 no change 4/31 no post-op measurement Extraocular muscles: 11/42(26%) normal 20/42(46%) improved 3/42 unchanged 1/42 worse 7/42 no post-op measurement. Proptosis: 23/38(61%) decrease in proptosis of 3mm or more soon after operation. 4/38(11%) no significant decrease. 8/38 no post-op measurements. Visual Fields: 13/18(72%) recovered field loss completely within one month 3/18 improved 2/18 not plotted post-op. External appearance: 39/41(94%) significant decrease of chemosis. 40/44(41%) decrease or disappearance of scleral injection 26/29(90%) decrease or disappearance of eyelid edema.	All of the patients had Graves' disease.

Historical Data: Exophthalmos Alternate Modes of Treatment (Continued)

Author, Year	Total # Patients	Treatment	Results	Notes
Jones, 1968	18	Metronidazole Double-blind, cross-over technique was used.	With Metronidazole: 8/18 exophthalmos increased. 6/18 exophthalmos unchanged. 4/18 exophthalmos decreased. With Placebo: 12/18 exophthalmos increased. 6/18 exophthalmos unchanged. The drug had no effect on irradiation, lachrymation, photophobia, diplogia, lid retraction, lid lag, periorbital edema, chemosis, conjunctival edema, or ophthalmoplegia.	Based on the results of this study metronidazole does not have any significant effect on human exophthalmos.
Crombie and Lawson, 1967	20	Guanethidine sulphate (10%)	18/20 subjective benefit. 4/6 periorbital edema improved. 4/18 significant decrease in exophthalmometer readings. 9/13 marked relief or abolishment of lid retraction. No effect on conjunctival edema, conjunctival infection, ophthalmoplegia, pupil, lens, fundus, and refractive errors.	Side effects: Superficial punctate keratitis (10) Local irritation on instillation (10)
Garber, 1966	15	Methylprednisone (subconjunctival or retrobulbar injection discomfort in all patients.)	Moderate to dramatic relief from symptoms of ocular discomfort in all patients.	Four patients had previously received orbital irradiation. Complications: Steroid glaucoma (1) completely reversible on withdrawal of treatment.
Gay and Wolkstein, 1966	7	Topical guanethidine (10%)	7/7 subjective symptomatic improvement. 6/7 lid fissures became more symmetrical 1 patient - decrease of 2mm in exophthalmometer readings.	All patients had endocrine lid retraction.
Werner, 1966	2	Prednisone	Cases: 1. Vision improved, scotomata disappeared. Function of external muscles of the eye restored to 85% of normal. Proptosis improved significantly in both eyes. 2. Muscles of the right eye almost normal. Left eye could be raised above the midline.	Both cases had far advanced eye changes and were treated with large doses.

Historical Data: Exophthalmos Alternate Modes of Treatment (Continued)

Author, Year	Total # Patients	Treatment	Results	Notes
Brown et al, 1963	19	Prednisone	10/19 extraocular movements improved substantially. 13/19 significant decrease (2mm or more exophthalmometer reading) in proptosis in at least one eye. 6/8 marked improvement of visual acuity. Four patients were considered therapeutic failures.	All patients had severe ophthalmic complications. Eleven had received prior therapy (orbital irradiation in 2). Major side effects: Peptic ulcer (3) Toxic psychosis (1) Some degree of relapse of ocular changes in 8/19 when steroid therapy was reduced or discontinued. Muscle recessions for persistent diplopia were later done in 4 patients. Four patients required orbital decompression.

References

1. Hurbli T, Char DH, Harris J, Weaver K, Greenspan F and Sheline G (1985) Radiation therapy for thyroid eye diseases. *Am J Ophthalmol* **99**: 633-637.
2. Olivotto IA, Ludgate DM, Allen LH and Rootman J (1985) Supervoltage radiotherapy for Graves' ophthalmopathy: CCABC techniques and results. *Int J Radiation Oncology Biol Phys* **11**: 2085-2090.
3. Ouwerkerk BM, Wijngaarde R. Hennemann G, van Andel JG and Krenning EP (1985) Radiotherapy of severe ophthalmic Graves' disease. *J Endocrinol Invest* **8**: 241-247.
4. Kinyoun JL, Kelina RE, Brower SA, Mills RP and Johnson RH (1984) Radiation retinopathy after orbital irradiation for Graves' ophthalmopathy. *Arch Ophthalmol* **102**: 1473-1476.
5. Brennan MW, Leone CR and Janaki L (1983) Radiation therapy for Graves' disease. *Am J Ophthalmol* **96**: 195-199.
6. Yamamoto K, Saito K, Takai T and Yoshida S (1983) Diagnosis of exophthalmos using orbital ultrasonography and treatment of malignant exophthalmos with steroid therapy, orbital radiation therapy, and plasmapheresis. *Prog Clin Biol Res* **116**: 189-205.
7. Yamamoto K, Saito K, Takai T and Yoshida S (1982) Treatment of Graves' ophthalmopathy by steroid therapy, orbital radiation therapy, plasmapheresis, and thyrokine replacement. *Endocrinol Jpn* **29**: 495-501.
8. Teng CS, Crombie AL and Ross WM (1980) An evaluation of supervoltage orbital irradiation for Graves' ophthalmopathy. *Clin Endocrinol (Oxf)* **13**: 545-551.
9. Trobe JD, Glaser JS and LaFlamme P (1978) Dysthyroid optic neuropathy. Clinical profile and rational for management. *Arch Ophthalmol* **96**: 1199-1209.
10. Covington EE, Lobes L and Sudarsanam A (1977) Radiation therapy for exophthalmos: Report of seven cases. *Radiology* **122**: 797-799.
11. Ravin JG, Sisson JC and Knapp WT (1975) Orbital radiation for the ocular changes of Graves' disease. *Am J Ophth* **79**: 285-288.
12. Ravin JG, Sisson JC and Knapp WT (1975) Correspondence. *Am J Ophth* **79**: 889.
13. Rubenzik R (1975) Orbital radiation in Graves' disease. *Am J Ophth* **79**: 888.
14. Clarke PR (1975) Proceedings of the society of British neurological surgeons. Endocrine exophthalmos treated by orbital decompression. *J Neurol Neurosurg & Psychiat* **38**: 822-829.
15. Donaldson SS, Bagshaw MS and Kriss JP (1974) Orbital radiotherapy for the ophthalmopathy of Graves' disease. *New Eng J Med* **290**: 805.
16. Gorman CA, DeSanto LW, MacCarty CS and Riley FC (1974) Optic neuropathy of Graves' disease. Treatment by transantral or transfrontal orbital decompression. *New Eng J Med* **290**: 70-75.
17. Gorman CA, DeSanto LW, MacCarty CS and Riley FC (1974) Orbital radiotherapy for the ophthalmopathy of Graves' disease. *New Eng J Med* **290**: 805.
18. Ogura JH and Lucente FE (1974) Surgical results of orbital decompression for malignant exophthalmos. *Laryngoscope* **84**: 637-644.
19. Donaldson SS, Bagshaw MS and Kriss JP (1973) Supervoltage orbital radiotherapy for Graves' ophthalmopathy. *J Clin Endocr & Metab* **37**: 276-285.
20. Haddad HM (1973) Pathogenesis and treatment of endocrine exophthalmos. *Int Surg* **58**: 482-484.
21. Asregadoo ER (1970) Guanethidine ophthalmic solution 5%. Use in the treatment of endocrine exophthalmos. *Arch Ophth* **84**: 21-24.
22. Burrow GN, Mitchell MS, Howard RO and Morrow LB (1970) Immunosuppressive therapy for the eye changes of Graves' disease. *J Clin Endocr & Metab* **31**: 307-311.
23. Cant JS (1970) The assessment and treatment of endocrine exophthalmos. *Proc Roy Soc Med* **63**: 783-786.
24. MacCarty CS, Kenefick TP, McConahey WM and Kearns TP (1970) Ophthalmopathy of Graves' disease treated by removal of roof, lateral walls and lateral spheroid ridge: Review of 46 cases. *Mayo Clin Proc* **45**: 488-493.
25. Jones DIR (1968) The effect of metronidazole on exophthalmos in man. *J Endocr* **41**: 609-610.
26. Crombie AL and Lawson AAH (1967) Long-term trial of

26. local guanethidine in treatment of eye signs of thyroid dysfunction of idiopathic lid retraction. *Br Med J* **4**: 592–595.
27. Garber MI (1966) Methylprednisone in the treatment of exophthalmos. *Lancet* **1**: 958–960.
28. Gay AJ and Wolkstein MA (1966) Topical guanethidine therapy for endocrine lid retraction. *Arch Ophth* **76**: 364–367.
29. Werner SC (1966) Prednisone in emergency treatment of malignant exophthalmos. *Lancet* **1**: 1004–1007.
30. Blahut RJ, Beierwaltes WH and Lampe I (1963) Exophthalmos response during roentgen therapy. *Am J Roent Rad Ther & Nuc Med* **90**: 261–268.
31. Brown J, Coburn JW, Wigod RA, Hiss JM and Dowling JT (1963) Adrenal steroid therapy of severe infiltrative ophthalmopathy of Graves' disease. *Am J Med* **34**: 786–795.
32. Furth ED, Becker DV, Ray BS and Kane JW (1962) Appearance of unilateral infiltrative exophthalmos of Graves' disease after the successful treatment of the same process in the contralateral eye by apparently total surgical hypophysectomy. *J Clin Endocr & Metab* **22**: 518–524.
33. Henderson JW (1958) Optic neuropathy of exophthalmic goiter (Graves' disease). *Arch Ophth* **59**: 471–480.
34. Lamberg BA (1957) Thyro-hypophyseal syndrome II. Roentgen irradiation of pituitary region in the treatment of hypophyseal eye signs (including exophthalmos) after thyroidectomy. *Acta Med Scand* **156**: 361–376.
35. Lamberg BA and Hernberg CA (1957) Thyro-hypophyseal syndrome III. Pituitary roentgen irradiation in the treatment of hypophyseal eye signs (including exophthalmos) during treatment of thyrotoxicosis with thyrostatic drugs. *Acta Med Scand* **156**: 377–390.
36. Lamberg BA (1957) Thyro-hypophyseal syndrome IV. Hypophyseal eye signs (including exophthalmos) without thyrotoxicosis (solitary thyro-hypophyseal syndrome) and their treatment by roentgen irradiation of the pituitary region. *Acta Med Scand* **156**: 391–402.
37. Gedda PO and Lindgren M (1954) Pituitary and orbital roentgen therapy in the hyperophthalmopathic type of Graves' disease. *Acta Radiol* **42**: 211–220.
38. Beierwaltes WH (1953) X-ray treatment of malignant exophthalmos: A report on 28 patients. *J Clin Endocr & Metab* **13**: 1090–1100.
39. Jones A (1951) Orbital x-ray therapy of progressive exophthalmos. *Br J Radiol* **24**: 637–646.

Immunosuppression, Lupus Nephritis, Multiple Sclerosis, and Organ Transplantation

The current use of Total Lymphoid Irradiation (TLI) as immunosuppressive therapy for non-malignant diseases is experimental and has been utilized *(1)* in preparation for allogeneic organ transplantation (i.e., kidney, pancreas, etc.; 26% of radiation oncologists in the national survey would not treat), *(2)* in the treatment of autoimmune diseases (i.e., rheumatoid arthritis, systemic lupus erythematosus, etc.; 94% of radiation oncologists in the national survey would not treat), and *(3)* in the treatment of neurological disorders considered to have an immune-mediated pathogenesis (i.e., multiple sclerosis, chronic demyelinating polyneuropathy, etc.; 93% of radiation oncologists in our national survey would not treat).

TLI is an effective and relatively non-toxic mode of immunosuppression in selected circumstances with the potential clinical advantages for patients who have advanced autoimmune diseases, and for preparation of high-risk patients for organ transplantation. It is an experimental treatment modality. Optimal fractionation schemes and total dose requirements are yet to be determined. Its use should be restricted to controlled clinical trials undertaken in major medical centers.

Homograft Rejection

Author, Year	Total # Pts.	Treatment	Results	Notes
Godfrey and Salaman, 1976	36	1. Standard form of rejection therapy (high doses of steroid drugs: 16 pts) 2. Standard form of rejection therapy plus radiotherapy (600r to the graft: 20 pts)	Minimum follow up of 1 year. 1. 50% rejection reversed within 4 weeks 50% transplants functioning at one year. 56% patients surviving one year. 2. 58% rejection reversed within 4 weeks. 25% transplants functioning at one year. 47% patients surviving one year.	Renal allografts. This study revealed no improvement among the treated group in the number of grafts or patients surviving, or the level of function achieved.

Historical Data: Homograft Rejection

Author, Year	Total # Patients	Treatment	Results	Notes
Hume and Wolf, 1967	4	Sublethal total body irradiation.	2/4 died as a direct consequence of irradiation. 2/4 still alive.	Renal transplants.
Woodruff, 1966	1	Two days prior to transplantation, the patient received 150r minimum central dose whole body irradiation plus 100-110r localized irradiation to the spleen and lower right abdomen. Eleven days after transplantation the patient was given an additional 50r whole body irradiation.	Sixteen days after irradiation there was a large drop in blood platelets. All types of leukocytes disappeared from the patient's blood. Patient developed a fatal septicemia.	Renal transplantation
	6	Chemotherapy (prolonged administration of an antimetabolite, Imuran) plus preoperative local irradiation of the spleen and graft site.	4/6 alive with functioning transplants. Of the two patients who died, one was severely ill at the time of transplantation. In the other, the transplant continued to function up until the time of death, and it is thought that death was due to the toxic effect of prolonged administration of Imuran.	
Hamburger et al, 1965	43	Irradiation alone and/or drug therapy (Imuran or 6-mercaptopurine). Some patients received a second transplant.	Irradiation alone: 12 early failures 2 lengthy tolerance and survival Irradiation plus drugs: 8 well, 1-34 months 1 progressive renal failure, second transplant at 22 months 3 died at 9-23 months. Drugs alone: 2 early failures 16 well at 1-10 months	Renal transplants
Morgan, 1964	6	Whole body irradiation (100-400r) prior to transplantation	3/6 died within 26 days 1/6 died at 3 months 2/6 still alive, one at 27 months	Renal transplantation
Hume et al, 1963	6	1. Total body irradiation (150-300r) plus post-op irradiation to the transplant (total dose 100-500r: 4 pts) 2. Post-op irradiation to the transplant only (600r/4F: 2pts)	1. 1/4 transplant function excellent at 5 months 2/4 died within 34 days 1/4 transplant function declining at 6 months 2. 2/2 transplant function died	Renal transplants
Shackman et al, 1963	6	Pre-op total body irradiation plus post-op local irradiation in 2 patients. Post-op local irradiation only in 2 patients. Pre-op total body irradiation only in 2 patients.	Prolonged survival in one patient	Renal transplants

Historical Data: Homograft Rejection (Continued)

Author, Year	Total # Pts.	Treatment	Results	Notes
Woodruff et al, 1963	6	Pre-op irradiation plus post-op administration of antimetabolite. Pre-op irradiation (100–200r to spleen and graft site; 2Mev or 4Mev)	4/6 alive (at 3–9 months, one patient has excellent renal function) 2/6 died, one at 2 months (Imuran intoxication) and one at 12 days post-op	Renal transplants
Hamburger et al, 1962	6	Total body irradiation. 430–460r (central dose)/5days (approximately 220r on 1st day and 220r on next 2–5 days). Transplantation was done on the day following the last irradiation treatment.	3/6 early rejection (25 hours – 21 days) 3/6 prolonged tolerance (6 months – 2.5 years)	Renal transplants
Murray et al, 1962	12	Total body irradiation 6–700r (2Mev) followed by bone marrow infusion in the two patients with absence of renal tissue. 200–450r (250Kv)/1–3F/ max of 8 days to the other 10 pts. Transplant was done on the day of or the day following the last x-ray treatment.	11/12 died (two receiving marrow transplants died from sepsis and infection; 5 others showed excellent early renal function, but there was rapid cessation of function in 3–6 days) 1/12 alive and well at 3.5 years.	Renal transplants. Two patients had absence of renal tissue following injury or removal of a solitary kidney. 10 patients were in a pre-terminal state from renal disease. 6 of the patients were reported previously.
Tubiana et al, 1961	5	Whole body irradiation 400–450r/1–2F. Some patients received additional irradiation to the spleen. 2 pts also received additional irradiation 2–3.5 months post-op.	3/5 alive with functioning kidney at 5–22 months 1/5 died from hepatic metastasis at 5 months, kidney was functioning 1/5 died at 50 days of complete medullary aplasia	

References

1. Godfrey AM and Salaman J (1976) Radiotherapy in the treatment of acute rejection of human renal allografts. *Lancet* **1**: 938–939.
2. Hume DM and Wolf JS (1967) Abrogation of the immune response: irradiation therapy and lymphocyte depletion. Modification of renal homograft rejection by irradiation. *Transplantation* **5**: 1174–1191.
3. Woodruff MF (1966) The management of patients given whole body irradiation or antimetabolites to promote the survival of a renal homotransplant. *Clin Radiol* **15**: 30–40.
4. Hamburger J, Crosnier J and Dormont J (1965) Experience with 45 renal homotransplants in man. *Lancet* **1**: 985–992.
5. Morgan R (1964) Clinical experience of whole body radiation in man as a preliminary to renal transplantation. *Clinic Radiol* **15**: 35–40.
6. Hume DM, Magee JH, Kauffman HM, Rittenbury MS and Prout GR (1963) Renal homotransplantation in man in modified recipients. *Ann Surg* **158**: 608–644.
7. Shackman R, Dempstu WJ and Wrong OM (1963) Kidney homotransplantation in the human. *Br J Urol* **35**: 222–225.
8. Woodruff MFA, Robson JS, Nolan B, Lambie AT, Wilson TI and Clark JH (1963) Homotransplantation of kidney in patients treated by preoperative local irradiation and postoperative administration of an antimetabolite (Imuran). Report of six cases. *Lancet* **2**: 675–682.
9. Hamburger J, Vayesse J, Crosnier J, Avvert J, Lalanne CM and Hopper J (1962) Renal homotransplantation in man after radiation of the recipient. *Am J Med* **32**: 854–871.
10. Murray JE, Merrill JP, Dammin GJ, Dealy JB, Alexandre GW and Harrison JH (1962) Kidney transplantation in modified recipients. *Ann Surg* **156**: 337–355.
11. Tubiana M, Lalanne CM and Surmont J (1961) Total body irradiation for organ transplantation. *Proc Roy Soc Med* **54**: 1143–1150.
12. Murray JE, Merrill JP, Dammin GH, Dealy JB, Walter CW, Brooke MS and Wilson RE (1960) Study on transplantation immunity after total body irradiation: clinical and experimental investigation. *Surg* **48**: 272–284.

Lupus Erythematosus (Lupus Nephritis)

Author, Year	Total # Pts.	Site and Age of Patient	Treatment	Results	Notes
Strober et al, 1987	15	Total lymphoid irradiation for diffuse lupus nephritis, moderate to high chronicity index on renal biopsy, and nephrotic syndrome	2000r in 4-6 weeks in sequential TLI	13/15 patients alive with stable renal function. Patients had improved renal function. 4 patients had steroids withdrawn with resolution of nephrotic syndrome	Update and extension of series reported by Strober et al *Ann Int Med* 1985
Ben-Chetrit et al, 1986	2	Total lymphoid irradiation. 23 and 34 year old patients who had failed conventional treatment	2000r in 200r fractions to mantle, followed by 2000r in 200r fractions to spleen and inverted Y	No beneficial clinical effects regardless of adequate immunosuppression. Proteinuria increased, creatinine clearance decreased.	After 800r subdiaphragmatic XRT in one pt treatment was discontinued. Both patients developed major complications and one died within 2 weeks of XRT from florid nephritis. Experimental therapy
Strober et al, 1985	10	Total lymphoid irradiation. 19-43 years of age with severe intractable glomerulonephritis	2000r in 200r fractions to mantle followed by 2000r in 200r fractions to inverted Y and spleen (pelvis omitted in females). Kidneys not irradiated	All patients had increase in serum albumin and decrease in serum anti-DNA antibodies with increase in serum complement levels. 8/10 patients had improvement for 12-44 months with decrease in serum creatinine in 3 and stabilization in 7 patients. All patients had less urinary leakage of albumin.	Side effects were minor. Experimental therapy

Multiple Sclerosis

Author, Year	Total # Pts.	Site and Age of Patient	Treatment	Results	Notes
Devereux et al, 1988	20	Total lymphoid irradiation in adults with mean age of 44 years and chronic progressive multiple sclerosis	1980r in 180r fractions to mantle and spleen followed by 1980r in 180r fractions to inverted Y (including pelvis)	TLI vs sham-treated: functional scale assessment 84% vs 45% ($p < 0.03$)-12 months 72% vs 37% ($p < 0.03$)-18 months 56% vs 26% (NS)-24 months 50% vs 13% (NS)-30 months Reduction in lymphocyte count 3 months post-irradiation ($p < 0.02$)	Update of paper by Cook et al *Lancet* 1986. Prospective, randomized, double-blind study compared against sham-irradiated controls

Multiple Sclerosis (Continued)

Author, Year	Total # Pts.	Site and Age of Patient	Treatment	Results	Notes
Cook et al, 1987	45	Total lymphoid irradiation Adults 20-60 years	1980r total lymphoid irradiation vs sham-TLI	Clinical effects: Patients with sustained lymphocyte counts <900mm^3 for prolonged periods after XRT had less rapid progression of disease over 3 years than patients with lymphocyte counts >900mm^3 ($p<0.01$)	Update of 1986 article All patients had chronic progressive multiple sclerosis Prospective, randomized double-blind study
Cook et al, 1986	20	Total lymphoid irradiation Adults with mean age 42.9 years having chronic progressive multiple sclerosis	1980r in 180r fractions to mantle, followed by 1980r in 180r fractions to inverted Y and spleen (pelvis excluded)	Clinical effects: Longer time to sustained progression than controls ($p<0.05$) and less functional decline, particularly in patients with sustained lymphocytopenia	Prospective, randomized, double blind study compared against sham-irradiated controls Minor side effects Experimental therapy
Kolar and Hornback, 1986	1	Total lymphoid irradiation Age 37	2000r in 200r fractions over 59 days	Progression of clinical course	Transient clinical improvement with transient normalization of OKT8/OCT4 cell ratio during irradiation, but overall progression
Tourtellotte et al, 1980	20	Cranial-spinal irradiation Ages 30-58	1200r or 1800r in 150r fractions	No neurological improvement, change in activity of the disease, or persistent adverse effects	Transient reduction in rate of de novo CNS IgG synthesis with 1200r; enhancement following 1800r

Organ Transplantation, TLI in Renal Transplantation and Heart Transplantation

Author, Year	Total # Pts.	Site and Age of Patient	Treatment	Results	Notes
Ang et al, 1985	17	Total lymphoid radiation for cadaveric renal transplantation (diabetes) Ages 26-55	20-30Gy in 1Gy fractions	6 patients survive more than 1 year and 7 patients survive less than a year with functioning kidney graft. Reduced amounts of steroids and azothioprine were required.	2/13 patients had repeated rejection episodes necessitating cyclosporin A. 4 patients died of pericardial tamponade infection and other causes.
Levin et al, 1985	28	Total lymphoid irradiation for cadaveric renal transplantation Ages 22-66	2000r in 100r fractions to mantle, spleen and inverted Y	25 patients were evaluable. Actuarial graft survival at 18 months was 77% 4 patients died and 6 grafts were lost	Patients managed with low dose maintenance prednisone
Waer et al, 1985	20	Total lymphoid irradiation for cadaveric renal transplantation	2000-3000r in 100r fractions	16/20 patients alive, 15 with functioning grafts in 2 year follow up	12 patients had rejection episode, managed with prednisone Other 8 patients had rejection episode requiring ATG, cyclosporin or azothioprine

Organ Transplantation, TLI in Renal Transplantation and Heart Transplantation (Continued)

Author, Year	Total # Pts.	Site and Age of Patient	Treatment	Results	Notes
Vanrenterghem et al, 1984	10	Total lymphoid irradiation for cadaveric renal transplantation Ages 32-51	2000-2500r in 100r fractions	All patients survived with 9/10 grafts functioning with 12 month follow up	Reduced need for steroids in most patients
Najarian et al, 1982	22	Total lymphoid irradiation for human renal transplantation Ages 5-55	1050-4050r in 100-125r fractions to mantle and inverted Y simultaneously	78% actuarial patient survival and 74% well functioning grafts at 2 year follow up	17 patients had complications requiring interruption of therapy and 4 patients died, 2 with lymphoma Recommend 2500r fractionated TLI followed by transplantation within 2 weeks of XRT

Local Field Irradiation in Renal Transplantation

Author, Year	Total # Pts.	Site and Age of Patient	Treatment	Results	Notes
Halperin et al, 1984	67	Renal allograft irradiation Mean age 37 years	300-1200r to kidney in 150r fractions Mean dose 600r	Of 53 kidneys irradiated because of failure of standard immunosuppression for acute rejection, 21% of allografts functioned 1 year after transplant	
Pilepich et al, 1983	62	(64 grafts) Renal graft irradiation in acute rejection, any age	methyl prednisolone XRT 34 grafts randomized to XRT 525r given in 175r fractions every other day	No difference in reversal of graft rejection or graft survival in the irradiated grafts as compared to sham controls.	A prospective randomized study
Peeples et al, 1982	44	Renal graft irradiation for rejection Ages 16-60 Mean age 41 years	600r/course 4 meV photons 150r fractions	Successful renal function was 52% among 29 patients who had 1 course of XRT 60% among 15 patients with 2-4 courses of XRT 60% among 50 patients with steroids only and no XRT	Non-randomized study
Besarab et al, 1982	83	(89 cadaver donor grafts) Prophylactic renal graft irradiation along with acute tubular necrosis (ATN) Average age 36 years	450r given in 3 150r fractions on alternating days, along with Imuran, prednisone, methyl prednisolone, and anti-lymphocyte globulin (AGC)	Prophylactic irradiation and ATN decreased graft survival, effects were additive	Prophylactic irradiation to recipients, alternated randomly, but not double-blind
Drenguis et al, 1977	178	Renal graft irradiation in acute rejection Ages 9-54 Mean age 27 years	4.5Gy given in three 1.5Gy fractions on alternate days along with systemic immunosuppressive therapy	Of the irradiated kidneys, 61% were functioning at 6 months, 58% at 12 months, and 49% at 18 months	

Local Field Irradiation in Renal Transplantation (Continued)

Author, Year	Total # Pts.	Site and Age of Patient	Treatment	Results	Notes
Godrey and Salaman, 1977	36	Renal graft irradiation at time of first rejection	One-half of patients received high doses of steroid drugs. One-half received 600r in 4 150r fractions on alternate days	At 3 years there was no difference in the two treatment groups in response to treatment, graft survival, or transplant function. No benefit from XRT was observed	Randomized study
Nakajima et al, 1977	158	(205 renal transplants 179 rejection episodes) Renal graft irradiation during acute rejection	i.v. methylprednisolone with and without XRT 600r given in 4 150r fractions	Local radiation did not contribute to improved graft survival or mortality	Significant sepsis was observed in those patients receiving more than 5gm methylprednisolone

Prospective randomized studies fail to demonstrate improvement in engraftment over non-irradiated controls. The continued use of this technique in non-protocol investigative studies is not warranted.

References

1. Devereux CK, Vidaver R, Hafstein MP, Zita G, Troiano R, Dowling PC, Cook SD (1988) Total lymphoid irradiation for multiple sclerosis. *Int J Radiation Oncol Biol Phys* **14**: 197-203.
2. Cook SD, Devereux C, Troiano R, Zito G, Hafstein M, Lavenhar M, Hernandez E, Dowling PC (1987) Total lymphoid irradiation in multiple sclerosis: blood lymphocytes and clinical course. *Annal Neurology* **22**: 634-638.
3. Strober S, Farinas C, Field E, Solovera JJ, Kiberc BA, Myers BD and Hoppe RT (1987) Lupus nephritis after total lymphoid irradiation: persistent improvement and reduction of steroid therapy. *Ann Intern Med* **107**: 689-690.
4. Ben-Chetrit E, Gross DJ, Braverman A, Weshler Z, Fuks Z, Slavin S and Eliakim M (1986) Total lymphoid irradiation in refractory systemic lupus erythematosus. *Ann Intern Med* **105**: 58-60.
5. Cook SD, Devereux C, Troiano R, Hafstein MP, Zito G, Hernandez E, Lavenhar M, Vidaver R and Dowling PC (1986) Effect of total lymphoid irradiation in chronic progressive multiple sclerosis. *Lancet* **1**: 1405-1409.
6. Kolar OJ and Hornback NB (1986) Total lymphoid irradiation in multiple sclerosis. *Lancet* **2**: 453.
7. Ang KK, Vanrenterghem Y, Waer M, Vandeputte M, Michielsen P and Van der Shueren E (1985) Kidney allograft tolerance in diabetic patients after total lymphoid irradiation (TLI). *Radiotherapy and Oncology* **3**: 192-199.
8. Levin B, Hoppe RT, Collins G, Miller E, Waer M, Bieber C, Girinsky T and Strober S (1985) Treatment of cadaveric renal transplant recipients with total lymphoid irradiation, antithymocyte globulin and low-dose prednisone. *Lancet* **2**: 1321-1325.
9. Strober S, Field E, Hoppe RT, Kotzin BL, Shemesh O, Engleman E, Ross JC and Myers BD (1985) Treatment of intractable lupus nephritis with total lymphoid irradiation. *Ann Intern Med* **102**: 450-458.
10. Waer M, Vanrenterghem Y, Roels L, Ang KK, Bouillon R, Lerut T, Gruwez J, Michielsen P, Van der Schueren F and Vandeputte M (1985) Total lymphoid irradiation in renal cadaveric transplantation in diabetes. *Lancet* **2**: 1354.
11. Halperin EC, Delmonico FL, Nelson PW, Shipley WU and Cosini AB (1984) The use of local allograft irradiation following renal transplantation. *Int J Radiat Oncol Biol Phys* **10**: 987.
12. Vanrenterghem Y, Waer M, Ang KK, Van der Schueren E, Gruwez J, Bouillon R and Michielsen P (1984) Cadaveric kidney transplantation in diabetes after total lymphoid irradiation (TLI). *Transplantation Proc* **16**: 636-639.
13. Pilepich MV, Sicard GA, Breaux SR, Etheredge EE, Blum J and Anderson CB (1983) Renal graft irradiation in acute rejection. *Transplantation* **35**: 208-211.
14. Besarab A, Jarrell B, Ihle BU, Colberg JE, Burke JF and Wesson L (1982) Adverse effects of prophylactic irradiation and acute tubular necrosis on renal graft function and survival. *Nephron* **31**: 347-353.
15. Najarian JS, Ferguson RM, Sutherland DER, Slavin S, Kim T, Kersey K and Simmonds RL (1982) Fractionated total lymphoid irradiation as preparative immunosuppression in high-risk renal transplantation: clinical and immunological studies. *Ann Surg* **196**: 442-452.
16. Peeples WJ, Wombalt DG, El-Mahdi AM and Turalba CIC (1982) Radiation therapy for renal transplant rejection reactions. *South Med J* **75**: 30-32.
17. Tourtellotte WW, Potvin AR, Baumhefner RW, Potvin JH, Ma BI, Syndulko K and Petrovich Z (1980) Multiple sclerosis de novo CNS IgG synthesis. Effect of CNS irradiation. *Arch Neurol* **37**: 620-624.
18. Drenguis B, Griffin T, Gerdes A and Marchioro T (1977) Effect of local irradiation on the acute rejection process in transplanted kidneys. *Acta Radiol Ther Phys Biol* **16**: 241-244.
19. Godfrey AM and Salaman JR (1977) Is graft irradiation of value in renal transplant rejection? *Transplant Proc* **9**: 1005-1006.
20. Nakajima N, Streepada Rao TK, Sakai A, Butt KH and Kountz SL (1977) Effects of intravenous bolus dosages of methylprednisolone and local radiation on renal allograft rejection and patient mortality. *Surg Gynecol Obstet* **144**: 63-66.

Infectious Disorders

Prior to the antibiotic era, cutaneous bacterial infections were often treated with small doses of radiotherapy at short intervals. This therapy apparently persists today in some European centers. Its use has been reserved for the rare cutaneous infections for patients who do not respond to traditional management techniques. Its use, however, remains controversial. In America there would seldom, if ever, be an indication for such treatment. Complications of the treatment, including radiation induced neoplasms, are now being appreciated.

Viral infections such as herpes simplex and zoster clearly should be treated with antiviral agents which now have proven efficacy. In regard to plantar warts and condyloma acuminata, there is evidence in the literature of significant response if the radiation dose is safely tailored. New antiviral agents which can be applied topically would now have to be compared for efficacy in order to justify use of radiation therapy. If all reasonable modalities have been utilized in the treatment of viral warts, with appreciation of the risk benefit ratio, there may be instances where radiation would be appropriate. One should realize in treating plantar warts, however, there is a 30-65% incidence of spontaneous remission. In addition reinfection can lead to recurrence.

The use of radiation in the treatment of chorioretinitis associated with ocular histoplasmosis remains experimental. Radioimmunotherapy using I^{131} labeled anti-cysticercus antibodies in patients with cerebral cysticercosis appears promising.

We strongly oppose the use of radiation in infectious disorders for the pediatric age group.

The results of the national survey indicate 97% of radiation oncologists would not treat fungal infections; 99% would not treat tuberculosis; 97% would not treat viral infections; 96% would not treat bacterial infections; 99% would not treat leprosy and other infections; and 73% of radiation oncologists would not treat viral warts.

Historical Data: Bacterial Infections

Author, Year	Total # Pts.	Site and Age	Treatment	Results	Notes
Fairris et al, 1984	6 pts 9 paired lesions	Palmoplantar Pustulosis involving palms and soles.	One site received 100r of superficial x-ray at 50Kv, and its pair received a placebo dose. Each dose administered 3 times, every 21 days.	At 6, 9, and 18 weeks there was no difference among x-ray treated lesions, and those treated by placebo.	Double-blind, placebo-controlled trials.
Gorrin-Yehudain, 1983	4	Acute suppurative perichondritis of the external ear	80r 150Kv x-ray for 3-4 fractions at 2 day intervals.	Regression of signs of inflammation with subsequent complete healing in patients with infection following a burn.	Cultures reveal pseudomonas aeruginosa and/or staphylococcus aureus. Presumably the irradiation inhibits the infection allowing healing.
Barker and Gould, 1978	2	Pyoderma faciale involving chin. Ages 45 and 43.	One treated with superficial x-ray (100r on 3 occasions) and sodium fusidate 2% ointment. The other was treated only with antiseptic solution, no x-ray.	Slow improvement, completely disappeared in 2 months. Resolved after three months.	Culture - coagulase negative staphylococci Culture - staphylococcus epidermidis.
Lukacs et al, 1978			Superficial x-rays 50-80r for 3-4 doses.	No data.	Used when adequate tissue levels of antibiotics cannot be achieved.
Webber, 1977		Radiation to children for pertussis (whopping cough)	3-4 treatments given at 2-3 day intervals approximately 300-600r.	Unclear therapeutic effect. Secondary cancers are now emerging.	

Historical Data: Viral Infections

Author, Year	Total # Pts.	Site and Age	Treatment	Results	Notes
Veien et al, 1982	1107	Warts on hands and feet, all ages.	3000r in a single dose, 29Kv, 25mA, 0.3mm Al filter. In 19% a repeat treatment was given after 4-6 weeks.	Sequelae occurred in 144 of 2980 sites (4.8%) that received one treatment, and 85 of 695 sites (12.2%) that received two treatments.	There were no malignant transformations, and no cases of osteotis or tendinitis.
Danoff et al, 1981	1	Condylomata acuminata of the male urethra, 36 years.	2000r in 2 1/2 weeks using 250r fractions by 4 MEV linear accelerator	Complete response, with no recurrence 3 years later.	Patient had failed previous treatment including: 5-fluorouracil, podophyllin, thiotepa, and transurethral resection.
Shair et al, 1978	427	Feet, ages 6-75.	1000-2700r by a 100Kv, 5ma machine with 0.5mm Al, in one treatment followed by salicylic acid plaster.	80% cure rate, which rose to 90% following 2-3 applications of topical medications.	No late effects with 25 years follow-up.
Lukacs et al, 1978		Plantar warts	Less than 1000r in doses of 200-300r at 1-3 week intervals HVL 0.3mm Al TSD 30cm.	No data on efficacy.	No late effects.
		Recurrent herpes simplex	Grenz rays of 10Kv 200r at 1-2 week intervals	80% improvement	
Macht and Cordero, 1977	531	Warts, all ages.	250KvP orthovoltage unit calibrated at 100KvP and HVL 2.1mm Al 100KvP superficial therapy unit. HVL 0.7mm Al 1000r (in air) in one treatment followed by a second 500r (treatment in 59 pts) and a third 500r treatment if needed (in 60 pts).	Average cures in the orthovoltage group was 89%, in contrast to 70% in the superficial group.	More younger patients were cured than older. No complications were seen.

Historical Data: Parasitic and Other Infections

Author, Year	Total # Pts.	Site and Age	Treatment	Results	Notes
Junaid, 1986	178	Cutaneous leishmaniasis Age: 1 mos to 60 years	Infrared heat wave length: 4000-7700mm (55c for 5 minutes) patient may be retreated 3 weeks later.	162 had only one application of infrared heat to the largest lesion, 15 patients had 2 applications and 1 required 3 applications.	It is thought that the heat destroys the parasite and provokes an immune response causing the other lesions to disappear in 5-6 weeks.

Historical Data: Parasitic and Other Infections (Continued)

Author, Year	Total # Pts.	Site and Age	Treatment	Results	Notes
Davidorf et al, 1983	32	Ocular histoplasmosis, chorioretinitis 21–63 years (mean age 38)	1000r by 5, 200r fractions using 4x4 cm lateral part ± corticosteroids	34% of irradiated pts were considered successes of the treatment (improvement of visual acuity to 20/100 or better and inactivation of the lesion at follow-up) as compared to 12.5% of the controls. $p = 0.05$	Average follow-up was 27 months (6–55 months) A controlled study. No complications were seen.
Skromne-Kadlubik and Celis, 1981	500	Cysticercosis of the nervous system	Radioimmuno treatment with anti-cysticercus antibodies labeled with I^{131}.	96% had good or excellent results, 4% had poor results.	

References

1. Fairris GM, Jones DH, Mack DP and Rowell NR (1984) Superficial x-ray therapy in the treatment of palmoplantar pustulosis. *Br J Dermatol* **111**: 499–500.
2. Gorrin-Yehudain J, Moscona AR and Hirshowitz B (1983) Treatment of acute suppurative perichondritis of the external ear by low dose x-ray irradiation. *Burns Incl Therm Inj* **10**: 140–144.
3. Barker DJ and Gould DJ (1978) A pustular eruption of the chin (a variant of pyoderma faciale?) *Acta Derm Verrol (Stockh)* **58**: 549–551.
4. Lukacs S, Braun-Falco O and Goldschmidt H (1978) Radiotherapy of benign dermatoses: Indications, practice and results. *J Dermatol Surg Oncol* **4**: 620–625.
5. Webber BM (1977) Radiation therapy for pertussis: A possible etiologic factor in thyroid carcinoma. *Ann Intern Med* **86**: 449–450.
6. Rook A (1986) Textbook of Dermatology, Fourth Edition.
7. Saner (1985) Manual of Skin Diseases.
8. Veien NK, Nrholm A, Hattel T and Justesen O (1982) Late effects of x-ray treatment of warts. *J Dermatol Surg Oncol* **8**: 275–281.
9. Danoff DS, Holden S, Thompson RW and David R (1981) New treatment for extensive condylomata acuminata: external radiation therapy. *Urology* **18**: 47–49.
10. Shair HM, Hanshaw WJ and Grayson CD (1978) Radiation therapy for plantar warts. *J Dermatol Surg Oncol* **4**: 635–637.
11. Lukacs S, Braun-Falco O and Goldschmidt H (1978) Radiotherapy of benign dermatoses: Indications, practice and results. *J Dermatol Surg Oncol* **4**: 620–625.
12. Macht SH and Cordero JM (1977) Superficial radiotherapy of warts: Results of treating 531 warts. *Radiology* **122**: 231–232.
13. Bunnly MH (1976) An assessment of method of treating warts by comparative treatment trials based on a standard design. *British J Dermatology* **94**: 667.
14. Sanders B and Stretcher Jr G (1976) Warts: Diagnosis & Treatment. *JAMA* **235**: 2859–2861.
15. Broughton RH (1974) A personal approach to the treatment of verrucae. *J Roy Naval Med Ser* **60**: 130–132.
16. Aguino JA (1972) Warts and radiotherapy. *Nova Scotia Med Bulletin.*
17. Dunham HH (1972) Radiation treatment of plantar warts. *J Ind State Med Assn.*
18. Linton WT (1970) Concepts on wart treatment. *Applied Therapeutics* **12**: 16–18.
19. Reymann F (1969) The sensitivity of plantar warts to roentgen radiation. *Acta Derm-Venereol* **49**: 171–175.
20. Hazel J and Bouchard J (1962) The value of radiation therapy in the treatment of verrucae plantar warts. *J Canad Assn Radiol* **13**: 70–71.
21. Vickers CFH (1961) Treatment of plantar warts in children. *British Med J:* 743.
22. Reeves RJ and Jackson MT (1956) Roentgen therapy of plantar warts. *Am J Roentgenol* **76**: 997–998.
23. Pipkin JL et al (1949) The treatment of plantar warts by single dose method of roentgen ray. *Southern Med J* **42**: 193.
24. Pendergrass EP and Hodes PJ (1941) Roentgen irradiation in treatment of inflammations. *Am J Roentgenol & Rad Therapy* **45**: 74–105.
25. Review of the Use of Ionizing Radiation for the Treatment of Benign Disease. U.S. DHEW, HEW Publication (FDA) 78–8043.
26. Junaid AJ (1986) Treatment of cutaneous leishmaniasis with infrared heat. *Int J Dermatol* **25**: 470–472.
27. Davidorf FH, Makley TA, Bruce RA, Batley F and Wasserstrom JP (1983) Irradiation of the central lesion of presumed histoplasmic chorioretinitis. *Int Ophthamol Clin* **23**: 101–109.
28. Skromne-Kadlubik G and Celis C (1981) Cysticercosis of the nervous system. Treatment by means of specific internal radiation. *Arch Neurol* **38**: 288.

Inflammatory Conditions

Arachnoiditis, Tendinitis, Sinusitis, Thyroiditis

Clearly, the risk/benefit ratio tends exceedingly toward risk and seems only of questionable benefit in considering radiotherapy for these inflammatory conditions. In the instances of tendinitis (cf. tendinitis, arthritis, synovitis) and thyroiditis, risk far exceeds potential benefit; benefit is difficult to establish. Regarding arachnoiditis, surgical and medical approaches outweigh suggested benefits cited in older literature (e.g., *Fed Am J Roentgen,* 1962). Serious consideration could only be given to radiation treatment of these conditions if a non-responsive group of patients with identifiable characteristics could receive randomized treatment. Finally, in the instance of sinusitis, lymphoid reduction observed in treated youths resulted at the risk of thyroid cancer and cancers of the nasopharyngeal region. Surgical removal of lymphoid tissue remains the procedure of choice, failing chronic antibiotic therapy. Results of the national survey indicate that radiation oncologists would not treat thyroiditis (93%), arachnoiditis (96%) or sinusitis (99%); 67% of radiation oncologists would not treat tendinitis.

Historical Data: Arachnoiditis, Optic Chiasm Arachnoiditis

Author, Year	Total # Patients	Treatment	Results	Notes
Jackson, 1974	1	Steroids and amphotericin B followed by surgical lysis of arachnoidal adhesions covering the chiasm. Patient received long-term low-dose steroid therapy post-op.	Visual fields and tangent screens improved. At 2 years post-op patient had only small paracentral scotomas in both eyes. She became pregnant and steroids were discontinued during pregnancy and for the following 3 years. Patient incurred some further deterioration of vision which improved with resumptive steroid therapy.	Case of optic chiasmatic arachnoiditis
Coyle, 1969	1	Surgery: Resection of the scar tissue binding down the chiasm and the optic nerves	Vision and visual acuity improved	Case of chiasmatic arachnoiditis
Cant and Harrison, 1968	1	Surgery: Brain and arachnoid were freed from the optic nerves	Vision improved rapidly Bi-temporal field constriction slowly improved	Case of chiasmatic arachnoiditis associated with growth failure
Dickmann et al, 1951	47	Surgery, followed by radiotherapy in some cases	Overall results: (37%): 6 improved 1 stationary (63%): 12 aggravated Operative mortality: 1(2%) Radiotherapy results: 3/4 improved with immediate post-op radiotherapy (1 remained stationary) 0/3 improved with late post-op radiotherapy	Opto-chiasmatic arachnoiditis Follow up obtained for only 19 pts

Inflammatory Conditions

Historical Data: Arachnoiditis and Spinal Arachnoiditis

Author, Year	Total # Patients	Treatment	Results	Notes
Duke and Hashimoto, 1973	1	Surgical excision followed by radiotherapy and corticosteroids for subsequent deterioration	Transient clinical improvement after excision Subsequent gradual deterioration No response to radiation therapy or corticosteroids	All were cases of spinal arachnoiditis occurring in the same family
	1	Surgical excision	Transient clinical improvement Subsequent gradual deterioration	
	2	No treatment	Died with complete paraplegia	
Savastano, 1968	12	Intrathecal corticosteroid injection	10/12 no improvement 2/12 favorable results, but requiring several injections All were cases of post-op spinal arachnoiditis	
Feder and Smith, 1962	17	Radiotherapy: 600-800r (air) in daily increments of 100-200r Area of cord involvement is irradiated through posterior ports, 8 x 10cm to 10 x 20 cm If more than one port is necessary, they are treated in rotation. Factors; 250 Kv, 0.5mm Cu filtration, HVL 1.7mm Cu, FSD 50cm. Course may be repeated at three month intervals	4/17 excellent response with return both of motor and sensory function 4/17 improved to a limited degree 5/17 arrest of the disease 4/17 no response and no arrest of progression	All of the patients had chronic adhesive spinal arachnoiditis and had been considered unsuitable for surgery
Selinsky, 1936	8	800r in fractions of 100-150r (air) Series repeated at intervals of 6 weeks if necessary Factors: 180 Kv, 4ma, 0.5mm Cu plus 1mm Al filtration	4/8 good results (relief of pain)	Disseminated spinal arachnoiditis

Historical Data: Arachnoiditis and Arachnoiditis Ossificans

Author, Year	Total # Patients	Treatment	Results	Notes
Nagpal et al, 1975	1	Treatment with large doses of steroids Surgery: removal of ossified arachnoid Second operation for aspiration of cyst was required	Signs became worse upon initial treatment with steroids Patient was discharged with a total spastic paraplegia, urinary incontinence and altered sensory loss	Case of ossification of spinal arachnoid with unrelated syringomyelia
Kaufman and Dunsmore, 1971	3	Surgery: Laminectomy and excision of ossification when possible	Slight improvement in 2d and 3d year	All three were cases of arachnoiditis ossificans. Author provides a review of reported cases in the literature Surgical results disappointing

Historical Data: Arachnoiditis and Arachnoiditis Ossificans (Continued)

Author, Year	Total # Patients	Treatment	Results	Notes
Wise and Smith, 1965	2	Laminectomy and surgical removal of plaques, bone encased in arachnoid, and adhesive arachnoidal tissue	Slight improvement in one patient. The other patient improved temporarily, but subsequently progressed to complete paraplegia	Both were cases of spinal arachnoiditis ossificans
Slager, 1960		Author reports a case of arachnoiditis ossificans found incidentally at autopsy		Literature review. With operative removal of the arachnoid bone 6/8 (75%) improved

References

1. Nagpal RD, Gokhale SD and Parikh VR (1975) Ossification of spinal arachnoid with unrelated syringomyelia. *J Neurosurg* **42**: 222-225.
2. Jackson FE (1974) Optic chiasmatic arachnoiditis: improvement of rapidly failing vision following surgical lysis of chiasmatic adhesions and postoperative steroid therapy. *Milit Med* **139**: 127-128.
3. Duke RJ and Hashimoto S (1973) Familial spinal arachnoiditis - a new entity. *Trans Am Neurol Assoc* **98**: 98-102.
4. Kaufman AB and Dunsmore RH (1971) Clinicopathological considerations in spinal meningeal calcification and ossification. *Neurology* **21**: 1243-1248.
5. Coyle JT (1969) Chiasmatic arachnoiditis. A case report and a review. *Am J Opth* **68**: 345-349.
6. Cant JS and Harrison MT (1968) Chiasmatic arachnoiditis with growth failure. *Am J Ophth* **65**: 432-434.
7. Savastano AA (1968) Operative arachnoiditis. *Rhode Island Med J* **51**: 337-343.
8. Wise BL and Smith M (1965) Spinal arachnoiditis ossificans. *Arch Neurol* **13**: 391-394.
9. Feder BH and Smith JL (1962) Roentgen therapy in chronic spinal arachnoiditis. *Radiology* **78**: 192-198.
10. Slager UT (1960) Arachnoiditis ossificans. Report of a case and review of the subject. *Arch Path* **70**: 322-327.
11. Dickmann GH, Cramer FC and Kaplan AD (1951) Optochiasmatic arachnoiditis. *J Neurosurg* **8**: 355-359.
12. Selinsky H (1936) Disseminated spinal arachnoiditis. Its diagnosis and treatment with roentgen rays. *Arch Neurol and Psychiat* **35**: 1262-1279.

Historical Data: Thyroiditis

Author, Year	Total # Patients	Treatment	Results	Notes
Papapetrov et al, 1972	12	Thyroxine (long term therapy average of 9.9 years)	Significant decrease in goiter size. In 4 patients the thyroid was not palpable. Six weeks after stopping therapy, 11 patients were clinically hypothyroid.	All were cases of Hashimoto's thyroiditis
Heimann, 1970	178	1. Surgery (58) 11 patients had also been treated by thyroid hormone. 2. Thyroid hormone (130) 3. No treatment (1)	1. Complications of surgery post-op growth of goiter (15.5%) Hypoparathyroidism (3.4%) Permanent unilateral vocal cord paralysis (3.4%) 2. Subacute cases 22.29 total regression of disease. Chronic cases 13% no change in status 87% regression of goiter	Chronic thyroiditis
Vagenakis et al, 1970	6	Prednisone	Dramatic and marked relief of symptoms in all cases. No recurrences when prednisone was continued until the I-131 uptake had returned to normal	All were cases of acute non-suppurative thyroiditis

Historical Data: Thyroiditis (Continued)

Author, Year	Total # Patients	Treatment	Results	Notes
Lindem and Clark, 1969	46	Surgery – near total thyroidectomy. Oral thyroid given after surgery in all patients	No follow up data	Type of thyroiditis: Hashimoto's disease (89%) Riedel's struma (4%) Granulomatous thyroiditis (7%) Indication for surgery was a mass with carcinoma as a possibility in 5%
Thomson et al, 1968	1	Steroids (betamethasone)	Good therapeutic response, but a hard goiter developed when an attempt to discontinue the steroid therapy was made. Steroids were restarted	Reidel's thyroiditis. *"In view of the satisfactory clinical response of the first patient, a trial of steroid therapy would seem indicated in this condition where surgical management may be hazardous."*
Varl et al, 1968	6	I-131 (diagnostic dose of 40-50uCi)	Immediate disappearance of pain, temperature decrease, thyroid became softer and signs of inflammation gradually regressed. Quick improvement in three cases of local thyroiditis and in two cases of a thyroiditis in a toxic thyroid nodule	All were cases of subacute diffuse thyroiditis
Blizzard et al, 1962	3	Cortisone	Within 20-40 days after cortisone treatment, all 3 patients became euthyroid and the glands were no longer palpable. The goiters recurred when the steroid dosage was reduced	Hashimoto's thyroiditis *"Signs and symptoms recur when therapy is discontinued. Desiccated thyroid remains preferable for the treatment of patients with this disease."*
Murray, 1958	3	Prednisone	3/3 rapid diminution in size of gland and an improvement in the associated biochemical abnormalities as long as treatment was continued. There was no change in the objective evidence of hyperthyroidism.	Hashimoto's thyroiditis. *"It is suggested that steroid therapy has little place in the treatment of this condition, but that if combined with the administration of thyroid it might be of value when rapid relief of symptoms due to pressure of an enlarged gland is required."*
Furr and Crile, 1954	62	1. Radiotherapy (after needle biopsy), 450-2400r (11 patients plus desiccated thyroid in 6 of those patients) 2. Desiccated thyroid (12 patients) 3. Cortisone (4 patients plus desiccated thyroid in 3 of those cases)	1. Occasionally a rapid decrease in size within a few days, but usually a progressive diminution, the goiter reduced 50% in two months 2. 1/12 decrease in size in less than 1 month In most cases size decreased 50% in 4-6 months 3. 4/4 decrease in size with 1-2 months	All were cases of struma lymphomatosa

Historical Data: Thyroiditis (Continued)

Author, Year	Total # Patients	Treatment	Results	Notes
Lindsay and Dailey, 1954	37	1. Surgery (25) 2. Nonoperative groups (12)	1. 10/13 became hypothyroid and required therapy with desiccated thyroid. No known recurrences of thyroiditis (follow up of 4 months, 15 years) 2. 5/12 completely free of pain/tenderness within 4 weeks The glands of 10 patients became essentially normal although slightly firm	Granulomatous or giant cell thyroiditis
Crile and Schneider, 1952				Authors state that they have employed radiotherapy with doses of 600-1000r as a standard therapy for subacute thyroiditis, which produces relief within 1-2 weeks. But they employ ACTH or cortisone in cases in which a quicker result (48 hrs) is desired. Struma of lymphomatosa is treated almost exclusively with desiccated thyroid.

References

1. Papapetrov Pd, Lazarus JH, MacSween RNM and Harden R (1972) Long-term treatment of Hashimoto's thyroiditis with thyroxine. *Lancet* **2**: 1045-1048.
2. Strahan RW, Calcaterra TC and Ward PH (1971) Thyroiditis. A classification and review. *Laryngoscope* **81**: 1388-1400.
3. Heimann P (1970) Treatment of thyroiditis. *Acta Med Scand* **187**: 323-329.
4. Vagenakis AG, Abreau, CM and Braverman LE (1970) Prevention of recurrence in acute thyroiditis following corticosteroid withdrawal. *J Clin Endocr and Metabol* **31**: 705-708.
5. Lindem MC and Clark JH (1969) Indications for survey in thyroiditis. *Am J Surg* **118**: 829-831.
6. Varl B, Kastelic B and Porenta M (1968) The therapeutic effect of a diagnostic dose of radioactive iodine on the subacute De Quervain thyroiditis. *Strahlentherapie* **36**: 162-169.
7. Thomson JA, Jackson IMD and Duguid WP (1968) The effect of steroid therapy on Riedel's thyroiditis. *Scot Med J* **13**: 13-16.
8. Blizzard RM, Hung W, Chandler, RW, Aceto T, Kyle M and Winship T (1962) Hashimoto's thyroiditis. *N Engl J Med* **267**: 1015-1020.
9. Murray JPC (1958) The effect of prednisone on Hashimoto's thyroiditis. *Scot Med J* **3**: 341-345.
10. Furr WE and Crile G (1954) Struma lymphomatosa: clinical manifestations and response to therapy. *J Clin Endocr and Metabol* **14**: 79.
11. Lindsay S and Dailey ME (1954) Granulomatous or giant cell thyroiditis. A clinical and pathologic study of thirty seven patients. *Surg Gyn Obst* **98**: 197-212.
12. Crile G and Schneider RW (1952) Diagnosis and treatment of thyroiditis with special reference to the use of cortisone and ACTH. *Cleveland Clin Qtly* **19**: 219-224.
13. Volpe R (1975) Thyroiditis. Current views of pathogenesis. *Med Clin N Am* **59**: 1163-1175.

Inverted Papilloma

Inverted papilloma is a rare lesion of the nasal cavity and paranasal sinuses which may transform into or be associated with a squamous cell carcinoma in the same location in 5–15% of cases. The primary treatment modality is surgery, although there is a substantial rate of recurrence. The experience with radiotherapy is limited but does suggest that high dose treatment is effective, providing regression and local control, although the regression rate is slow. Radiotherapy has been condemned by some authors for fear of malignant transformation. However, there are no firm data to support the contention that radiation therapy in this circumstance causes malignant transformation. In the national survey, eighty-one percent of radiation oncologists would not treat inverted papilloma.

Inverted Papilloma

Author, Year	Total # Pts.	Site and Age	Treatment	Results	Notes
Mendenhall et al, 1985	5	Nasal cavity and paranasal sinuse ages 40–53.	Radiation alone or in combination with surgical resection 4715–6920r.	Four of five pts are alive and disease free 3,3, 4 and 11 years following treatment. One of five patients died of intercurrent disease 9 years after therapy with no evidence of disease.	Two patients had pure inverted papilloma; 1 had inverted papilloma with a focus of squamous cell carcinomas; 2 had cylindrical cell papillomas.
Levendag et al, 1984	1	Nasal cavity and paranasal sinuses.	Extensive surgery with residual disease, followed by post-operative radiotherapy. Total dose 64 Gy.	Patient controlled with radiotherapy; NED at one year follow-up.	Inverted papilloma with in situ carcinoma.

References

1. Mendenhall WM, Million RR, Cassisi NJU and Pierson KK (1985) Biologically aggressive papillomas of the nasal cavity: the role of radiation therapy. *Laryngoscope* **95**: 344–347.
2. Levendag PC, Annyas AA, Escajadillo JR and Elema JD (1984) Radiotherapy for inverted papilloma: A case report. *Radiotherapy and Oncol* **2**: 13–17.

Keloid

Post-operative radiotherapy prevents keloid formation and should be given with superficial energy. Ninety-four percent of radiation oncologists would treat keloids post-operatively, according to the national survey.

Keloid Survey: Sixteen Centers (1976)

Kv	Dose and Time	Field Size	Organ at Risk
100 Kv	1200r/2 RX/8 days	2.5	Ear lobes
250 Kv	1500r/2 RX/18 days	5 x 9 10 x 11	Shoulder
140 Kv	1000r/3 days	Adequate	Thyroid

Keloid Survey: Sixteen Centers (1976) (Continued)

Kv	Dose and Time	Field Size	Organ at Risk
80 Kv	400r/2-8 days	2 x 7	Skin
100 Kv	300r x 3 400r x 3 500r x 3 600r x 2	From 2 x 4 to 23 x 12	Skin
90 Kv	1200r/3 F 1200r/3 F 900r/3 F	Chest wall Abdominal wall Parotid	Parotid
75 Kv	1200r/3 F	5 x 2	None
100 Kv	900r/3 F/1 week		Skin
50-140 Kv	1000r/1 F	To cover scar	
280 Kv	1500r/3 F		
180 Kv	900r/3 F		
100 Kv	1000r/3 F	As needed.	Skin
300 Kv	(600r/1 or 2 X's) 600-1200r	Variable	
6-8 Mev Electrons	1200r/3 F	Variable	Variable
Electrons or 85-100 Kv	1000r/3 F	To cover site with 3mm margin.	Skin
200 Kv	1000r/1 F	Mean 3 x 1	Marrow, thyroid and breast.
150 Kv	1200r/4 days	To keloid	Whatever lies beneath.

Keloids

Author, Year	Technical Details	Total Dose/Fractions/Time	Results	Notes
Enhamre and Hammar, 1983	47 patients, with 62 keloids.	Excision and post-operative superficial x-ray 1000-1500r fractionated or 1000-1200r single dose of 1200-1500r in 3 fractions.	88% good to excellent results.	Follow up 6 months to 9 years. Side effect: Hyperpigmentation in 16 of 47 patients.
Ollstein et al, 1981	40 patients with 68 keloids. 28 Females and 12 males, Ages 3-53 years.	1500r in 3 equal doses. First within several hours of surgery; rest at 2-3 day intervals.	72% control.	
Levy et al, 1976	37 patients	300r fractions to 1500-1800r. Treatment started within 24-48 hours of excision.	88% control.	
Malaker et al, 1976	30 patients	Iridium implant 2000r within 2.5mm from wire	80% control.	

Keloids (Continued)

Author, Year	Technical Details	Total Dose/Fractions/Time	Results	Notes
Cosman and Wolff, 1974	None given.	800r/24F beginning within 14 days post-op.	Excision plus radiotherapy: 26/46(37%) good results. 36% recurrence rate. Excision alone: 3/20(15%) good results. 63% recurrence rate.	All earlobe keloids.
Edsmyr et al, 1974	45 Kv, 10ma, 0.55mm Al filter or 100 Kv, 8ma, 1.70mm Al filter.	500-2400r/1-14 days beginning 1-22 days post-op.	Excision plus radiotherapy: 82/103(80%) no recurrence. Radiotherapy alone: 2/17 total regression. 14/17 amelioration of symptoms. Excision only: 12/12 recurred.	92.4% of the patients were Africans.
Inalsingh, 1974	60-90 Kv, no filtration lead cutouts used to shield all but the keloid area.	400r, single dose, monthly beginning approximately one week post-op. Number of treatments dependent on clinical response. (Radiotherapy alone was used in some cases - shoulder and sternal areas, small keloids).	383/501(76.5%) complete success. 76/501(15%) symptomatic success.	
Hintz, 1973	200 Kv, HVL 0.6-0.8mm Cu, FSD 50cm or 85 Kv (machine was not available until Feb '72).	1500-1800r/5-6F/7-12 days. 7/53 patients did not have keloidectomy prior to irradiation but had recent post-surgical keloid.	46/64(72%) good to excellent response.	Response rate of scars of the anterior thorax was statistically inferior to other sites.
Jaworski, 1973		Triamcinolone acetamide injection.	22/49(44%) good results. 18/49(37%) moderate results.	Some lesions with good results were later surgically removed because of persistent hyper-pigmentation.
Singleton and Gross, 1971		Excision followed by injection with a steroid (methyl-prednisolone acetate in most cases) monthly for 12 months post-op.	37/54(69%) good results.	
Greer and Vickers, 1970	100-135 Kv, HVL 1mm Al to 0.33mm Cu. Suture line plus needle holes and a margin of 1/2 cm are included in the field.	1600r(air)/4F/4 weeks beginning 24 hours post-op.	49/80(61%) lesions cleared. 31/80(39%) recurrences.	If lesions are large and require grafting rather than primary closure, only the suture line and not the center of the graft is treated.
King and Salzman, 1970	Low megavoltage (2.5 Mev) electron beam.	1000-1200r single dose within 10 days post-op.	Electron beam only: 15/57(26%) success. Excision plus electron beam: 23/32(74%) success.	Some selection of patients - older patients with large keloids would receive electron beam only.

Keloids (Continued)

Author, Year	Technical Details	Total Dose/Fractions/Time	Results	Notes
Weaver and Berliner, 1970		Fluocinolone acetonide – topical application to post-op wounds.	Decreased scar formation in 84%.	
Griffith, 1966		1100–1400r.	Excision only: 1. 5/7 no recurrences. Excision plus radiotherapy: 1. 4/4 no recurrences. Excision, radiotherapy and steroids (3 months course): 1. 2/3 no recurrences.	
		Triamcinolone acetonide (Kenalog) injection.	Intralesional Kenalog only: 1. 20/37(59%) symptoms eliminated. Excision plus Kenalog at operation: 1. 4/5(80%) symptoms eliminated. Excision plus Kenalog at operation and post-op: 1. 12/14(86%) symptoms eliminated.	
Ketchum et al, 1966		Triamcinolone acetonide injection.	183/200(19.5%) moderate marked atrophy of scar tissue.	Excessive atrophy in some patients. Depigmentation of the skin surrounding the scar (1).
Craig and Pearson, 1965	100 Kv shielding of adjacent skin with lead 1mm thick.	800r single dose within 48 hours post-op.	13/16(81%) cured. 3/16(19%) recurred.	
Wilson, 1965		Dexamethasone and lidocaine injection just prior to excision. Lidocaine injection prior to excision.	306/400(76.5%) good-excellent results. Poor results in all 101 cases.	
Brown and Brumberg, 1963	100 Kv, HVL 1.0–2.0mm Al, FSD 30cm.	1500r air/3F/7–10 days beginning within 3 weeks post-op.	18/30(60%) no regrowth. 10/30(33%) partial regrowth.	
Murray, 1963		Excision and Kenalog (triamcinolone acetamide) injection. Kenalog ointment massage post-op and 800r/4F.	1/7 good results.	
		Excision and Kenalog injection, revision with Kenalog ointment dressing, Kenalog ointment massage post-op and 800r/4F.	9/13 good results.	
		Excision and Kenalog injection and Kenalog ointment massage post-op.	1/4 fair results.	

Keloids (Continued)

Author, Year	Technical Details	Total Dose/Fractions/Time	Results	Notes
Murray, 1963 (continued)		Surgical abrasion, excision, revision with Kenalog ointment dressings, and massage with Kenalog ointment post-op.	17/25 good results.	
Cosman et al, 1961	None given.	800r/4F/4–8 weeks	Pre- plus post-op radiotherapy: 53/91(58%) success. Pre-op radiotherapy only: 2/5 success. Post-op radiotherapy only: 35/66(53%) success. Excision only: 10/22(46%) success.	Results further divided into early and late pre- and post-op therapy. (Early equals two weeks before or after operation). Best results with late pre-op and early post-op (74% success).
		Excision, Kenalog injection, revision with Kenalog ointment dressing, and Kenalog ointment massage post-op.	15/29 good results.	
		Excision, revision with Kenalog ointment dressings, and Kenalog ointment massage post-op.	6/9 good results.	
Conway et al, 1960	None given.	None given.	Excision only: 1. 12/22(55%) cured. Excision plus radiotherapy: 1. 12/22(55%) cured. Excision plus injection: 1. 36/56(64%) cured. Excision plus injection plus radiotherapy: 1. 27/38(71%) cured.	85% success in 7 patients treated with excision and cortisone.
Van den Brenk and Minty, 1960	None given.	400–1000r single dose or 1000–3000r/3F/ 2–9 months. Radiotherapy only.	Single dose: 1. 9/56(16%) good response. Fractionated dose: 1. 4/28(14%) good response.	Three cases of radionecrosis with the single doses.
	None given.	Excision followed by 500 – greater than 1000r/9 days – 4 weeks, or Excision followed by 600–1700r/4 days – 8 weeks, or Combined pre/post-op dose: 275r/1800r or 320r/3204r	Single dose: 1. 9/15(60%) no recurrence. Fractionated dose: 1. 2/6 no recurrence. Combined pre/post-op doses: 1. 2/2 no recurrences.	One case of radionecrosis with single dose of 1700r.
	Radium plaques, radon molds or interstitial needle implants (with or without additional x-rays).	No excision.	1/23 good response. 11/23 partial response.	Radionecrosis (4). Severe atrophy (11). Disturbance of bone growth (3).

Keloids (Continued)

Author, Year	Technical Details	Total Dose/Fractions/Time	Results	Notes
Arnold and Graver, 1959	140 Kv, 5ma, no filter, HVL 2mm Al, FSD 25cm. Skin is shielded right up to the line of incision using bismuth putty. This is then overlaid with a sheet of lead rubber.	1. 450-1200r/3F/1 month, repeated 2-4 times. 2. 1000-3000r/2-6F/10-30 days. Radiation following removal of sutures.	X-rays only: 1. 13/20(65%) fair-good results. 2. 33/39(84.6%) fair-good results. Excision and X-rays: 1. 19/28(67.9%) fair-good results. 2. 19/22(86.4%) fair-good results. Injection (hyaluronidase hydrocortisone): 1. 2/7 fair-good results Excision only: 1. 3/14(21.4%) fair-good results. No treatment: 1. 5/17(29.4) fair-good results.	Mild telangiectasia (4).
Belisario, 1957	HVL 1.5mm Al.	1200r/3F/1 month or 200r/1F/2 weeks repeated up to maximum of 1200r or 150r/week up to maximum of 1200r Radiotherapy begun immediately after surgery.	Radiotherapy alone: 1. 5/10(50%) good-improved. Excision plus radiotherapy: 1. 6/12(50%) good-improved. Injections (hyaluronidase/hydrocortisone alone: 1. 17/30(57%) good-improved. Excision plus injection: 1. 9/16(56%) good-improved. Excision plus injection plus radiotherapy: 1. 25/30(84%) good-improved.	

References

1. Enhamre A and Hammar H (1983) Treatment of keloids with excision and post-operative x-ray irradiation. *Dermatologica* 167: 90-93.
2. Ollstein RN, Siegel HW, Gillooley JF and Barsa JM (1981) Treatment of keloids by combined surgical excision and immediate post-operative x-ray therapy. *Ann Plast Surg* 7: 281-285.
3. Levy DS, Salter MM and Roth RE (1976) Post operative irradiation in the prevention of keloids. *Am J Roentgenol* 127: 509-510.
4. Malaker A, Ellis F and Paine CH (1976) Keloid scars A new methods of treatment combining surgery with interstitial radiotherapy. *Clin Radiol* 27: 179-183.
5. Cosman B and Wolff M (1974) Bilateral earlobe keloids. *Plast Reconst Surg* 53: 540-543.
6. Edsmyr F, Larsson LG, Onyango J, Wanguro S and Wood M (1974) Radiation therapy in the treatment of keloids in east Africa. *Acta Radiol [Ther]* 13: 102-106.
7. Inalsingh CHA (1974) An experience in treating five hundred and one patients with keloids. *Johns Hopkins Med J* 134: 284-290.
8. Ketchum LD, Cohen IK and Masters FW (1974) Hypertrophic scars and keloids. *Plast Reconstr Surg* 53: 140-154.
9. Hintz BL (1973) Radiotherapy for keloid treatment. *J Natl Med Assoc* 65: 71-75.
10. Jaworski S (1973) Kenacort a in the treatment of hypertropic scars and keloids in children. *Acta Chir Plast* 15: 206-215.
11. Singleton MA and Gross CW (1971) Management of keloids by surgical excision and local injections of a steroid. *South Med J* 64: 1377-1381.
12. Greer JL and Vickers B (1970) Combined surgical and x-ray therapy of keloids. *J La State Med Soc* 122: 107-109.
13. King GD and Salzman FA (1970) Keloid scars. *Surg Clin North Am* 50: 595-598.

14. Peacock EF Jr, Madden JW and Trier WC (1970) Biologic basis for the treatment of keloids and hypertrophic scars. *South Med J* **63**: 755-760.
15. Weaver RG and Berliner DL (1970) The action of fluocinolone acetonide upon scar tissue formation. *J Urol* **104**: 591-595.
16. Griffith BH (1966) The treatment of keloids with triamcinolone acetonide. *Plast Reconstr Surg* **38**: 202-208.
17. Ketchum LD, Smith J, Robinson DW and Masters FW (1966) The treatment of hypertrophic scar, keloid and scar contracture by triamcinolone acetonide. *Plast Reconst Surg* **38**: 209-218.
18. Craig RDP and Pearson D (1965) Early post-operative irradiation in the treatment of keloid scars. *Br J Plast Surg* **18**: 369-376.
19. Wilson WW (1965) Prophylaxis against postsurgical keloids: Results in 500 patients. *South Med J* **58**: 751-753.
20. Brown JR and Brumberg JH (1963) Preliminary studies on the effect of time - dose patterns in the treatment of keloids. *Radiology* **80**: 298-300.
21. Murray RD (1963) Kenalog and the treatment of hypertrophied scars and keloids in negroes and whites. *Plast Reconst Surg* **31**: 275-280.
22. Cosman B, Crikelair GF, Gavlin JC and Lotles R (1961) The surgical treatment of keloids. *Plast Reconst Surg* **27**: 335-358.
23. Conway H, Gillette R, Smith JW and Findley A (1960) Differential diagnosis of keloids and hypertrophic scars by tissue culture technique with notes on therapy of keloids by surgical excision and decadron. *Plast Reconst Surg* **25**: 117-132.
24. Van Den Brenk HAS and Minty CCJ (1960) Radiation in the management of keloids and hypertrophic scars. *Br J Surg* **47**: 595-605.
25. Arnold HL and Graver FH (1959) Keloids: Etiology and management of excision and intensive prophylactic radiation. *Arch Derm* **80**: 772-777.
26. Belisario JC (1957) The treatment of keloids. *Acta Dermovener* **37**: 165-181.

Lethal Midline Granuloma

Polymorphic Reticulosis/Lymphomatoid Granulomatosis

Polymorphic reticulosis/lymphomatoid granulomatosis complex is the preferred term for lethal midline granuloma. Lethal midline granuloma includes a spectrum of etiologic possibilities, including bacterial, fungal, neoplastic, and unknown origins. When lethal midline granuloma is localized to the upper airways it is termed polymorphic reticulosis. It may produce erosion of the upper airway and face. When localized, it responds to radiotherapy. Differentiation from malignant lymphoma, bacterial infection, fungal infection and Wegener's granulomatosis is essential for proper management.

In the national survey we believe it was not recognized that lethal midline granuloma and polymorphic reticulosis are the same disorder. Ninety-three percent of radiation oncologists when asked if they would treat lethal midline granuloma would treat this disorder; when asked about polymorphic reticulosis, however, 86% would not treat the disorder. Responses such as these indicate the importance both of nomenclature and familiarity with the name of the disorder.

Lethal Midline Granuloma Radiotherapy

Author, Year	Total # Patients	Treatment	Results	Notes
Smalley et al, 1988	34	33/34 radiation therapy. Median age 44 years; 24 males, 10 females	94% nasal obstruction 12 relapse 3 diffuse histiocytic lymphoma 67% NED 5 years 62% NED 10 years 43% NED 20 years 33% in-field failure	Minimum dose 4200r lymph nodes + 4000-5000 rad Marginal failure 20% Use larger volumes
Robinson et al, 1984	1	Para-nasal 5mm nose, palate. Age 39 years. 50Gy irradiation.	Regression of lesion.	Important to differentiate from Wegener's granulomatosis.
Halperin et al, 1982	2	Upper aerodigestive passages. Ages 27 and 29 years. 45 Gy Cobalt irradiation.	One patient did well and had no disease 2 1/2 years follow up. The second patient developed lesions outside of irradiated area and died.	Disease also called lethal midline granuloma.

Historical Data: Lethal Midline Granuloma Radiotherapy

Author, Year	Total # Patients	Treatment	Results	Notes
DeRemar et al, 1980	40	Nasal cavity nasopharynx palate. Ages: 15-80 years (average 45). The twenty patients with disease isolated to upper respiratory tract received radiotherapy.	3 of 20 living free of disease 1 1/2-19 years after therapy.	Four patients developed large cell lymphoma.
Fauci et al, 1976	11	Radiotherapy: 4000-5000 rad (tissue dose) /5 weeks. Co^{60} or 2 MEV. Wide field irradiation encompassing the nasal and palatal areas and the accessory sinuses.	8/10 apparent complete remission. 2/10 initial brief remission.	Disease activity was limited to the upper airway in all patients. There was no evidence of disseminated disease in any patient.
Harrison, 1974	14	1. Deep x-ray therapy (3 pts) 2. Corticosteroids (3 pts) 3. Deep x-ray therapy plus corticosteroids (3 pts) 4. Deep x-ray therapy plus intra-arterial methotrexate (1 pt) 5. Intra-arterial methotrexate (2 pt) 6. Azathioprine, cyclophosphamide, corticosteroids. Radiotherapy dosage varied from 800-1000 rad/6 days to a full curative dose of Co^{60}.		Cites three cases of patients with malignant granuloma who developed malignant lymphoma and eleven patients with Wegener's granulomatosis.
Friedman, 1971	5	1. Irradiation (3) 2. Steroids (1) 3. Steroids plus irradiation (1)	1. 2/3 alive at 8 years and 14 years. 1/3 dead at 12 years. 2. Dead at 2 years. 3. Dead at 6 years.	These cases were taken from the ENT Tumor Registry.
Kassell et al, 1969	1	Corticosteroids followed by oral methotrexate and radiotherapy, 1000r/6 days (2 Mev). Steroid therapy was continued. Approximately three months later he received another course of radiotherapy, 1000r/4 days (250 Kv).	Short term response to the first x-ray treatment. Patient died of disease 2.5 months following second treatment.	Authors also report on a case of Wegener's granulomatosis.
Friedman, 1964	15	Deep x-ray therapy.	6/15 survived from 8-15 years.	
Feder et al, 1963	4	1. Massive antibiotics (patient was acutely ill) followed later by prednisolone (1 pt). 2. Radiotherapy 450r/ 1 month (1 pt) or 900-975r/ 2.5-3 months (1 pt) or 2550r/3.5 months (1 pt) 300 KV, 0.75mm Cu filtration HVL 1.9mm Cu, FSD 70cm.	1. Favorable response lasted three months. Patient expired from disease. 2. Two patients well at 2.5-4 year follow up (one later died of coronary occlusion).	One patient has been observed for less than one year. One patient died of disease (this was the patient who had received 2550r).

Historical Data: Lethal Midline Granuloma Radiotherapy (Continued)

Author, Year	Total # Patients	Treatment	Results	Notes
Wildermuth, 1962	2	Prednisone and radiotherapy, 3000–3700r/24–48 days. 250 Kv.	Some response to treatment in both cases. Both patients are still under treatment.	
Merrill, 1961	1	Radiotherapy, 1100r(air)/15 days, 250 Kv, to the mass.	Painless swelling in right parotid gland. Original dx of chronic parotitis. After radiotherapy the size of the mass decreased and it was no longer detectable. Nine months later the patient had granulomatous lesions of the lateral pharynx, mucosal hypertrophy, and superficial ulceration of the aryepiglottic folds. She has been receiving prednisone and was now given a further course of radiotherapy. The patient's symptoms subsided. Patient died two months later of respiratory obstruction.	
Dickson, 1960	7	1. Radiotherapy plus surgery in some cases (3 pts). 2. Radiotherapy plus steroids, plus surgery in some cases (3 pts). 3. Steroids only (1 pt) Radiotherapy used was low dose in most cases.	1. 2/3 dead in one year 1/3 alive at 3 years. 2. 2/3 died within 2 years. 1/3 alive at 11 years. 3. Died at 4 months.	
Blatt et al, 1959	124	Surgery, steroids, or radiotherapy.	6/124 survived, 5 of these had received radiotherapy, one had been treated surgically. 9/124 remissions, all had been treated by steroids and x-ray therapy.	
Glass, 1955	4	Radiotherapy, 400–1200r/5–8 weeks	Good response to radiotherapy in all 4 cases.	
Ellis, 1955	1	Radiotherapy, 300r/1 month	Margins of the ulcer became clean. Mucosal junction between the oral and nasal surfaces of the palate healed. No further evidence of activity.	

References

1. Smalley SR, Cupps RE, Anderson JA, Ilstrup DM, McDonald TJ, Weiland LH and DeRemee RD (1988) Polymorphic reticulosis limited to the upper aerodigestive tract - natural history and radiotherapeutic considerations. *Int J Radiat Oncol Biol Phys* **15**: 599–605.
2. Robinson ACR, Fraser I, Bailey D and O'Halloran MJ (1984) Idiopathic midline destructive disease - case report and review of the literature. *Postgrad Med J* **60**: 471–473.
3. Halperin EC, Dosoretz DE, Goodman M and Wang CC (1982) Radiotherapy of polymorphic reticulosis. *Br J Radiol* **55**: 645–649.
4. DeRemar RA, Weiland LH and McDonald TJ (1980) Respiratory vasculitis. *Mayo Clin Prac* **55**: 492–498.
5. Fauci AS, Johnson RE and Wolff SM (1976) Radiation therapy of midline granuloma. *Ann Int Med* **84**: 140–147.
6. Schechter SL, Bole GG and Walker SE (1976) Midline granuloma and Wegener's granulomatosis: clinical and therapeutic considerations. *J Rhematol* **3**: 241–250.
7. Harrison DFN (1974) Non-healing granulomata of the upper respiratory tract. *Br Med J* **4**: 205–209.

8. Friedman I (1971) The changing pattern of granuloma of the upper respiratory tract. *J Laryngol & Ostol* **85**: 631-682.
9. Jarrett JE and Lehman RH (1971) Lethal midline granuloma. A review of the literature. *Rocky Mt Med J* **68**: 40-45.
10. Kassel SH, Echevarria RA and Guzzo FP (1969) Midline malignant reticulosis (so-called lethal midline granuloma). *Cancer* **23**: 920-935.
11. Eichel BS and Mabery TE (1968) The enigma of the lethal midline granuloma. *Laryngoscope* **78**: 1367-1386.
12. Friedman I (1964) Midline granuloma. *Proc R Soc Med* **57**: 289-297.
13. Feder BGH, Shramek JH and Ikeda TS (1962) Large field radiotherapy in lethal midline granuloma. *Radiology* **81**: 293-299.
14. Wildermuth O (1962) Lethal midline granuloma. *Radiology* **78**: 269-271.
15. Merrill MD (1961) Roentgen therapy in Wegener's granulomatosis. A case report. *Am J Roentg Rad Ther & Nucl Med* **85**: 96-98.
16. Dickson RJ (1960) Radiotherapy of lethal midline granuloma. *J Chronic Disease* **12**: 417-427.
17. Blatt IM, Seltzer HS, Rubin P, Furstenberg AC, Maxwell JH and Schull WJ (1959) Fatal granulomatosis of the respiratory tract. *Arch Otolaryngol* **70**: 707-757.
18. Ellis M (1957) Malignant granuloma of the nose. *Ann Otol Rhinol & Laryngol* **66**: 1002-1008.
19. Ellis M (1955) Malignant granuloma of the nose. *Br Med J* **1**: 1251-1253.
20. Glass EJG (1955) Malignant granuloma. *J Laryngol & Otol* **69**: 315-320.

Lymphoid Hyperplasia - Pseudotumor

Lymphoid hyperplasia occurs predominantly in the orbit, Waldeyer's ring, and skin. It has also been observed in patients with AIDS. In the pediatric age group with tonsillar/nasopharyngeal hyperplasia, surgical or medical management is appropriate; radiation therapy is not (see section titled Otitis Media). In orbital pseudotumor, once the obvious potential for lymphoma has clearly been eliminated, carefully applied simulation and treatment planning and the delivery of 2000 rad achieves a high complete response rate. There has been as high as a thirty percent incidence of lymphoma among patients with an earlier history and pathologic diagnosis of pseudotumor. In cutaneous lymphoid hyperplasia with the same clinical and histological provisos, remission can be achieved with similar doses of radiation. In AIDS, although formal reports are not available, 2000 rad has alleviated pain and discomfort and caused masses to remit. In the national survey, fifty-one percent of radiation oncologists would not treat lymphoid hyperplasia of the larynx and fifty-four percent would not treat lymphoid hyperplasia of the nasopharynx, whereas eighty-one percent would treat lymphoid hyperplasia of the orbit which is often referred to as pseudotumor of the orbit.

Lymphoid Hyperplasia - Pseudotumor

Author, Year	Total # Pts.	Sex/Age	Treatment	Results	Notes
Austin-Seymour et al 1985	20 (Orbit)	Ages 25-80 years. Mean 55 years. 13 Females and 7 Males.	2000-3600 rad.	15/20 complete resolution.	No complications.
Meyers and Hakami, 1985	1 (Orbit)	Age 14 years. Male	750 rad	Regression, with eighteen month follow-up.	Patient had hemophilia. Table with seven reports of radiation for pseudotumor of hemophilia is provided.
Olson et al, 1985	4 (Skin)	Ages 28-67 years. 1 Female and 3 Males.	1500 rad in 5 fractions.	Complete regression in all cases. One marginal recurrence spontaneously remitted.	Eight months - seven years follow-up.
Jereb et al, 1984	5	Ages 23-76 years. 4 Females and 1 Male	2000-2500 rad	All with no evidence of disease	
Sergott et al, 1981	19 (21 Orbits)	Ages 23-83 years. 12 Females and 7 Males.	1000-2000 rad	Fifteen orbits responded favorably. Six orbits did not respond.	Fifteen had failed previous steroids. Mean follow-up - 25 months.

References

1. Austin-Seymour MM, Donaldson SS, Egbert PR, McDougall IR and Kriss JP (1985) Radiotherapy of lymphoid diseases of the orbit. *Int J Rad Oncol Biol Phys* **11**: 371-379.
2. Meyers L and Hakami N (1985) Pseudotumor of hemophilia in the orbit. *Am J of Hematology* **19**: 99-104.
3. Olson LE, Wilson JF and Cox JD (1985) Cutaneous lymphoid hyperplasia: Results of radiation therapy. *Radiology* **155**: 507-509.
4. Jereb B, Lee H, Jakobiec FA and Kutcher J (1984) Radiation therapy of conjunctival and orbital lymphoid tumors. *Int J Radiation Oncol Biol Phys* **10**: 1013-1019.
5. Sergott RC, Gaser JS and Charyulu K (1981) Radiotherapy for idiopathic inflammatory orbital pseudotumor: Indications and results. *Arch Ophthalmol* **99**: 853-856.

Meningioma

The primary treatment for non-malignant meningioma is surgical excision. If there is any question about surgical margins, the high recurrence rates and the recognized effectiveness of radiotherapy would indicate the early use of post-operative radiotherapy. When the base of the skull or other critical sites are involved and surgical attempts would produce high morbidity, radiation alone is then appropriate. Finally, when there is recurrence of meningioma following surgical excision, radiation therapy is still effective, but not as effective as in the immediate post-operative period. The radiation oncologist and neurosurgeon as a team must weigh the risks and benefits of a repeat surgical excision followed by radiotherapy compared to radiotherapy alone. Evidence indicates that marginal recurrence can be avoided by using wide fields. Minimal tumor doses of 5000-5500 rad are generally recommended. In the national survey, ninety-one percent of radiation oncologists would treat meningioma.

Meningioma

Author, Year	Total # Pts.	Sex/Age	Treatment	Results	Notes
Petty et al, 1985	12	Median Age - 48 years. (One 15 year old child) 8 Females and 4 Males.	Post-operative. Radiotherapy - 4800-6080 rad.	Nine remissions. Three recurred (two at margin).	All incompletely resected. Follow-up 54.5 months.
Carella et al, 1982	68	Ages 25-80 years. 49 Females and 19 Males.	43 - Surgery followed by radiotherapy. 14 - Radiation for recurrence. 11 - Radiation as primary treatment.	41 of 43 remissions. 5 of 14 remissions. 9 of 11 improved.	Radiation doses 5000-6500 rad.

References

1. Mirimanoff RO, Dosoretz DE, Linggood RM, Ojemann RG and Martuza RI (1985) Meningioma: Analysis of recurrences and progression following neurosurgical resection. *J Neurosurg* **62**: 18-24.
2. Petty AM, Kun LE and Meyer GA (1985) Radiation therapy for incompletely resected meningioma. *J Neurosurg* **62**: 502-507.
3. Carella RJ, Ransohoff J and Newall J (1982) Role of radiation therapy in the management of meningioma. *Neurosurgery* **10**: 332-339.
4. Wara WM, Sheline GE, Newman H, et al (1975) Radiation therapy of meningiomas. *AJR* **123**: 453-458.

Mikulicz Syndrome

Mikulicz syndrome is a benign lymphoepithelial lesion usually involving the salivary glands. It is imperative that malignant lymphoma, malignant lymphoepithelioma, and malignant epithelial tumors be excluded as diagnostic possibilities. Further, the clinical diagnosis without complete pathologic support may be exceedingly dangerous. Infectious diseases must be considered. Culturing as well as histology is mandatory. We have observed a case of actinomycosis bovis, referred as Mikulicz syndrome, which after careful histopathologic study and culture was treated approximately and not with radiation. However, if the diagnosis of Mikulicz benign lymphoepithelioma is unequivocally established and the lesion or lesions cause signs and symptoms, modest doses of radiation have been reported to lead to remission. Eighty-three percent of radiation oncologists would not treat Mikulicz syndrome according to the national survey.

Survey of Mikulicz Syndrome: Four Centers (1976)

Kv	Dose and Time	Field Size	Organ at Risk
255 Kv or Co^{60}	2000 rad/10 F 2 weeks	Gland and small margin. 8 x 8	Skin, salivary gland.
Co^{60}	150 rad x 4	6 x 8	
200 Kv	1000 rad/5 F 1 week	8 x 10	Thyroid
10 Mev Electrons	3000 rad/3 weeks	8 x 8	Skin

Mikulicz Syndrome

Author, Year	Total # Patients	Treatment	Results	Notes
Causey, 1976	1	Prednisone Chlorambucil	Response to prednisone was poor and was discontinued. Chlorambucil rapidly reduced the size of the involved glands. This regression persisted during gradual reduction in dose, and was maintained with small intermittent doses. Therapy was discontinued after two years without clinical evidence of relapse.	The patient had a well documented benign lymphoepithelial lesion. One year after discontinuation of chlorambucil therapy, the patient had enlarged cervical, axillary, inguinal, femoral, and iliac nodes without changes in the parotid and submaxillary glands. Biopsy showed malignant lymphocytic-histocytic lymphoma.
Kelly et al, 1975	10	Parotidectomy (9 pts, 3 of these were bilateral procedures). One patient was biopsied only.	Two patients no progression of disease. Four patients developed arthritis (one patient also had xerostomia and Sjogren syndrome). Three patients died from other causes. One patient developed systemic amyloidosis and recent systemic lymphoma (7 years post-op). This case which was originally diagnosed as benign lymphoepithelial lesion was rediagnosed two years later as nodular lymphosarcoma.	Benign lymphoepithelial lesions of the salivary glands. Authors recommend that mild symptomatic diffuse enlargements be managed conservatively. They do not consider radiation therapy as a good mode of treatment in patients already having a tendency toward dry mouth problems. They recommend total parotidectomy with preservation of the facial nerve for recurrent severe infections.
Leban and Stratigos, 1974	1 Male, age 28 years.	Treated with 250r x 4 fractions	Response to treatment.	Histopathology is reviewed.

Mikulicz Syndrome (Continued)

Author, Year	Total # Patients	Treatment	Results	Notes
Gravanis and Giansanti, 1970	2	Partial parotidectomy followed 1-3 years later by a total parotidectomy sacrificing the facial nerve for a recurrent lesion (2 patients).	Case #1. Patient is without clinical evidence of recurrence at one year following the second procedure. Case #2. A destructive process involving most of the wing of the sphenoid bone, pterygoid plate, and hamulus and enlarged nodes were discovered six months following the second procedure. This was treated with radiation. There was clinical improvement with resolution of the nodes. One and a half years later the patient returned with another mass which was found to be infiltrating anaplastic carcinoma with a lymphoid stroma. The patient had recurrences over the next eight years. He died of other causes.	Original pathology report. Case #1. Lymphoepithelial lesion of the right parotid. Case #2. Benign lymphoepithelial lesion of left parotid gland.
Pinkus and Dekker, 1970	1	Bilateral superficial lobe parotidectomies.	Post-op follow up – slight enlargement of right lacrimal gland, but this was not evident during subsequent examinations. One and a half years later a mass in the left inguinal areas was noted. Biopsy revealed acute inflammation and granulation tissue. Nine months later right inguinal mass had enlarged. Superclavicular and axillary adenopathy were present. Both parotids were enlarged. Biopsy of cervical node revealed probable malignant lymphoma, from which she eventually died.	
Schindel and Levie, 1969	1	Biopsy followed two years later by partial left parotidectomy. Radiotherapy, 1600r/9 days (200 Kv, 0.5mm Cu, FSD 50cm). Radiotherapy, 1600r, one year later to the left parotid gland.	Nodules on the right parotid gland disappeared completely. No recurrence to date. Follow up examination one year later showed a nodule of the left parotid gland. This was treated with radiotherapy. No recurrences to date.	Pathology report: Benign lymphoepithelial lesion.
Sprinkle and Yarrington, 1968				Authors report success in treating moderately symptomatic patients with small doses of radiotherapy. Some of their patients are five years post therapy without a recurrence. They had used 500-700r/3 weeks for children, and 500-700r/10-14 days for adults.

Mikulicz Syndrome (Continued)

Author, Year	Total # Patients	Treatment	Results	Notes
Lancaster and Hughes, 1963	1	Surgical excision of the mass in the hard palate and the entire right submaxillary gland. Acute swelling and discomfort treated with antibiotics.	Patient returned seven months later with acute swelling and discomfort of both parotid glands with a purulent discharge. Following antibiotic treatment the swelling subsided. There was no further recurrence during the next two months.	Mikulicz disease involving multiple salivary glands.
Bhaskar and Bernier, 1960	73			Authors provide a review of the clinical features, histology, and histogenesis of Mikulicz disease. They recommend that treatment be conservative (partial or complete parotidectomy). X-irradiation, and radium implantation should not be employed in its management.
Morgan and Castleman, 1953	18	Surgical excision alone (11) or excision plus irradiation (5). Two patients received no treatment.	17/17 no recurrence of disease locally or spread to other organs (three patients died of apparently non-related causes).	
Heaton and Shannon, 1948	1	Radiotherapy, 1200r/6F, to both parotids (200 Kv, 0.5mm Cu plus 1mm Al filtration).	Regression of the lesions. The glands returned to normal size. Bilateral recurrences 1.5 years later were again treated with radiotherapy resulting in rapid subsidence of swelling.	Mikulicz disease.

References

1. Causey JQ (1976) The benign lymphoepithelial lesion - a harbinger of neoplasia. *Southern Med J* **69**: 60-63.
2. Kelly DR, Spiegel JC and Maves M (1975) Benign lymphoepithelial lesions of the salivary glands. *Arch Otol* **101**: 71-75.
3. Leban SG and Stratigos GT (1974) Benign lymphoepthelial sialoadenopathies. The Mikulicz/Sjogren controversy. *Oral Surg Oral Med & Oral Path* **38**: 735-748.
4. Meyer D, Yanoff M and Hanno H (1971) Differential diagnosis in Mikulicz's syndrome, Mikulicz's disease and similar disease entities. *Am J Opth* **71**: 516-524.
5. Gravanis MB and Giansanti JS (1970) Malignant histologic counterpart of the benign lymphoepithelial lesion. *Cancer* **26**: 1332-1342.
6. Pinkus GS and Dekker A (1970) Benign lymphoepithelial lesion of the parotid glands associated with reticulum cell sarcoma. Report of a case and review of the literature. *Cancer* **25**: 121-127.
7. Schindel J and Levie B (1969) Benign lymphoepithelial lesion of the parotid gland. Mikulicz's disease. *Arch Otolaryngol* **90**: 496-499.
8. Bark CJ and Perzik S (1968) Mikulicz's disease, sialoangiectasis and autoimmunity based upon a study of parotid lesions. *Am J Clin Path* **49**: 683-689.
9. Sprinkle PM and Yarrington CI (1968) Disease of the salivary glands and benign lymphoepithelial lesion. *Southern Med J* **61**: 971-974.
10. Lancaster JE and Hughes KW (1963) Mikulicz's disease involving multiple salivary glands. Report of a case. *Oral Surg Oral Med & Oral Path* **16**: 1266-1269.
11. Bdhaskar SN and Bernier JL (1960) Mikulicz's disease. Clinical features, histology and histogenesis. *Oral Surg Oral Med & Oral Path* **13**: 1387-1399.
12. Morgan WS and Castleman B (1953) A clinopathologic study of Mikulicz's disease. *Am J Path* **29**: 471-503.
13. Godwin JT (1952) Benign lymphoepithelial lesion of the parotid gland. *Cancer* **5**: 1089-1103.
14. Heaton TG and Shannon EH (1948) Mikulicz's disease. *Canad Med Assoc J* **58**: 368-370.

Myasthenia Gravis and Thymus Gland Abnormalities

Myasthenia gravis is clearly related to the production of autoantibody to acetyl choline. Its pathologic association with malignant thymoma leads to surgical excision in those presenting with the tumor. It has also been associated with follicular hyperplasia of the thymus which has led to thymic radiation in the past, even without the presence of tumor. New research suggests that both drug management and the possibility of immunosuppressive radiation need to be investigated. The role of radiotherapy in the post-operative incompletely resected malignant thymoma appears appropriate with doses of 4500 rad or greater. In the non-tumor situation, the role of radiation therapy to the mediastinum has not been scientifically established. In the national survey sixty-seven percent of radiation oncologists would treat thymoma with myasthenia gravis.

Thymoma in Myasthenia Gravis

Author, Year	Total # Patients	Treatment	Results	Notes
Currier et al, 1983	28 Median Age 40 years. Ages 11–74 years. 19 Females and 9 Males.	3000r to mediastinum.	16 – improved. 4 – improved on steroids. 4 – no change. 4 – died.	Without thymoma: Median follow up eight years. All had failed previous optimum anti-cholinesterase therapy.
King Engel et al, 1981	5 Females	Splenic irradiation 100r given up to 1000r.	1 – failed. 1 – subjective response. 3 – objective response.	All failed thymectomy and drug treatment response four months.
	2 Females	Total body irradiation. 150r over 5 weeks. Two 15r fractions/week.	Dramatic and sustained improvement.	
Salyer and Eggleston, 1976	26	Apparent complete surgical removal in most cases. 14 patients – treated. 9 patients – no treatment.	1/14 alive without tumor or syndrome. 2/14 alive with syndrome, without tumor. 10/14 dead with syndrome with or without tumor. 3/14 post-op death.	All had myasthenia gravis and thymoma.
Goldman et al, 1975	26	1. Radiotherapy (1000–6061r) either alone or in combination with a steroid preparation or cytotoxic agent or both (10 pts). 2. Prednisone or ACTH, either alone or in combination with radiation therapy and/or cytotoxic agents (11 pts). 3. High dosage alternate days, prednisone and radiation therapy (2 pts). 4. Cytotoxic agents in association with either radiation therapy and/or steroid preparation (3 pts).	1. 4/10 alive, average life duration of 7.5 years since onset of illness. 2. 7/11 alive, average life duration of 6.25 years since onset of illness. 3. 2/2 alive, average life duration of 4 years since onset of illness. 4. 3/3 alive, average life duration of 8.5 years since onset of illness.	All patients had myasthenia gravis and invasive thymoma. Malignancy was removed at thoracotomy if this could be done safely. All patients received some form of anticholinesterase during their illness. There was no difference in tumor response to radiation or chemotherapy in reference to tissue type.

Thymoma in Myasthenia Gravis (Continued)

Author, Year	Total # Patients	Treatment	Results	Notes
DeSevilla et al, 1974	1	Radiotherapy: 3680r anteriorly and 1040r posteriorly to mediastinal mass (midline dose of 2430r)/2 weeks, Co^{60}. 3000r/2 weeks to left ilium.	The anterior mediastinal mass slowly decreased in size and patient was well for approximately six months when patient was readmitted with weakness and increasing dyspnea. No response of red cell aplasia to steroids or cyclophosphamide.	Metastatic thymoma with myasthenia gravis and pure red cell aplasia in a 55 year old man.
Mulder et al, 1974	27	Thymectomy.	Without tumor (73): 62/73(85%) remission or improvement. With tumor (27): 8/13(61%) improved.	Thymoma (27 pts). No thymoma (40). 7 early post-op deaths.
Weissberg et al, 1973	15	1. Resection with or without radiotherapy (11 pts). 2. Radiotherapy alone (3 pts).	1. 5/11 significant remission of myasthenia. 2. 1/3 significant remission of myasthenia. No patient experienced a permanent remission.	Thymoma and myasthenia gravis. Tumor was benign in eight patients, malignant in seven. Duration of remission varied between three months and five years.
Levasseur et al, 1972	74	Thymectomy.	With thymoma: 16/26(64%) good results. Without thymoma: 30/39(79%) good results.	Thymoma (28). No thymoma (46).
Vessey and Doll, 1972	382	Minimum of three years follow up. Five patients died from extra-thymic tumors, 5.5 would have been expected based on the national experience. Five others developed non-fatal extra-thymic tumors.	Thymoma (65). No thymoma (317). These data provide no evidence that adult thymectomy is followed by an increased risk of neoplastic disease.	
Wolfe et al, 1972	42	Thymectomy.	2/42 operative deaths. 3/42 late deaths, two in patients with a malignant thymoma. 11/42 stable and receiving no medications. 19/42 improved and require less medication.	9/42 had thymoma (6 benign, 3 malignant).
Braitman et al, 1971	17	Thymectomy.	7/17(44%) good-excellent results (objective improvement of symptoms).	All had myasthenia gravis and thymomas. 8/17(47%) invasive lesions.
Papatestas et al, 1971	185	Without thymoma (111): 28/111(25.2%) remission. 56/111(50.4%) improvement. With thymoma (61): 6.5% in remission. 18.6% improvement.	Without thymoma (111). With thymoma (74). At five year follow up 90% of patients well in remission or were improved.	
Schulz and Schwab, 1971	72	1. Thymic irradiation only. 2. Thymic irradiation and thymectomy.	1. Without tumor: 19/35(54%) improved. With tumor: 6/10(60%) improved. 2. Without tumor: 13/19(68%) improved. With tumor: 5/8(62%) improved.	Without thymoma (45). With thymoma (27).

Thymoma in Myasthenia Gravis (Continued)

Author, Year	Total # Patients	Treatment	Results	Notes
	128	1. Thymectomy without irradiation (63). 2. Thymectomy with irradiation (65).	1. 44/63(70%) improved. 2. 57/65(88%) improved.	These data include patients from the current study and from a previous study by one of the authors (Schwab).
Seybold et al, 1971	102	Medical treatment alone (54). Medical treatment plus thymectomy (48).	With thymectomy: 37.5% in remission 18.8% died No thymectomy: 24.1% in remission 20.4% died These results are not statistically significant.	All were cases of juvenile myasthenia gravis. These results suggest, but fail to prove, the effectiveness of thymectomy in inducing remission or decreasing the mortality rate.
Zeldowicz and Saxton, 1969	68	Without Thymoma (60): 1. Medical treatment (30). 2. Thymectomy (30). With Thymoma (8): 3. Medical treatment or thymectomy.	Without thymoma: 1. 50% moderate to good improvement over mean follow up of 11 years. 10% died from myasthenia gravis. 2. 83% good to excellent improvement. With Thymoma: 3. No significant difference between the medically and surgically treated patients. 50% moderate improvement during mean follow up of five years. 50% after initial improvement deteriorated later and died from myasthenia 3-4 years after thymectomy.	Without thymoma (60). With thymoma (8).
Kreel et al, 1967	127	With Thymoma: 1. No treatment (15). 2. X-ray only (16). 3. Surgery only (23). 4. Surgery and x-ray (13). With Benign Hyperplasia: Thymectomy.	With Thymoma: 1. 4/15(27%) living longer than 1 year. 2. 7/16(44%) living longer than 1 year. 3. 10/23(44%) living longer than 1 year. 4. 5/13(38%) living longer than 1 year. With Benign Hyperplasia: 42/60 remission or improvement.	With benign hyperplasia (60). With thymoma (36). Authors concluded that radiotherapy as the sole form of treatment is of limited use. Also pre-operative radiotherapy did not seem to be useful.
Phillips and Buschke, 1967	7	Radiotherapy, 3000-5500r, to the thymus.	Initial response: 6/7 complete remission or improvement. Present state: 3/7 complete remission or improvement. 2/7 died of tumor.	4/7 had a thymic neoplasm.
Wolfe, 1966	1	Partial excision of tumor plus post-op irradiation (3000r) plus drug therapy.	Patient improved. Almost complete remission of myasthenia at ten month follow up.	Patient had myasthenia gravis and thymoma.

References

1. Currier RD, Routh A, Hickman BT and Douglas MA (1983) Thymus irradiation for myasthenia gravis. *Radiology* **146**: 199-201.
2. King Engel W, Lichten AS and Dalakas MC (1981) Splenic and total-body irradiation treatment of myasthenia gravis. *Ann NY Acad Sci* **377**: 744-754.
3. Salyer WR and Eggleston JC (1976) Thymoma - a clinical and pathological study of 65 cases. *Cancer* **37**: 229-249.
4. DeSevilla E, Forrest JV, Ziunuska FR and Sagel SS (1975) Metastatic thymoma with myasthenia gravis and pure red cell aplasia. *Cancer* **36**: 1154-1157.
5. Goldman AJ, Herrman C Jr, Keesey JC, Mulder DG and Brown WJ (1975) Myasthenia gravis and invasive thymoma: A 20 year experience. *Neurology* **25**: 1021-1025.
6. Cohn HE, Solit RW, Schatz & Schlezinger N (1974) Surgical treatment in myasthenia gravis. *J Thorac & Cardiovas Surg* **68**: 876-885.
7. Mulder GG, Herrman C and Buckberg GD (1974) Effect of thymectomy in patients with myasthenia gravis. *Ann Surg* **128**: 202-206.
8. Weissberg D, Goldberg M and Pearson FG (1973) Thymoma. *Ann Thorac Surg* **16**: 141-147.
9. Levasseur P, Noviant Y, Miranda, AR, Merlier M and LeBrigand H (1972) Thymectomy for myasthenia gravis. *J Thorac & Cardiovas Surg* **64**: 1-5.
10. Vessey MP and Doll R (1972) Thymectomy and cancer. A follow up study. *Br J Cancer* **26**: 53-58.
11. Wolfe WG, Sealy WC and Young WG (1972) Surgical management of myasthenia gravis. *Ann Thoracic Surg* **14**: 645-649.
12. Braitman H, Li W, Herrmann C Jr, and Mulder DG (1971) Surgery for thymic tumors. *Arch Surg* **103**: 14-16.
13. Papatestas AE, Alpert LI, Osserman KE and Kark AE (1971) Studies in myasthenia gravis. Effects of thymectomy. *Am J Med* **50**: 465-474.
14. Perlo VP, Arnason B, Poskanzer D, Castleman B, Schwab RS, Osserman KE, Paptestis A, Alpert L and Kark A (1971) The role of thymectomy in the treatment of myasthenia gravis. *Ann New York Acad Sci* **183**: 308-315.
15. Schulz MD and Schwab RS (1971) Results of thymic (mediastinal) irradiation in patients with myasthenia gravis. *Ann New York Acad Sci* **183**: 303-307.
16. Seybold ME, Howard FM, Duane DD, Payne WS and Harrison EG Jr (1971) Thymectomy in juvenile myasthenia gravis. *Arch Neurol* **25**: 385-392.
17. Cohn LH and Grimes OF (1970) Surgical management of thymic neoplasms. *Surg Gyn & Obst* **131**: 206-215.
18. Kirschner PA (1969) Studies in myasthenia gravis. Transcervical total thymectomy. *JAMA* **209**: 906-910.
19. Zeldowicz LR and Saxton GD (1969) Myasthenia gravis. Comparative evaluation of medical and surgical treatment. *Canad Med Assoc J* **101**: 609-613.
20. Kreel I, Osserman KE, Genkins G and Kark AE (1967) Role of thymectomy in the management of myasthenia gravis. *Ann Surg* **165**: 111-117.
21. Phillips TL and Buschke F (1967) The role of radiation therapy in myasthenia gravis. *Calif Med* **160**: 282-289.
22. Perlo VP, Poskanzer DC, Schwab RS, Viets HR, Osserman KE and Genkins G (1966) Myasthenia gravis. Evaluation of treatment in 1355 patients. *Neurology* **16**: 431-439.
23. Wilkins EW, Edmunds LH Jr and Castleman B (1966) Cases of thymoma at the Massachusetts General Hospital. *J Thorac & Cardiovasc Surg* **52**: 322-330.
24. Wolfe SM (1966) The relationship between thymoma and myasthenia gravis. *Bull Los Angeles Neurol Soc* **31**: 107-113.
25. Latles R (1962) Thymoma and other tumors of the thymus. An analysis of 107 cases. *Cancer* **15**: 1224-1260.
26. Grob D (1953) Course and management of myasthenia gravis. *JAMA* **153**: 529-532.
27. Aring CD (1943) Treatment of myasthenia gravis with the roentgen ray. *Ohio State Med J* **39**: 241-243.

Neurofibroma

Benign neurofibroma most often occurs in association with von Recklinghausen disease, but may also occur independently. In von Recklinghausen disease sarcomatous changes occur without previous irradiation. Critical location and recurrence are the most common reasons for treatment of benign neurofibroma. Definitive radiation may be used in circumstances such that complete excision is not feasible, or where debulking plus radiation therapy may lead to control, or when excision to any extent is severely limited. High dose radiation therapy is then recommended. The limited literature for this condition is worthy of review prior to considering treatment. The usual proviso for risk-benefit and informed consent should be followed. Seventy-three percent of radiation oncologists in the national survey would not treat neurofibroma.

Neurofibroma

Author, Year	Total Cases	Site and Age	Treatment	Results	Notes
Tepper and Suit, 1985	8		Radiation therapy 6400-6600cGy in shrinking field technique	100% actuarial local control and survival at 5 years	
Smalley et al, 1984	1	(L) sciatic nerve	Surgical excision, post-operative radiation of 4500r to pelvis, 540r sacral boost, 1000r intra-operative radiation to (L) pelvic sidewall plus 500r boost.	Relief of discomfort. Developed metastatic disease 10 months after radiation; treated with chemotherapy. 20 months after irradiation, while on chemotherapy had apparent local control.	
Suit and Russell, 1975	1	Right, premaxillary space; 12 years old	Surgical resection and post-operative radiation, 4600r external beam followed by 2600r radium needle implant, total 7200r.	Free of tumor and asymptomatic at 2 years post treatment.	
Greenberg et al, 1981	3	Supraclavicular hip neck	4800-6400r one patient hyperfractionated	Two out of three controlled	5500r or more based on limiting tissue.

References

1. Tepper JE and Suit HD (1985) The role of radiation therapy in the treatment of sarcoma of soft tissue. *Cancer Invest* **3**: 587-592.
2. Smalley SR, Rubin J and Leifermann KM (1984) Neurofibrosarcoma and the sign of Leser-Trelat. *Ca* **34**: 295-298.
3. Greenberg HM, Goebel R, Weichselbaum RR, Greenberger JS, Chaffey JT and Cassady JR (1981) Radiation therapy in the treatment of aggressive fibromatosis. *Int J Radiat Oncol Biol Phys* **7**: 305-310
4. Suit HD and Russell WO (1975) Radiation therapy of soft tissue sarcoma. *Cancer* **36**: 759-764.

Optic Nerve Glioma

Tumors of the visual pathways - optic nerve, optic chiasm and optic tract - may have a long natural history. Controversies exist as to their appropriate management. Some believe therapy should be reserved until a patient has progressive symptoms, although others argue for early treatment to minimize visual deterioration. Depending on the location of the tumor, surgery, combined modalities and radiotherapy alone may be used in the treatment of this disorder. Some argue that attempt at surgical removal, even just biopsy, may make vision worse. Most of the literature recommends radiation doses of at least 4500-5000 rad. Improvements in vision are frequently seen following radiotherapy. Vascular occlusion is a late risk of high fractionated dose and high total dose radiation. Ninety-one percent of radiation oncologists would treat optic glioma according to the national survey.

Optic Nerve Glioma

Author, Year	Total # Pts.	Site and Age	Treatment	Results	Notes
Beyer et al, 1986	3	Optic chiasm 16 months, 13 months and 3 years.	2 and 4 MeV megavoltage treatments Dose: 4560-5537 rad to optic chiasm.	Vascular occlusion occurring 5-6 years after completion of treatment.	
Hirata et al, 1985	2	Optic chiasm and hypothalamus. 5 years and 21 years.	4700 rad/6 weeks in 150 rad fractions, 5000 rad/5 weeks in 200 rad fractions.	Good effect from radiotherapy but vascular occlusion occurring 8 months and 5 years after treatment.	Review article of 20 similar patients.
Horwich and Bloom, 1985	30	Optic nerve and chiasm. 9 months - 56 years.	45-40 Gy in 5-8 weeks. 2 patients received 55 Gy in 7 weeks megavoltage radiation.	43% had improvement in visual acuity. 18% had increase in visual field. 90%(26/29) remained free of disease progression. 10-15 year survival - 93%.	29 of 30 patients had progressive disease when treated. Median follow-up 10 years. Treatment early in the course minimizes visual deficit.
McFadzean et al, 1983	9	Optic chiasm glioma. 4-49 years (mean 19 years)	Craniotomy, followed by radiotherapy 3000-5000 rad.	8 of 18 eyes showed improvement in vision	Follow-up 3 months to 13.5 years (mean - 3.9 years)
Packer et al, 1983	21	Chiasmatic glioma, median age 4.	Radiotherapy in 18 patients (4000-6000 rad), chemotherapy in 2 patients, observation in 1.	5 year survival - 89% but only 60% in 10 years. 48% had disease recurrence, or visual and/or neurologic deterioration 6 years after diagnosis.	
Gaini et al, 1982	57	Optic nerve and chiasm. Children and adults.	Surgery - 27 Radiotherapy - 15.	Patients analyzed as to site: optic nerve, chiasm and diencephalo - chiasmatic tissues. Best results were with surgery and radiation.	
Giuffre et al, 1982	28	Anterior optic pathways. Children and adults.	Surgery and radiotherapy in 20 of 28 cases.	20 of 28 living.	Review articles. Treatment should be individualized.
Sung, 1982	43	Optic chiasmal gliomas. All children.	42 had primary radiotherapy 3500-6000 rad in 3.5-7 weeks.	10 year survival anterior optic chiasmal gliomas - 72% and posterior optic chiasmal glioma - 40%. Quality of survival - active normal life: 36% - anterior lesions 75% - posterior lesions Improvement in vision in: 32% - anterior lesions 67% - posterior lesions	36 - anterior lesions 7 - posterior lesions

Historical Data: Optic Nerve Glioma

Author, Year	Total # Pts.	Site and Age	Treatment	Results	Notes
Tenny et al, 1982	104	Optic nerve glioma 11 months - 64 years	Surgery and/or radiotherapy	Anterior lesions - 85% survival Posterior lesions - 50% survival	Neurofibromatosis present in 14%.
Parker et al, 1981	1	Chiasmal glioma, 16 years.	4680 rad in 5 weeks.	Stability of visual function.	
Danoff et al, 1980	18	Optic nerve glioma. Ages 2-12 years (mean - 5.9 years).	Radiotherapy 5000-6000 rad in 5-6.5 weeks.	83% 5 year survival and 73% 10-year survival. Visual status was maintained or improved in 78%.	Follow up is 1-19 years.
Dosoretz et al, 1980	20	Optic nerve and chiasm. Ages 6 months - 40 years (median - 6 years).	Limited tumors were operated; the advanced tumors received post-operative radiotherapy 4500-5000 rad.	Of 8 resected patients, 6 stabilized. Of 12 advanced patients 10 were stable, 7 with no major complications.	
Robertson and Brewin, 1980	10	Optic nerve glioma involving chiasm. Ages 0-50 years.	Radiotherapy 3000-5000 rad.	Vision improved in 4 of 10 patients. None died from tumor.	
Brand and Hoover, 1979	16	Optic tract glioma Ages 4 months - 15 years.	All received radiotherapy 4000-6000 rad post-operatively (average - 5000 rad).	9 survived with average survival 1-5.5 years after treatment.	
Harter et al, 1978	8	Intracranial nerves and optic chiasm.	Exploration followed by radiotherapy.	Patients with tumors of optic nerve and/or chiasm did well 7-10 years. Of 6 patients with tumor extension beyond chiasm, 3 recurred within 1 year of treatment and died. Vision improved with radiotherapy.	
Heiskanen et al, 1978	24	Optic pathways. Ages 10 months - 16 years. (mean - 5 years)	Optic nerve: excision plus/or minus radiotherapy. Anterior chiasm: biopsy plus radiotherapy.	Patients with optic nerve tumors did well. Patients with anterior chiasmal tumors in 13 survivors, the vision was stable or improved. Posterior chiasmal tumors fared poorly.	Mean follow-up 10 years.
Lowes et al, 1978	13	Optic glioma Ages 20 months - 24 years (average - 14 years).	Craniotomy - 12 of 13 received post-operative radiotherapy 4000-5500 rad.	4 patients had stable or improved vision. 3 patients died.	
Servo and Puranen, 1978	1	Optic glioma Age 1.5 years	4200 rad/4 weeks post-operative	Did well until age 12 - panhypopituitarism was diagnosed. At age 15 he developed occlusion and stenosis of internal carotid arteries.	

Historical Data: Optic Nerve Glioma (Continued)

Author, Year	Total # Pts.	Site and Age	Treatment	Results	Notes
Montgomery et al, 1977	16	Optic nerve Ages 10 months – 49 years (mean age 13.3 years)	All received radiation therapy, none had surgical extirpation. Doses 3500–6500 rad (average – 5000 rad) supervoltage.	Vision improved in all who survived. No patient receiving 5000r recurred. 4 of 7 with doses < 5000r, recurred.	Mean follow up 6.3 years.
Chutorian et al, 1976	2	Optic nerve glioma (multicenter origin) Ages 2 and 3	4500 rad/5.5 weeks	Excellent result with improvement in vision at 5 year and 3 months follow up.	

References

1. Beyer RA, Paden P, Sobel DF and Flynn FG (1986) Moyamoya pattern of vascular occlusion after radiotherapy for glioma of the optic chiasm. *Neurology* **36**: 1173–1178.
2. Hirata Y, Matsukado Y, Mihara Y, Kochi M, Sonoda H and Fukmura A (1985) Occlusion of the internal carotid artery after radiation therapy for the chiasmal lesion. *Acta Neurochir* **74**: 141–147.
3. Horwich A and Bloom HJ (1985) Optic gliomas: Radiation therapy and prognosis. *Int J Radiat Oncol Biol Phys* **11**: 1067–1079.
4. McFadzean RM, Brewin TB, Doyle D and Grossart K (1983) Gliomas of the optic chiasm and its management. *Trans Ophthalmol Soc UK* **103**: 199–207.
5. Packer RJ, Savino PJ, Bilaniuk LT, Zimmerman RA, Schatz NJ, Rosenstock JG, Nelson DS, Jarrett PD, Bruce DA and Schut L (1983) Chiasmatic gliomas of childhood. A reappraisal of natural history and effectiveness of cranial irradiation. *Child's Brain* **10**: 393–403.
6. Gaini SM, Tomei G, Arienta C, Zaranone M, Giovanelli M and Villani R (1982) Optic nerve and chiasm gliomas in children. *J Neurosurg Sci* **26**: 33–39.
7. Giuffre R, Bardelli AM, Tarerniti L and Barberi L (1982) Anterior optic pathways gliomas. The dilemma of treatment. *J Neurosurg Sci* **26**: 61–72.
8. Sung DI (1982) Suprasellar tumors in children. A review of clinical manifestations and managements. *Cancer* **50**: 1420–1425.
9. Tenny RT, Laws ER, Younge BR and Rush JA (1982) The neurosurgical management and optic glioma. Results in 104 patients. *J Neurosurg* **57**: 452–458.
10. Parker JC, Smith JL, Reyes P and Vuksanovic MM (1981) Chiasmal optic gliomas after radiation therapy. Neuro-ophthalmologic/pathologic correlation. *J Clin Neuro-Ophthalmol* **1**: 31–43.
11. Danoff BF, Kramer S and Thompson N (1980) The radiotherapeutic management of optic nerve gliomas in children. *Int J Radiation Oncol Biol Phys* **6**: 45–50.
12. Dosoretz DE, Blitzer PH, Wang CC and Linggood RM (1980) Management of glioma of the optic nerve and/or chiasm. An analysis of 20 cases. *Cancer* **45**: 1467–1471.
13. Robertson AG and Brewin TB (1980) Optic nerve glioma. *Clin Radiol* **31**: 471–474.
14. Brand WN and Hoover SV (1979) Optic glioma in children. Review of 16 cases given megavoltage radiation therapy. *Child's Brain* **5**: 459–466.
15. Harter DJ, Caderao JB, Leavens ME and Young SE (1978) Radiotherapy in the management of primary gliomas involving the intracranial optic nerves and chiasm. *Int J Radiation Oncol Biol Phys* **4**: 681–686.
16. Heiskanen O, Raitta C and Torsti R (1978) The management and prognosis of gliomas of the optic pathways in children. *Acta Neurochir* **43**: 193–199.
17. Lowes M, Bojsen Mller M, Vorre P and Hedegaard O (1978) An evaluation of gliomas of the anterior visual pathways. A 10-year survey. *Acta Neurochir* **43**: 201–206.
18. Servo A and Puranen M (1978) Moyamoya syndrome as a complication of radiation therapy. Case report. *J Neurosurg* **48**: 1026–1029.
19. Montgomery AB, Griffin T, Parker RG and Gerdes AJ (1977) Optic nerve gliomas: The role of radiation therapy. *Cancer* **40**: 2079–2080.
20. Chutorian AM, Housepian EM and Hilal S (1976) Optic gliomas of multicentric origin with favorable response to radiotherapy. *Trans Am Neurol Assoc* **101**: 229–232.

Osteoblastoma/Osteoid Osteoma

Surgical removal is the treatment of choice for these benign bone lesions. The role of radiotherapy is controversial and the histologic diagnosis difficult. As the number of patients reported is limited, our ability to evaluate radiation therapy in this disorder is similarly limited. For nonresectable tumors, radiotherapy has been associated with long term local control.

In the national survey 91% of radiation oncologists would not treat osteoid osteoma.

Osteoblastoma/Osteoid Osteoma

Author, Year	Total # Pts.	Site and Age	Treatment	Results	Notes
Capanna et al, 1986	2	Sacrum, age 17, 20	Curettage and radiotherapy	Disease free at 9 and 25 years follow-up.	
Mitchell and Ackerman, 1986	2	Ilium, age 15.	Curettage, XRT, 6000 rad	Palliation of pain, but no tumor response. Died with metastatic osteosarcoma	Difficulties in differentiating histologically: osteoblastoma, aggressive osteoblastoma and osteoblastoma-like osteosarcoma osteoid osteoma.
		Femur, age 12	Excision local recurrence. Rebiopsy 2500 rad/2 weeks.	Symptoms decreased. No evidence of disease at 14 year follow-up.	
Jackson, 1978	3	Recurrence: Reexcision and radiotherapy. Details not given.	Two of three were without recurrence three and four years later.	Review article, all lesions were recurrent.	
	3	Sacrum, ilium	Recurrence – treated with radiotherapy only	Two of three lesions persisted requiring further surgery	

References

1. Capanna R, Cayala A, Bertoni F, Picci P, Calaeroni P, Gherlinzoni F, Betelli G and Campanacci M (1986) Sacral osteoid osteoma and osteoblastoma: a report of 13 Cases. *Arch Orthop Trauma Surg* **105**: 205–210.
2. Mitchell ML and Ackerman LV (1986) Metastatic and pseudomalignant osteoblastoma: A report of two unusual cases. *Skeletal Radiol* **15**: 213–218.
3. Jackson RP (1978) Recurrent osteoblastoma. A review. *Clin Orthop* **131**: 229–233.

Otitis Media

Radium applications to the nasopharynx for treatment of bilateral serous otitis media, conductive hearing loss, and glue-ear were commonly employed in the 1950's. Therapeutic response with follow up normal hearing, normal drums and no subsequent otitis were common. With long term follow up, however, secondary solid tumors are now reported, even following presumed low doses of radiation to small volume. Such treatment is inappropriate today.

Otitis Media

Investigator, Year	Cases	Site, Age	Treatment	Results	Notes
Sofferman and Heisse, 1985	1	Nasopharynx; 31 yrs	50 mgm Crowe-Burnam radium application 12.5 min to each side of nasopharynx in 3 treatments over 2 wks (~4000r ranging to 320r 1mm from source)	23 years later, found to have adenoid cystic carcinoma of the nasopharynx	Used for bilateral serous otitis media. Not conclusive, but likely is a radiation-induced malignancy

Otitis Media (Continued)

Investigator, Year	Cases	Site, Age	Treatment	Results	Notes
Loeb, 1979	41	Nasopharynx; 1yr to 30+	"Crowe" applicator 50 mg radium 12 min to each side of nasopharynx for 3 treatments in 2 wks	Of 28 patients with long term follow up: 24 had good results 2 had fair result 2 had poor result No secondary tumors	Patients had recurrent serous otitis, conductive hearing loss, and visible lymphoid tissue in the nasopharynx Follow up 15-30 yrs after therapy

References

1. Sofferman RA and Heisse JR (1985) Adenoid cystic carcinoma of the nasopharynx after previous adenoid irradiation. *Laryngoscope* **95**: 31-41.
2. Loeb WJ (1979) Radiation therapy of the nasopharynx: a 30 year view. *Laryngoscope* **89**: 16-21.

Pancreatic Fistulae

There is no evidence of the beneficial effect of radiation in the treatment of pancreatic fistulae. Spontaneous healing can occur independently or in close association with a course of irradiation. The use of radiation, thus, is unwarranted as an approach to this disorder. The so-called "experience" or "empiricism" in pancreatitis and in pancreatic fistulae is probably best related to similar impressions in the treatment of bursitis and tendinitis where critical randomized studies proved "no benefit."

Pancreatitis

As recently as 1973 there were reports of supervoltage radiation treatment for pancreatitis of 2000 rad, although the evidence of a positive effect is far from convincing. We do not reference this condition, since 92% of radiation oncologists in the national survey would not treat pancreatitis. Further, it is important to note that those physicians who fail to demand tissue diagnosis for cancer of the pancreas may face the possibility of treating pancreatitis. Physicians undertaking such therapy must observe stringent criteria for treatment and must fully inform their patients of the risks involved. (See section *"Standard of Care"*).

Paraganglioma (Chromaffin Positive)
(Chromaffin Negative - see Chemodectoma)

This rare tumor is more often reported as non-chromaffin positive, when it is referred to as chemodectoma. Even more rare is the chromaffin positive paraganglioma which must be reviewed separately. In this section, we review the chromaffin positive tumors. Conclusions are that radiation therapy has not been established in the management of these tumors and a definitive opinion cannot be given. When asked if they would treat paraganglioma-chemodectoma, 93% of radiation oncologists would treat. In the same national survey when asked if they would treat chromaffin tumors, 53% would not treat. Realization that chromaffin positive tumors are not chemodectoma may aid radiation oncologists in their determinations.

Paraganglioma (Chromaffin Tumors)

Author, Year	Total # Patients	Treatment	Results	Notes
Arom and Nicoloff, 1976	1	Excision	Patient well at two year follow up.	Intrathoracic paraganglioma arising from an aorticosympathetic ganglion.
	5	Excision	3/5 alive and well at 3.5 months-6 years after surgery. 1/5 died during anesthesia for thoracotomy. 1/5 recurrence at primary site suspected after treatment.	These are five cases of thoracic paraganglioma at the costovertebral sulcus reported in the literature and reviewed in this report by Arom and Nicoloff.
Kay et al, 1975	1	Excision.	No evidence of recurrence at 7.5 month follow up.	Paraganglioma located over the thyroid cartilage.
Horoupian et al, 1974	1	Laminectomy and excision.	Patient doing well at 1 year.	Paraganglioma of cauda equina.
Miller et al, 1972	1	Cholecystectomy and wedge resection of liver.	No follow up reported.	Paraganglioma of the gallbladder.
Leestma and Price, 1971	24	Treatment ranged from initial transurethral biopsy and attempted resections but usually led to an open operative procedure such as a wedge resection of the bladder.	12/17 alive and well 6 months to 17 years post-op. 2/17 died in the post-op period. 2/17 died free of tumor 1/17 died 14 years post-op of CVA and severe hypertension. Chromaffin tumor of the organ of Zuckerkandl was present at autopsy.	Paraganglioma of the urinary bladder.
	34	Excision.	8/34 recurrence, failure to totally remove the lesion, or a second tumor near the original.	These 34 cases are a result of the authors' survey of the literature for bladder paragangliomas.
Kepes and Zachanias, 1970	2	Excision.	No recurrences.	Gangliocytic paragangliomas of the duodenum. These tumors differ from chemodectomies of the carotid body or glomus jugulare and may be a transitional form of tumor between gangliocytomas and nonchromaffin paragangliomas.
Cardenas et al, 1970	1	Adrenalectomy.	No recurrence at 5 years post-op.	Adrenal medullary paragangliomas producing Cushing's syndrome.
Brantigan and Katase, 1969	3	1. Surgery plus radiotherapy (1 pts). 2. Surgery only (1 pt). 3. Radiotherapy only (1 pt).	1. Good initial response but metastases noted two years later. 2. Patient was hypertensive without recurrence or metastases noted; lost to follow up 8 years later. 3. Patient remained normotensive for two years until he died. At autopsy tumor of the organ of Zuckerkandl was found.	Paragangliomas of the organ of Zuckerkandl.

References

1. Arom KV and Nicoloff DM (1976) Intrathoracic paraganglioma arising from aorticosympathetic paraganglion. *Arch Surg* **111**: 275–279.
2. Kay S, Montague JW and Dodd RW (1975) Nonchromaffin paraganglioma (chemodectoma) of thyroid region. *Cancer* **36**: 582–585.
3. Horoupian DS, Kerson LA, Saiontz H and Valsamis M (1974) Paraganglioma of cauda equina. *Cancer* **33**: 1337–1348.
4. Miller TW, Weber TR and Applebaum HD (1972) Paraganglioma of the gallbladder. *Arch Surg* **105**: 637–639.
5. Kepes JJ and Zacharias DL (1971) Gangliocytic paragangliomas of the duodenum. *Cancer* **27**: 61–70.
6. Leestma JE and Price EB Jr. (1971) Paraganglioma of the urinary bladder. *Cancer* **28**: 1063–1073.
7. Cardenas F, Coffey RJ and Meloni R (1970) Cushing's syndrome secondary to a benign paraganglioma. *Am Surg* **36**: 283–289.
8. Brantigan CV and Katase RY (1969) Clinical and pathologic features of paragangliomas of the organ of Zuckerkandl. *Surg* 898–905.

Parotitis

The mortality for postoperative suppurative parotitis was significant in medicine before the advent of antibiotics. The Mayo Clinic non-randomized study of 1936 indicated increased survival with radium treatment. Early use of antibiotics such as sulfonamides, however, did not significantly alter the use of radiation treatment. Buschke and Cantril, notable and respected radiation oncologists, reported regression of postoperative parotitis without suppuration in 1944, and, although it could not be determined if worst case selection for combined therapy was used, those patients receiving concomitant sulfonamides before or after radiation seemed to have more complicated courses. These physicians concluded that sulfonamides were unnecessary for remission of the parotitis when using radiation.

Citation of benefit from radiation treatment continues to appear in the scientific literature through the 1960's, usually indicating orthovoltage to decrease postoperative parotitis. The pediatric literature in particular, however, began to reflect concern for late effects of radiation treatment, especially growth retardation or retardation in the mandibular region and possible malignant transformation. Although historically appropriate, radiation treatment for parotitis is not indicated today. 52% of radiation oncologists would not treat parotitis.

Parotitis Radiotherapy

Author, Year	Total # Patients	Treatment	Results	Notes
Yonkers et al, 1972	11	Radiation: 3784r/16 days	Antibiotics only: 4/7 required incision and drainage Radiation plus antibiotics: 0/2 required incision and drainage No specific treatment 0/2 required incision and drainage	Surgical parotitis
Leake et al, 1971	28	Pediatric parotitis: (Individual treatment with/without antibiotics) 1. Sialography 2. Incision and drainage 3. Biopsy 4. Irradiation 5. Excision 6. No treatment	Recurrences: 1/4 0/2 1/5 1/6 1/6 0/5	In acute suppurative parotitis irradiation is not indicated, since most organisms are sensitive to one or more antibiotics. Chronic suppurative parotitis is somewhat less responsive to irradiation.

Historical Data: Parotitis Radiotherapy

Author, Year	Total # Patients	Treatment	Results	Notes
Leake and Leake, 1970	10	Neonatal parotitis: Antibiotics and/or low dose radiotherapy (75-100r/1-3F)	Antibiotics only: 5/6 improved Radiotherapy only: 1/1 improved Antibiotics and radiotherapy: 1/3 improved (1 death; a patient with congenital heart disease and pneumonia)	All cases neonatal suppurative parotitis.
Larsen et al, 1963	20	(17) radiation + supplemental medical care (1) radiation + incision and drainage (2) medical care alone	13/17 resolution within 15 days	Surgical parotitis
Krippaehne et al, 1962	80	Radiation alone or radiation plus antibiotics (no details provided)	Radiation: 10/40 died Radiation + antibiotics: 9/40 died	Acute suppurative parotitis (majority of geriatric patients) "Many factors influenced the decision to use irradiation and from these data it is impossible to draw conclusions regarding effectiveness." Authors recommend radiation only for the relief of pain in the first 24 hours.
Spratt, 1961	206	No specific therapy Radiation only Radiation plus antibiotics or sulfonamides Antibiotics only Drainage only Radiation and delayed drainage Radiation, delayed drainage and antibiotics or sulfonamides Drainage and antibiotics or sulfonamides	Infection subsided without producing a septic complication or death: 35/69 4/5 10/20 13/16 36/64 6/8 5/11 11/13	Technical details of radiotherapy: maximum dose 400-600r/8-12F/8-12 days (200-250Kv) "The continued use of irradiation on acute bacterial infections of the parotid gland is a therapeutic anachronism."
Gilchrist and McAndrew, 1958	7	75r/day	1/7 resolution. 6 remaining subsequently underwent surgical decompression	Surgical parotitis.
Gustafson, 1951	83	Radiation: 250-750r/2-5 days (150Kv, unfiltered, HVL 0.25mm Cu, or 200Kv, 1mm Al plus 0.5mm Cu filtration HVL 0.9mm Cu).	Radiation: 52/68 (76%) prompt resolution without abscess formation Radiation plus antibiotics: 11/15 prompt resolution	Acute parotitis results are better if treated early 51/80 followed operation.
Neuhauser and Ferris, 1945	4	300r/2F/2 days An additional 150r on third day if necessary. Patients also received penicillin or sulfonamides	4/4 parotid involvement disappeared in 2-6 days with no recurrence	Acute suppurative parotitis (3 neonatal cases)

Historical Data: Parotitis Radiotherapy (Continued)

Author, Year	Total # Patients	Treatment	Results	Notes
Buschke and Cantril, 1944	26	50-100r/day as needed	17/26 (65%) parotitis healed	Surgical parotitis: All cases leading to suppuration received sulfonamides in addition to roentgen therapy, either preceding or immediately following irradiation. Only 1/12 with uncomplicated recoveries had received sulfonamides in addition to radiotherapy.
Fricke and Madding, 1942	190	Radium Therapy: 900-100r to the parotid. Radium sulfate was used. Other measures: heat, cold compresses, gentian violet, sulfonamide, *etc*.	Radium: 84/111 (75%) parotitis healed; 9/111 (8%) incision and drainage necessary; 13/111 (22.7%) died, parotitis uncontrolled; 5/111 abscesses ruptured spontaneously. Other measures: 59/79 (73%) parotitis healed; 15/79 (19%) incision and drainage necessary; 6/79 (7.6%) died, parotitis uncontrolled	Surgical parotitis. Radium therapy was often used as a last resort when other treatment had failed, or when the patient was critically ill.
Pendergrass and Hodes, 1942	47	400-500r/3-4F/3-5 days	32/47 (68%) pts benefitted	Acute postoperative parotitis
McCormick, 1942	20	300-400r(air)/2F/1 day (200 Kv, 0.5mm Cu plus 3mm Al or 1mm Cu plus 4mm Al filtration, FSD 50cm)	12/20 completely cured	Suppurative parotitis (16 post operative cases). Results were much better if treated within 16 hours of onset.
Latchmore and La Touche, 1940	11	100r daily or 200r on alternate days to total of 500-600r (skin). (200 Kv, 1mm Cu filter, FSD 23cm)	6/11 complete resolution (Resolution was taking place in an additional patient when the patient died from other causes)	Acute suppurative parotitis. (8 post operative cases). Results were better (5/7) in cases treated immediately.

References

1. Garvar LR and Kingstein GJ (1974) Recurrent parotitis in childhood. *J Oral Surg* **32**: 373-376.
2. Leban SG and Stratigos GT (1974) Benign lymphoepithelial sialoadenopathies. *Oral Surg* **38**: 735-748.
3. Schwartz AE and Friedman EW (1973) Salivary gland disorders. *New York State J Med* **73**: 297-302.
4. Batsakis JG and McWhirter JD (1972) Non neoplastic diseases of the salivary glands. *Am J Gastroent* **57**: 226-247.
5. Spiers CF and Mason DK (1972) Acute septic parotitis: incidence, aetiology and management. *Scot Med J* **17**: 62-66.
6. Yonkers AJ, Krous HF and Yarington CT (1972) Surgical parotitis **82**: 1239-1247.
7. Hemeway WG (1971) Chronic punctate parotitis. *Laryngoscope* **81**: 485-509.
8. Leake DL, Krakowiak FJ and Leake RC (1971) Suppurative parotitis in children. *Oral Surg* **31**: 174-179.
9. Patey DJ (1971) Recurrent swelling of the parotid gland (recurrent parotitis). *Modern Trends Surg* **3**: 261-283.
10. Leake D and Leake R (1970) Neonatal suppurative parotitis. *Pediatrics* **46**: 203-207.
11. Sprinkle PM and Yarington CT (1968) Disease of the salivary glands and benign lymphoepithelial lesion. *South Med J* **61**: 971-974.
12. Diamant H and Enfors B (1965) Treatment of chronic recurrent parotitis. *Laryngoscope* **75**: 153-160.
13. Blatt IM (1964) On sialectasis and benign lymphosialadenopathy. *Laryngoscope* **74**: 1684-1746.
14. Larsen RR, Sawyer RM and Sawyer KC (1963) Surgical parotitis. *Postgrad Med* **33**: 149-152.
15. Krippaehne WW, Hunt TK and Dunphy JE (1962) Acute suppurative parotitis. *Ann Surg* **156**: 251-257.

16. Spratt JS (1961) The etiology and therapy of acute pyogenic parotitis. *Surg Gynec Obstet* **112**: 391–405.
17. Diamant H (1958) Ligation of the parotid duct in chronic recurrent parotitis. *Acta Otolaryngol* **49**: 375–380.
18. Gilchrist RK and McAndrew JR (1958) Surgical parotitis. *Arch Surg* **76**: 863–867.
19. Gustafson JR (1951) Acute parotitis. *Surgery* **29**: 786–801.
20. Neuhauser EBD and Ferris BG (1945) The treatment of acute suppurative parotitis in infants. *J Pediat* **27**: 589–590.
21. Buschke F and Cantril ST (1944) The course of postoperative parotitis under radiation therapy. *West J Surg Obstet Gynecol* **52**: 21–28.
22. Hare HF (1944) The management of acute postoperative parotitis. *Surg Clin North Am* **24**: 603–606.
23. Fricke RE and Madding GF (1942) Further observations on the radium treatment of postoperative parotitis. *Radiology* **38**: 294–298.
24. Madding GF and Fricke RE (1942) Secondary or postoperative parotitis. *Surgery* **11**: 45–47.
25. McCormick NA (1942) Suppurative parotitis. *Canadian Med Assoc J* **47**: 29–33.
26. Pendergrass EP and Hodes PJ (1942) Acute postoperative parotitis. *Radiology* **38**: 307–312.
27. Latchmore AJC and La Touche AAD (1940) Acute suppurative parotitis. *Lancet* **I**: 497–499.
28. Bowing HH and Fincke RE (1936) Radium treatment of postoperative parotitis. *Radiology* **25**: 37–40.

Peptic Ulcer

The era of widespread use of cimetidine (Tagamet) and ranitidine (Xantac) as medical treatment for peptic ulcer would suggest that radiation may no longer be seriously considered in treating this condition. Thirty-two percent of radiation oncologists participating in the national survey, however, would treat peptic ulcer with radiation. It is of particular interest to note that two internists, Cocco and Mendeloff, in publishing their experience with 463 patients in 1979, supported selection of certain patients for radiation treatment.

Unlike other benign diseases where the efficacy of radiation remains unestablished, supportive data exist for this treatment, although significant precautions and stringent criteria are indicated. The following review of the literature therefore includes cautions concerning radiation nephritis and reviews of appropriate techniques. Finally, Griem's caution that a 2.5-fold increase exists for adenocarcinoma of the pancreas and colon and for stomach cancers twenty years after treatment with 1600 rad irradiation to the stomach speaks to restricting use of such radiation to select and appropriate patients. The patient experience for second tumors represents 40 patients of 2049 treated. It is recommended that radiation treatment be undertaken only after a very careful review of alternate methods of treatment, a thorough review of the literature, an assessment of risk/benefit, and the careful documentation of informed consent. Sixty-eight percent of radiation oncologists in the national survey would not treat peptic ulcer.

Peptic Ulcer Radiotherapy

Author, Year	Total # Pts.	Technical Details	Total Dose/ Fraction/Time	Results	Complications/ Comments	Notes
Lieber et al, 1985	2049		1600–1700r	2 sarcomas predicted: 3 occurred, some question of relationship		This study needs to be followed; presently not conclusive
Cocco and Mendeloff, 1979	463	Of 463 selected ulcer patients, 207 were duodenal, 82 were gastric and 174 had both	1500–2000r 250Kv upper two-thirds stomach	90% control 14 year FU	No renal injury was documented	Elderly requiring ulcerogenic drugs for other disorders and poor operative risks; no tumors post treatment; cost analysis performed

Historical Data: Peptic Ulcer Radiotherapy

Author, Year	Total # Pts.	Technical Details	Total Dose/Fraction/Time	Results	Complications/Comments	Notes
Findlay et al, 1974	24	6-Mev; opposed anterior and posterior fields	Initial doses of 650-900r; doses later standardized to 1500r/10F/12 days	16/24 complete symptomatic relief. 3/24 partial symptomatic relief. 5/24 failures (3 of these had further radiotherapy and ultimately received full symptomatic relief). Maximum acid output was reduced to 30% of the pretreatment value at a mean of 10.7 months after therapy, 58% of the pretreatment value at 230 months.	none	83% of pts were 60 yrs or older Dx: Gastric ulcer (3) Duodenal ulcer (4) Jejunal ulcer (3) Oesophageal ulcer (2) Oesophagitis (15) Second-part duodenal ulcer (1)
Anselm and Schuman, 1972	36	Co60 One anterior and one posterior portal covering the upper portion of the stomach	2000r/10 days (100r daily to each portal)	25/36 good results – no recurrence in 2 yr follow up 12/15 no basal HCL after treatment 3/15 completely achlorhydric within 3 weeks	none	29/36 were over 60 yrs of age. Dx: Gastric ulcer (14) Duodenal ulcer (11) Stomal ulcer (6) Esophagitis (5)
Levin, 1972	47	250 Kv, 30ma, Thoreus 3 filter, HVL 3.25mm Cu, FSD, 50-70cm	1900-2000r (mid plane dose)/10-14F	Duodenal ulcer: 16.2% recurrence Gastric ulcer: 4/7 no recurrence in 2-8 year follow up Gastric and duodenal ulcer: 3/3 symptom free for 3-16 yrs following therapy		Duodenal ulcer (37) Gastric ulcer (7) Both duodenal and gastric ulcer (3) All patients were 60 yrs of age or older
Cocco and Mendeloff, 1970	33	Co60 One anterior and one posterior field centered over the upper two-thirds of the stomach	2000r/8-10/F to each portal	28/33 asymptomatic at 3 yr follow up 94% showed achlorhydria or greater than 50% reduction of acid response (Key test) after 6 months	Vomiting (6) Nausea (13)	Ages ranged from 57 to 85 years All were cases of duodenal ulcers
Clayman et al, 1968	145	250 Kv, 1mm Cu plus 1mm Al filter, HVL 1.5mm Cu, focus distance 50cm Field size: 13 x 13cm or 10 x 17cm. Anterior and posterior fields	1600-1700r (depth dose)/10-12 days Depth dose is estimated in a plane 1/3 of the distance from the anterior surface of the body and 2/3 of the distance from the posterior surface	640/1485 (44%) achlorhydria or greater than 50% reduction in acid for 1 year or more	Pericarditis (1) Other minimal side effects	Duodenal ulcer (1251) Gastric ulcer (154)

Historical Data: Peptic Ulcer Radiotherapy (Continued)

Author, Year	Total # Pts.	Technical Details	Total Dose/Fraction/Time	Results	Complications/Comments	Notes
Cooper et al, 1968	20	not given	1600r/10F/10 days to *each* portal	10/16 good-excellent symptomatic results (long term) 5/12 achlorhydria or greater than 50% reduction in stimulated (Histalog) acid output	Transient increased dysphagia (2)	All were cases of peptic esophagitis. All patients were continued on a standard medical program after irradiation
Brown et al, 1962	121	Co60 One anterior and one posterior field centered over the upper two-thirds of the stomach	2000r/6-8F to *each* portal	87/121 good results - no evidence of recurrent ulcer. 90% achlorhydria or greater than 50% reduction in basal gastric secretion in the first 6 months. 55% achlorhydria or greater than 50% reduction in stimulated (Histalog) acid secretion in the first 6 months.	Vomiting (11) Nausea (11)	Supplemental medical treatment was also used. Duodenal ulcer (80) Gastric ulcer (23) Marginal ulcer (18)
Klein and Berman, 1961	50	250 Kv, 30 mg, Thoreus 3 filter, HVL 3.25 mm Cu, FSD 50-40 cm. Alternating anterior and posterior fields. Field size: 12 x 8 cm to 14 x 9 cm	1700-2000r (midplane dose)/10-14F	27/50 (54%) excellent results 11/50 (22%) good results	Some nausea and vomiting Chondritis (1) Radiation pneumonitis (1)	All were cases of duodenal ulcers. No medical therapy of any type was given after irradiation
Kiefer and Smedal, 1959	23	2 meV, HVL 12.8 mm Cu, target midplane distance of 125 cm Alternating anterior and posterior fields Field size: 10 x 10 cm	1800r (tissue dose/10F/2weeks)	18/23 clinically satisfactory results after 1-3 courses of therapy 11/12 free acid level was reduced (achlorhydria in 5) at 2-6 months after therapy	Nausea (4) Renal cell carcinoma (1) (left kidney) - possible relationship to radiation therapy	All were cases of stoma ulcer occurring after subtotal gastrectomy
Brown and Wood, 1956; Brown et al, 1952	52		Antroduodenectomy and irradiation (2000r tissue dose/3 weeks)	46/52 (83%) very good results Remaining 6 developed recurrent ulcer	Long term follow up revealed radiation nephritis in a significant number	All were cases of duodenal ulcer
	48		Antroduodenectomy only	37/48 very good results 5/48 moderately good result		
	10		Irradiation only (2000r/3 weeks)	4/10 free from symptoms 2/10 minor symptoms		

Historical Data: Peptic Ulcer Radiotherapy (Continued)

Author, Year	Total # Pts.	Technical Details	Total Dose/ Fraction/Time	Results	Complications/ Comments	Notes
Holman and Lewis, 1941	15	400 Kv, 4.25 mm Cu plus 1 mm Al filtration, HVL 4.5 mm Cu, FSD 80 cm. Circular anterior and posterior ports, 12.3 cm diameter	500–700r (depth dose)	All cases showed a reduction in level of free HCL, but this reduction was variable in amount and duration		All were cases of duodenal ulcer.
Eichorn et al, 1961	4	No details given Field size: 15 x 8 cm.	2000r through an anterior field to the lower two-thirds of the stomach	All patients showed a reduction in gastric acidity		Esophageal varices with bleeding (2) Hiatal hernia (1) Post-operative esophagitis (1)
Teplitz et al, 1961	6	Beta irradiation with Ru-Rh^{105} from an intragastric point source centered in a balloon inflated with 515 cc of air	200–1000 rep at the surface of the mucosa	3/6 abolition or substantial decrease in basal acid secretion (all pts received doses of 450 rep or greater)	Gastric ulcer of the lesser curvature (1)	The single dose method used is not satisfactory
McGeorge, 1950	32	Radium needles	2000–3000 mg-hrs	10/32 good symptomatic results 6/32 significant symptomatic improvement 14/18 maximum free acidity and free acid production (Histamine) below initial level	Nausea in some	All were cases of duodenal ulcer Impossible to estimate the dosage in rads to the gastric mucosa

References

1. Lieber MR, Winans CS, Griem ML, Mossa R, Elmer VM and Franklin WA (1985) Sarcomas arising after radiotherapy for peptic ulcer disease. *Dig Dis Sci* **30**: 593–599.
2. Cocco AE and Mendeloff AI (1979) Gastric irradiation of peptic ulcer. *Amer J Gastroenterol* **71**: 577–581.
3. Findlay JM, Newaishy GA, Sircus W and McManus JPA (1974) Role of gastric irradiation in management of peptic ulceration and oesophagitis. *Br Med J* **3**: 769–771.
4. Griem ML (1974) External irradiation at the University of Chicago. In: Gastric Irradiation in Peptic Ulcer WL Palmer (ed) Chicago: University of Chicago Press, pp 39–44.
5. Palmer WL and Griem ML (1974) Adverse effects of gastric irradiation. In: Gastric Irradiation in Peptic Ulcer WL Palmer (ed) Chicago: University of Chicago Press, pp 89–93.
6. Anselm K and Schuman BM (1972) Gastric irradiation for complicated peptic ulcer in geriatric patients. *J Am Geriatr Soc* **20**: 14–16.
7. Levin E (1972) Peptic ulcer in the aged. *Geriatrics* **27**: 83–90.
8. Anselm K, Schuman BM and Cook CA (1971) The mucosal response to gastric irradiation. *Gastroent Endosc* **17**: 105–106.
9. Thompson PL, Mackay IR, Robson GSM and Wall AJ (1971) Late radiation nephritis after gastric x-irradiation for peptic ulcer. *Qrtly J Med* **40**: 144–155.
10. Cocco AE and Mendeloff AI (1970) Effects of gastric irradiation in duodenal ulcer patients: gastric secretory response to maximal histamine stimulation during a three year period. *Johns Hopkins Med J* **126**: 61–68.
11. Thompson PL, Mackay IR, Robson GSM and Wall AJ (1969) Radiation nephritis after gastric irradiation for gastric ulcer. *Gastroenterology* **56**: 816–817.
12. Clayman CB, Palmer WL and Kirsner TB (1968) Gastric irradiation in the treatment of peptic ulcer. *Gastroenterology* **55**: 403–407.
13. Cooper JN, Gelzayd EA and Kirshner JB (1968) Mild gastric fundal irradiation in the treatment of peptic esophagitis. *Gastroent Endosc* **14**: 222–224.
14. Kirsner JB (1964) Long-term evaluation of mild gastric irradiation as adjunctive therapy. *Am J Dig Dis* **9**: 726–728.
15. Brown CH, Sahba M and Levin E (1962) Irradiation with Cobalt 60 teletherapy in the treatment of complicated peptic ulcer. *Am J Gastroent* **38**: 278–289.
16. Eichorn RD, Wolever TH and Leite O (1961) New and expanded uses of gastric irradiation therapy. *South Med J* **54**: 662–665.
17. Teplitz R, Fox BW, Littman MS and Littman A (1961) In-

tragastric beta irradiation with Ru-RH[106] in human subjects: results with single doses. *J Nucl Med* **2**: 187-199.
18. Klein JC and Berman NE (1961) Gastric radiation-nonsurgical treatment for the surgical ulcer. *JAMA* **176**: 98-101.
19. Brown CH (1959) Therapeutic principles in management of peptic ulcer. *Am J Dig Dis* **4**: 1066-1072.
20. Kiefer ED and Smedal MI (1959) Radiation therapy for stoma ulcer occurring after subtotal gastrectomy. *JAMA* **169**: 447-451.
21. Brown CH and Hays RA (1957) Cobalt-60 teletherapy for complicated peptic ulcer. *Cleveland Clin Qrtly* **24**: 17-25.
22. Levin E, Clayman CB, Palmer WL and Kirsner JB (1957) Observations on the value of gastric irradiation in the treatment of duodenal ulcer. *Gastroenterology* **32**: 42-51.
23. Brown G and Wood IJ (1956) Treatment of chronic duodenal ulcer by antroduodenectomy and x-irradiation. *Lancet* **2**: 169-171,
24. Carpender JWJ, Leven E, Clayman CB and Miller RF (1956) Radiation in the therapy of peptic ulcer. *Am J Roent Rad Ther Nucl Med* **75**: 374-379.
25. Brown G and Wood IJ (1955) Antroduodenectomy and x-ray irradiation in the treatment of duodenal ulcer. *Australian and New Zealand J Surg* **24**: 260-267.
26. Brown G (1954) Surgical technique in the treatment of duodenal ulcer by antroduodenectomy and x-ray irradiation. *Br J Surg* **41**: 359-365.
27. Levin E, Palmer WL and Kirsner JB (1954) Observations on the diagnosis, treatment and course of gastric ulcer. *JAMA* **156**: 1383-1389.
28. Brown G, Scott RK, Homan WP, Wood IJ, Finckh ES, Weiden S and Davis P (1952) Antroduodenectomy and x-ray irradiation in the treatment of duodenal ulcer. *Lancet* **2**: 1145-1149.
29. McGeorge M (1950) Results of treatment of gastric hyperacidity by radium with special reference to duodenal ulceration. *Qrtly J Med* **19**: 111-128.
30. Ricketts WE, Palmer WL, Kirsner JB and Hamann A (1948) Radiation therapy in peptic ulcer: an analysis of results. *Gastroenterology* **11**: 189-805.
31. Holman WP and Lewis RA (1941) Some observations on the effects of selective irradiation on the stomach in cases of chronic nonobstructive duodenal ulcer with hyperchlorhydria. *Med J Aust* **2**: 735-740.

Perifolliculitis Capitis Abscedens et Suffodiens

Perifolliculitis capitis abscedens et suffodiens is an inflammatory scalp condition with folliculitis and perifolliculitis resulting from occlusion of the hair follicles and secondary bacterial infection. The disease spreads horizontally and forms sinus tracts, resulting in abscess formation, alopecia and scarring. To date only 50 patients in the American literature have been treated with epilating doses of irradiation. The mechanism of action of irradiation in controlling the chronic inflammatory process is unclear. Apparently, responses following scalp epilation are seen with temporary control of the inflammatory process. No long term data are provided. Thus, treatment with radiation should not be used generally, as data relating to long term efficacy and complication rates are *not* available. Grenz ray treatments have been used in the treatment of psoriasis of the scalp. Short term responses can be produced, but long term complications may outweigh its use. In the national survey 95% of radiation oncologists would not treat perifolliculitis.

Perifolliculitis Capitis Abscedens Radiotherapy

Investigator, Year	Cases	Site, Age	Treatment	Results	Notes
Kumar et al, 1976	4	Scalp; ages 22-37 yrs	300-600r using 85Kv machine with 1mm Al filter and 2mm Al HVL, using Kienbock-Adamson technic, or with a 4 Mev linear accelerator rotational treatment	Complete scalp epilation and pustular lesions subside Lesions subsided	Patients were all Blacks Duration of disease prior to x-ray epilation was 10 mos-8yrs All patients failed prior topical and systemic antibiotics Follow up of short duration 1 of 4 pts recurred
Johannesson and Lindelof, 1985	16	Psoriasis lesions of scalp; ages 27-71 yrs	Grenz ray: 11 Kv, 10mA, HVL, 0.03mm Al 4 Gy given on 6 occasions at 1 wk intervals	14/16(87.5%) complete healing on the grenz ray treated scalp after 6 weeks 9 pts were still free of lesions of scalp 3 mos after start of treatment Grenz rays were significantly better than placebo (p<0.0001)	Double blind trial One side of scalp received active treatment, the other side was treated with placebo

References

1. Kumar PP, Henschke UK and Kovi J (1976) Perifolliculitis capitis abscedens et suffodiens. *J Natl Med Assoc* **68**: 9-13.

2. Johannesson A and Lindelof B (1985) The effect of grenz rays on psoriasis lesions of the scalp: a double blind bilateral trial. *Photodermatol* **2**: 388-391.

Peyronie's Disease

The pathogenesis of this idiopathic penile disease is associated with pain, sexual dysfunction, penile deformity and single or multiple indurated plaques. Evaluation of the natural course of the disorder is made difficult by spontaneous resolution as well as by severe progression. It seems clear that relief of pain in disease of modest duration (5 months or less) can be accelerated by fractionated external radiation of 900-1200 rad. Using either external radiation or an isotopic mold for relief of deformity or resolution of induration, however, is less hopeful when the disease has been prolonged. Finally, there is some suggestion that a higher dose, 1200 rad, may enhance plaque resolution. Other issues of consideration are gonadal dose, gonadal protection, realistic expectation of results, and possible remission independent of the treatment. Patients should be fully informed of these facts, and the patient/physician understanding should be documented and accompanied by a detailed permission slip (see *Informed Consent*).

Peyronie's Disease

Author, Year	Total # Patients	Treatment/Results
Carson and Coughlin, 1985	40 patients: 32 patients failed vitamin E, or para-aminobenzoate	900r average 30 plaque (4 improved) 32 curvature (2 improved) 14 pain (4 improved) 2 erectile (no improvement) impotence
Alth, Koren, Gasser and Edler, 1985	636 patients 21% Dupuytren's	Radium mold, gonadal shield 6.6 to 8.2 Gy (Relief) Induration 70-85% Deviation 33-53% Pain 83-90%
Mira, Chabazian and del Regato, 1980	56 patients	1000-1400r CR PR Induration 6% 38% Curvature 5% 33% Pain 51% 28% (More than 5 months less benefit)
Tynan, 1976	12 patients: 2 worse (no Rx) 2 improved (no Rx) 8 patients treated	5/8 definite improvement 1-2 months

Peyronie's Disease Radiotherapy

Author, Year	Total # Pts.	Treatment	Results	Complications	Notes
Furlow et al, 1975	41	250–600r single dose (130Kv, HVL 0.3mm Cu-250Kv, HVL 1.5mm Cu) Field size: entire shaft of penis through a single dorsal port.	One treatment: 11/22 (50%) improvement of curvature 12/22 (55%) improvement of plaque Two treatments: 7/18 (39%) improvement of curvature 8/19 (44%) improvement of plaque		Improvement of painful intercourse or erections in average of 9 months.
	23	Other treatment (vitamin E, potassium para-aminobenzoate, steroids, radium therapy, or surgery), alone or in combination with orthovoltage radiotherapy.	18/23 (78%) improved		
	26	No treatment	12/23 (52%) improvement of curvature 15/26 (58%) improvement of plaque		Improvement of painful intercourse or erections in average of 16 months.
Bystrom et al, 1972	12	1200r (to central part of corpus of the penis) 7 days (140–170Kv, 4mm Al or 1/2 mm Cu plus 1mm Al, FSD, 40–50cm).	1/12 improved		
	7	Radiotherapy plus vitamin E	3/7 improved		
	17	Vitamin E alone	1/17 improved		
	11	Local cortisone injections (prednisolone) plus vitamin E	3/11 improved		
	30	Local cortisone injections alone	9/30 improved		
	7	No treatment	3/3 improvement of pain 2/5 improvement of curvature 5/7 improvement of plaque		
Helvie and Ochsner, 1972	40	900r/5 days (280Kv, 20ma, HVL 1.5mm Cu) Additional treatments of 300r at 4–6 wks to max of 2400r if clinically warranted. 3 pts received 900–1000r at 50Kv, 25ma, HVL, 75mm Al. Field direct anteroposterior port with field centered to plaque.	72% relief of pain 35% decreased size of plaque 29% decreased penile angulation.		13/16 (81%) who had previously received other forms of treatment improved.

Historical Data: Peyronie's Disease Radiotherapy

Author, Year	Total # Pts.	Treatment	Results	Complications	Notes
Martin, 1972	77	2100r/8 days (200–260Kv) If no improvement, second series in 4–7 months is advised.	26/77 (33.8%) completely cured. Of remaining 51: 43/51 (84.3%) relief of pain 32/51 (62.7%) improvement of curvature 39/51 (76.4%) improvement of plaque		17 well after 1 series, 10 were well in less than one year.
Feder, 1971	46	600–800r/4 F/10 days or 900–1200r/6–12 F/3 wks (250Kv, HVL 0.5mm Cu)	29/36 (80.5%) fair-good relief of pain 18/46 (39%) fair-good improvement of deformity.		
Dunlop and Lathem, 1969	23	1000r(air)/10F/ 10 weeks 220Kv, HVL 0.5mm Cu Field centered to plaque	21/23 (90%) decreased pain 15/23 (65%) angulation improved, plaque diminished		
Williams and Thomas, 1970	9	600–1600r/6 days	7/9 improved or cured		None showed improvement in less than 12 months.
	12	No treatment	9/12 improved or cured		
Aquino et al, 1967	32	700r single dose (Co^{60}) Special cube made of plaster and bolus material was used.	23/28 (82%) relief of pain 20/31 (64.5%) deformity improved 18/29 (62%) plaque diminished	Transient urethritis (1)	
Griff, 1967	17	600–1800r/3–6F (250Kv, HVL 1.85–2.05mm Cu) or radium mold treatment of 1500mg delivering 1200r to the skin in 10 hours.	8/9 relief of pain 3/9 decreased plaque formation.		
Duggan, 1964	87	800–1000r(skin)/4–5F/ 10–12 day (270Kv, 20ma, HVL 1.2mm Cu) Right and left lateral ports, one port treated daily. Second course given in 10 patients (400r to one port, 600r to the other in a total of 5 days).	High dose (46 pts): 83% symptom free or improved. Low dose (41 pts)		Average time for improvement was 6 months.
Ashworth, 1960	8	500r single dose repeated 2–3 times at intervals of a few months or 800–1000r/ 8–10F/8–10 weeks (250Kv)	1/8 normal function 3/8 relief of pain 4/8 no benefit		

Historical Data: Peyronie's Disease Radiotherapy (Continued)

Author, Year	Total # Pts.	Treatment	Results	Complications	Notes
	5	Cortisone	1/5 normal function 1/5 relief of pain		
	8	No treatment	None have normal function		

Historical Data: Peyronie's Disease Alternate Modes of Treatment

Author, Year	Total # Pts.	Treatment	Results	Complications	Notes
Chesey, 1975	23	Local corticosteroid (dexamethasone) injection	19/23 (83%) improved.		Response in 6–12 months.
	47	Local corticosteroid injections plus vitamin E	37/47 (79%) improved.		
	16	Local corticosteroid injections plus vitamin E plus Prednisolone.	15/16 (94%) improved.		
	79	Vitamin E	48/79 (61%) improved.		
	28	Vitamin E plus prednisolone	19/28 (68%) improved.		
	5	Surgical removal of plaques	2/5 improved.		Advised only when plaques are extensive and calcified.
	24	Procarbazine	15/24 (62.5%) improved.	Experimental evidence of damage to germinal epithelium.	Blood counts done weekly. Restrict use of drug to pts who do not plan a family.
Morales and Bruce, 1975	12	Intralesional injection of parathyroid hormone.	6/12 (50%) relief of pain 8/12 (66%) improvement of curvature 8/12 (66%) decreased size of plaque		
Oosterlinck and Renders, 1975	10	Procarbazine	1/10 completely cured.	Nervous tension and insomnia (1). Rash with edema of eyes and face and disturbance of equilibrium (1).	Regular blood counts.
Winter and Khanna, 1975	21	Dermo-jet injection of dexamethasone (6–10 injection). Patients return monthly for a total of six treatments.	18/21 (86%) relief of pain 16/21 (76%) improvement of curvature 16/21 (76%) improvement of plaque	Minimal discomfort and ecchymosis	71% of the patients had tried other methods and were unsuccessful.

Historical Data: Peyronie's Disease Alternate Modes of Treatment (Continued)

Author, Year	Total # Pts.	Treatment	Results	Complications	Notes
Devine and Horton, 1974	7	Surgical treatment with a dermal graft. Vitamin E for 3-6 months pre-op and 6 months-1 year post-op.	7/7 improvement to the degree that intercourse is possible.		All had disease refractory to other modes of treatment.
Bystrom et al, 1973	13	Excision and dermo-fat grafting.	10/13 good-excellent results	Minor haematomas (2) Slight flap necrosis (1) Urethritis (1) Impaired erection present, 6 months post-op in some patients.	Patients considered for operation should have a well circumscribed plaque and distinct angulation of the penis. Also should have previously tried some other form of therapy or be observed for 1/2-1 year before operation.
Poutasse, 1972	36	Surgical excision of plaque	All are able to accomplish satisfactory sexual relations	Numbness of gland (1) Flail penis (2)	All patients observed for at least one year prior to surgery.
Frank and Scott, 1971	25	Ultrasound (intensity of 1.5 watts/cm^2) Treatments on consecutive days except weekends (average of 12 treatments)	23/25 (92%) subjective improvement 19/25 (76%) decrease in plaque size		Earlier cases also received vitamin E
Tokus, 1971	5	Surgical exposure of plaque. Direct dermo-jet injection of triamcinolone acetate	5/5 improved		
Desanctis and Furey, 1967	14	Steroid (dexamethasone) injection	12/14 (85%) improved		
	6	Steroid injection plus vitamin E	6/6 improved		
	3	Steroid injection plus potassium para-aminobenzoate	3/3 improved		
Heslop et al, 1967	9	Ultrasound (intensity increasing to 3 watts/cm^2 for 10 min). Average of 6 treatments.	9/9 relief of pain 8/9 improvement of plaque	Superficial blistering (1)	
Persky and Stewart, 1967	13	Dimethyl sulfoxide external topical application.	6/13 improved	Garlic like odor of breath	
Rothfield and Murray, 1967	12	Iontophoresis of 21 esterified glucocorticoids	9/9 relief of pain 7/8 improvement of curvature 12/12 improvement of plaques		

References

1. Alth G, Koren H, Gasser G and Edler R (1985) On the therapy of indurated penis plastica by means of radium moulages. *Strahlentherapie* **161**: 30–34.
2. Carson CC and Coughlin PWF (1985) Radiation therapy for Peyronie's disease: Is there a place? *J Urol* **134**: 684–686.
3. Mira JG, Chabazian CM and del Regato JA (1980) The value of radiotherapy for Peyronie's disease: Presentation of 56 new case studies and review of the literature. *Int J Rad Onc Biol Phys* **6**: 1661–1666.
4. Tynan AP (1976) Peyronie's disease. *Brit J Urol* **48**: 151–152.
5. Martin CL (1972) Long time study of patients with Peyronie's disease treated with irradiation. *Amer J Roentgenol* **114**: 492–497.
6. Billing R, Baker R, Immergut M and Maxted W (1975) Peyronie's disease. *Urology* **6**: 409–419.
7. Chesey J (1975) Peyronie's disease. *Brit J Urol* **47**: 209–218.
8. Furlow WL, Swenson HE and Lee RE (1975) Peyronie's disease: A study of its natural history and treatment with orthovoltage radiotherapy. *J Urol* **114**: 69–71.
9. Morales A and Bruce AW (1975) The treatment of Peyronie's disease with parathyroid hormone. *J Urol* **114**: 901–902.
10. Oosterlinck W and Renders G (1975) Treatment of Peyronie's disease with procarbazine. *Br J Urol* **47**: 219–220.
11. Winter CC and Khanna R (1975) Peyronie's disease: Results with dermo-jet injection of dexamethasone. *J Urol* **114**: 898–900.
12. Devine CJ and Horton CE (1974) Surgical treatment of Peyronie's disease with a dermal graft. *J Urol* **111**: 44–49.
13. Bystrom J, Alfthan O, Johansson B and Korlof B (1973) Induratio penis plastica (Peyronie's disease). *Scand J Plast Reconstr Surg* **7**: 137–140.
14. Bystrom J, Johansson B, Edsmyr F, Korlof B and Nylen B (1972) Induratio penis plastica (Peyronie's disease). Scand J Urol *Nephrol* **6**: 1–5.
15. Helvie WW and Ochsner SF (1972) Radiation therapy in Peyronie's disease. *South Med J* **65**: 1192–1196.
16. Martin CL (1972) Long time study of patients with Peyronie's disease treated with irradiation. *Am J Roent Rad Ther Nucl Med* **114**: 492–497.
17. Poutasse EF (1972) Peyronie's disease. *J Urol* **107**: 419–422.
18. Feder BH (1971) Peyronie's disease. *J Am Geriat Soc* **19**: 947–955.
19. Frank IN and Scott WW (1971) The ultrasonic treatment of Peyronie's disease. *J Urol* **106**: 883–887.
20. Tokus E (1971) Peyronie's disease: A method of treatment. *J Urol* **105**: 523–524.
21. Williams JL and Thomas GG (1970) The natural history of Peyronie's disease. *J Urol* **103**: 75–76.
22. Dunlop JA and Lathem JE (1969) X-ray therapy in Peyronie's disease. *Southern Med J* **62**: 1485–1486.
23. McRoberts JW (1969) Peyronie's disease. *Surg Gynec Obstet* **129**: 1291–1294.
24. Aquino JA, Cunningham RM and Filbee JF (1967) Peyronie's disease. *J Urol* **97**: 492–493.
25. Desanctis PN and Furey CA Jr (1967) Steroid injection therapy for Peyronie's disease: A 10-year summary and review of 38 cases. *J Urol* **97**: 114–116.
26. Griff LC (1967) Peyronie's disease. The role of radiation therapy and a general review. *Am J Roent Rad Ther Nucl Med* **100**: 916–919.
27. Heslop RW, Oakland DJ and Maddix BT (1967) Ultrasonic therapy in Peyronie's disease. *Brit J Urol* **39**: 415.
28. Persky L and Stewart BH (1967) The use of dimethyl sulfoxide in the treatment of genitourinary diseases. *Ann NY Acad Sci* **141**: 551–554.
29. Rothfield SH and Murray W (1967) The treatment of Peyronie's disease by iontophoresis of C^{21} esterified glucocorticoids. *J Urol* **97**: 874–875.
30. Duggan HE (1964) Effect of X-ray therapy on patients with Peyronie's disease. *J Urol* **91**: 572–573.
31. Ashworth A (1960) Peyronie's disease. *Proc Roy Soc Med* **53**: 692–694.
32. Burford EH and Burford CE (1957) Combined therapy for Peyronie's disease. *J Urol* **78**: 265–268.
33. Dahl O (1954) The treatment of plastic induration of the penis (Peyronie's disease). *Acta Radiol* **41**: 290–301.
34. Reeves RJ (1953) Peyronie's disease. *NC Med J* **14**: 245–246.
35. Trostler IS (1948) Peyronie's disease. *Miss Valley Med J* **70**: 234.
36. Schourup K (1945) Plastic induration of the penis. *Acta Radiol* **26**: 313–323.

Pinealoma

This germ cell tumor is highly treatable by radiation; results are available in standard texts. Ninety-two percent of radiation oncologists would treat pinealomas according to the national survey.

References

1. Onoyama Y, Abe M, Takahashi M, Yahumoto E and Sakamato T (1975) Radiation therapy of brain tumors in children. *Rad* **115**: 687–693.
2. Sheline GE (1975) Radiation therapy of tumors of the central nervous system in childhood. *Cancer* **35**: 957–964.
3. Backlund E, Rahn T and Sarby B (1974) Treatment of pinealomas by stereotactic radiation surgery. *Acta Rad (Ther)* **13**: 368–376.
4. Tod PA, Porter AJ and Jamieson KG (1974) Pineal tumors. *Am J Roent Rad Ther & Nuc Med* **120**: 19–26.
5. Borden S, Wever AL, Toch R and Wang CC (1973) Pineal germinoma. Long term survival despite hematogenous metastases. *Am J Dis Child* **126**: 214–216.
6. Conway LW (1973) Stereotactic diagnosis and treatment of intracranial tumors including an initial experience with cryosurgery for pinealomas. J Neurosurg **38**: 453–460.
7. DeGiralami U and Schmidek H (1973) Clinicopathological study of 53 tumors of the pineal region. *J Neurosurg* **34**: 455–462.

8. Bradfield JS and Perez CA (1972) Pineal tumors and ectopic pinealomas. *Radiology* **103**: 399-406.
9. El-Mahdi Am, Philips E and Lott S (1972) The role of radiation therapy in pinealoma. *Radiology* **103**: 407-412.
10. Luccarelli G (1972) Ectopic pinealomas of the optic nerves and chiasms. Report of two personal cases. *Acta Neurochir* **27**: 205-221.
11. Cole H (1971) Tumors in the region of the pineal. *Clin Rad* **22**: 110-117.
12. Jamieson KG (1971) Excision of pineal tumors. *J Neurosurg* **35**: 550-553.
13. Kageyama N (1971) Ectopic pinealoma in the region of the optic chiasm. Report of five cases. *J Neurosurg* **35**: 755-759.
14. Stern WE, Batzdorf U and Rich JR (1971) Challenges of surgical excision of tumors in the pineal region. *Bull Los Angeles* Neurol Soc **36**: 105-118.
15. Suzuki J and Hori S (1969) Evaluation of radiotherapy of tumors in the pineal region of ventriculographic studies with iodized oil. *J Neurosurg* **30**: 595-603.
16. Poppen JL and Marino R (1968) Pinealomas and tumors of the posterior portion of the third ventricle. *J Neurosurg* **28**: 357-364.
17. Simson LR, Lampe I and Abell MR (1968) Suprasellar germinomas. *Cancer* **22**: 533-544.
18. Maier JG and DeLong D (1967) Pineal body tumors. *Am J Roent Rad Ther & Nuc Med* **99**: 826-832.
19. Matsuoka K & Uozumi T (1966) Long surviving cases of pineal body tumors treated by radiation. *Neruologia* **8**: 73-79.
20. Rubin P and Kramer S (1965) Ectopic pinealoma: A radiocurable neuro-endocrinologic entity. *Radiology* **85**: 512-523.
21. Suzuki J and Iwabuchi T (1965) Surgical removal of pineal tumors (pinealomas and teratomas): experience in a series of 19 cases. *J Neurosurg* **23**: 565-571.
22. Cummins FM, Taveras JM and Schlesinger EB (1960) Treatment of gliomas of the third ventricle and pinealomas. *Neurol* **10**: 1031-1036.
23. Horrax G (1950) Treatment of tumors of the pineal body. *Arch Neurol Psychiat* **64**: 227-242.

Pituitary Adenomas

These benign tumors cause endocrine abnormalities as well as mechanical injury such as blindness. Surgical decompression, resection and radiation therapy have become standard methods of treatment. Although this disorder will not be extensively reviewed, the following brief analysis of chromophobe adenoma is offered.

Headache, visual field loss, extraocular palsies and diabetes insipidus are manifestations that lead to consideration of treatment for this benign tumor. Currently, computer axial tomographs and magnetic resonance account for the majority of diagnostic evaluations. Surgery plus radiation may be expected to yield 96% recurrence-free survival. This tumor, although histologically benign, is treated with radiation due to its critical location. Attention is given to avoiding the orbit, delivering in 180 rad fractions 4500 rad by rotation, wedged arc rotation and multiple fixed fields. Fraction size and dose can also lead to injury, and must be carefully assessed. In the national survey, 97% of radiation oncologists would treat pituitary adenomas. Standard texts and references should be reviewed before treatment.

Pituitary Adenomas

Author, Year	Total Cases	Treatment	Results	Notes
Pistenma et al, 1975	62	1. Radiotherapy alone (29) 2. Post-op irradiation (33) Radiotherapy: 4400r/4.5wks to 7000r/7wks	Recurrence free after initial treatment: 1. 58.6% 2. 81.8% Total control: 1. 89.6% 2. 84.9%	
Berti et al, 1974	11	All pts treated surgically: (10) transcranial approach (1) stereotaxic transsphenoidal aspiration (3) Radiotherapy following surgery	3/11 total recovery 4/11 improved 2/11 improved (blindness right eye 1 pt; left optic nerve sacrificed at surgery 1 pt) 2/11 died 2 wks and 5 mos post-op.	Pituitary apoplexy (acute) hemorrhagic necrosis of a pituitary adenoma

Pituitary Adenomas (Continued)

Author, Year	Total Cases	Treatment	Results	Notes
Sheline, 1974	140	1. Radiotherapy alone 2. Surgery alone (surgical decompression with biopsy and partial removal of the adenoma) 3. Partial surgical resection plus radiotherapy	5 year determinate control rates: 1. 14/15 (93%) 2. 9/24 (38%) 3. 65/68 (96%)	Nonfunctioning chromophobe adenomas of the pituitary. Op mortality 8/37 (22%) in those pts treated by surgery alone
Wirth et al, 1974	160	1. Radiotherapy alone (17) 2. Surgery alone (66) 3. Post-op radiotherapy (77)	1. 11/17 subsequently underwent operation (3 required urgent surgical decompression) 2. 17/66 (25.8%) recurrences 3. 9/77 (11.7%) recurrences	Operation mortality 11%
Carlson and Marsh, 1971		1. Radiotherapy alone 2. Post-op irradiation Radiotherapy: 3160r/17 days to 5850r/76 days, Co-60	Overall control: 1. 85% 2. 83% Total overall control rate of 90% (4/8 patients responded to further surgery)	
Hayes et al, 1971		1. Radiotherapy alone (23) 2. Post-op irradiation (19) 3. Surgery alone (29) Radiotherapy: 4500-5000r/4.5wks	Success: 2-16 yr follow-up 1. 18/23 (78%) 2. 14/19 (74%) Recurrences: 1. 22% 2. 21%	Operation mortality 12.5%
Kramer, 1968		1. Radiotherapy alone (20) 2. Post-op irradiation Radiotherapy	1. 11/20 (55%) alive and well at 1-9 yr follow-up 2/20 recurrences 2. 31/39 (79%) 2/39 recurrences	
Chang and Pool, 1967	51	Radiation alone 4000-5000r	Percent and duration of visual improvement 78%	
Bouchard, 1966	56	1. Radiation alone 2. Post-op radiotherapy Radiotherapy: 4500-5000r/5-6wks	Success: 1. 20/28 (71%) 2. 25/28 (82%)	Operation mortality 3-5%

References

1. Fuks Z, Glatstein E, Marsa GW, Bagshaw MA and Kaplan HS (1976) Long term effects of external radiation on the pituitary and thyroid glands. *Cancer* 37: 1152-1161.
2. Pistenma DA, Goffinet DR, Bagshaw MA, Hanbery JW and Eltringham JR (1975) Treatment of chromophobe adenomas with megavoltage irradiation. *Cancer* 35: 1574-1582.
3. Berti G, Hersey WG and Dohn DF (1974) Pituitary apoplexy treated by stereotactic transsphenoidal aspiration. *Cleve Clin Qtly* 41: 163-175.
4. Sheline GE (1974) Treatment of nonfunctioning chromophobe adenomas of the pituitary. *Am J Roent Rad Ther Nuc Med* 120: 553-561.
5. Wirth FP, Schwartz HG and Schwetschenau PR (1974) Pituitary adenomas: factors in treatment. Clin Neurosurg 21: 8-25.
6. Kramer S (1973) Indications for and results of treatment of pituitary tumors by external radiation. In: Kohler PO and Ross GT (eds) Diagnosis and Treatment of Pituitary Tumors, New York Excerpta Medica: NY, p 217.
7. Carlson DH and Marsh SH (1971) Cobalt 60 teletherapy of pituitary adenomas. *Radiology* 98: 655-659.
8. Hayes TP, Davis RA and Raventos A (1971) The treatment of pituitary chromophobe adenomas. *Radiology* 98: 149-153.
9. Sheline GE (1971) Untreated and recurrent chromophobe adenomas of the pituitary. *Am J Roent Rad Ther Nuc Med* 112: 768-773.
10. Kramer S (1968) The value of radiation therapy for pituitary and parapituitary tumors. *Canad Med Assoc J* 99: 1120-1127.
11. Chang CH and Pool JL (1967) The radiotherapy of pituitary chromophobe adenomas. *Radiology* 89: 1005-1016.
12. Bouchard J (1966) Radiation Therapy of Tumors and Dis-

Plantar Fibromatosis

This condition is often associated with Dupuytren's contracture (see that section) and evidence for treatment is not convincing. Eighty percent of radiation oncologists in the national survey would not treat this disorder.

Plantar Fibromatosis

Author, Year	Total # Patients	Treatment	Results	Notes
Benninghoff and Robbins, 1954	1	Excision followed by 600r/2 weeks.	Right foot: Recurrence five years later. Additional 1300r given, free of recurrence for three years. Left foot: Recurrences six and eight years later (at different sites). 600r given in both instances.	No recurrence at four year follow up.
Stout, 1954	3	Excision.	2/3 recurred at six months in one and at seven years in the other.	All three cases were previously reported by Pickren. Authors stated that such growths remain small and symptomless and should probably be ignored after biopsy to prove that they are not malignant.
Pickren et al, 1951	16	Local excision (14).	13/14 recurred at two weeks to 4.5 years.	

References

1. Benninghoff D and Robbins R (1964) The nature and treatment of desmoid tumors. *Am J Roentg Rad Ther & Nuc Med* **91**: 132-137.
2. Stout AP (1954) Juvenile fibromatosis. *Cancer* **7**: 953-978.
3. Pickren JW, Smith AG, Stevenson TW and Stout AP (1951) Fibromatosis of the plantar fascia. *Cancer* **4**: 846-856.

Plasmacytoma (Solitary)

This localized malignancy may be cured by irradiation. Standard texts and references are available. Ninety-seven percent of radiation oncologists in the national survey would treat solitary plasmacytomas.

Plasmacytoma (Bone & Extramedullary)

Author, Year	Total # Patients	Treatment	Results	Notes
Dobson, 1975	1	Radiotherapy: 5500r/22F/ 5 weeks 6 Mev.	Complete clearing of the sinus and reconstruction of its bony walls.	Solitary extramedullary plasmacytoma of the head and neck.
Jacobson et al, 1975	10	Radiotherapy: 3500-5000r (tumor dose). Co^{60} or megavoltage irradiation period. If abnormal serum ^{M}component persisted for three months after radiation therapy, chemotherapy was administered until the patient was in complete remission. Two patients also had excision (partial or total) prior to radiotherapy.	Follow up of six months to seven years. 7/10 alive and in complete remission. 2/10 developed multiple myeloma, are alive and receiving chemotherapy. 1/10 died six months after onset of paraplegia from vertebral lesions.	Location of lesions: Ilium (3) Manubrium sterni (3) Maxilla or frontal bone (4) 5/5 serum and urine protein electrophoresis returned to normal after radiation therapy. Three patients developed myeloma at twenty-six months to seven years after presentation with solitary lesions.
Noorani, 1975	3	Radiotherapy: 1800r (middle ear tumor) to 4000r.	3/4 good response, no signs of recurrence. 1/4 unsatisfactory response, tumor was subsequently excised.	Plasmacytoma of the middle ear (1), nasal cavity (1), and nasal cavity and maxillary sinus (1>).
Kutcher et al, 1974	2	Surgery (partial excision) followed by radiotherapy 3000-4000r.	Both patients are alive with no evidence of systemic myeloma at two year follow up.	Plasmacytoma of the calvaria with dural involvement. One patient developed a left hemiplegia post-op which partially resolved.
Catalona and Biles, 1974	1	Laparotomy, post-operative radiotherapy to the right renal fossa followed by parenteral cyclophosphamide therapy.	No follow up.	Renal plasmacytoma. Patient had undergone temporal lobectomy followed by 3400r Co^{60} eight years previously for a plasmacytoma of the right temporal lobe.
Meyer and Shulz, 1974	12	Radiotherapy (11): 4000-5000r initially to the primary site. Surgical removal (1).	Radiotherapy: 4/11 recurred locally (all four patients had received an initial dosage of 3000r or less). 5/11 local control recurred at another site 2/11 local control, no recurrence at five years and twelve years following diagnosis. Surgery: Patient survived seven years with no evidence of dissemination. Died two years later of multiple myeloma.	Location of lesion: Vertebra (5) Pelvis (3) Femur (2) Rib (1) Scapula (1) 9/11 eventually developed multiple myeloma.

Plasmacytoma (Bone & Extramedullary) (Continued)

Author, Year	Total # Patients	Treatment	Results	Notes
Griffiths and Brown, 1974	1	Radiotherapy: 6000r/6 weeks/ to the larynx by opposing fields.	Slow tumor reponse. At three months after irradiation the biopsy showed no evidence of tumor. Follow up at three years showed no residual tumor and no evidence of systemic spread of disease.	Extramedullary plasmacytoma of the larynx.
Castro et al, 1973	21	Primary cases (15): 1. Resection of maxilla (5). 2. External radiation (orthovoltage and/or radon seed implants (7). 3. Chemotherapy alone (1) or plus radiotherapy (1). 4. Excision followed by radiotherapy (1). Secondary cases (6): 5. Resection of the maxilla plus orbital exenteration in one (5). 6. Coagulation/evacuation of tumor and radon implant and external radiation (orthovoltage).	Primary cases: 1. 4/5 died of generalized disease at six months, one year and five years. 2. 2/7 dead at two years of disseminated disease. 3/7 free of disease at 15-23 years. 2/7 died of other causes. 3. 2/2 died of disease at 2 years and 13 years. 4. Alive with disease at 18 months. Secondary cases: 5. 2/5 died of generalized disease at six months and eleven months. 1/5 no evidence of disease at 15 years. 1/5 died of other causes without evidence of disease at 13 years. 1/5 lost to follow up. 6. No evidence of disease at 13 years.	All were cases of plasmacytoma of the paranasal sinuses and nasal cavities.
Van Wart et al, 1973	1	Radiotherapy: 4800r	Patient presented with headache, abducens paralysis, and left nasal obstruction. After radiotherapy, vision returned to normal and no tumor was present at two year follow up.	Plasmacytoma of the paranasal sinuses.
Gromer and Duvall, 1973	6	1. Excision plus radiotherapy, 1800-4000r, (2 patients, 1 of these also received a short course of 5FU). 2. Radiotherapy only, 3500-4500r (2 patients). 3. Surgical excision only (2 patients).	1. One died of disease at 23 months. One is alive and free of disease at 15 years. 2. One died at nine months (autopsy showed retroperitoneal and mesenteric plasmacytoma, no local tumor was found). One is alive and free of disease at 8 years. 3. Both died of other causes.	Plasmacytoma of the head and neck.
Kotner and Wang, 1972	20	1. Radiotherapy (17): 2200-800r/14-85 days. 2. Surgery (2). 3. No treatment (1).	1. 9/17 (52%) alive without disease. 2/17 dead without disease. 2. 1/2 alive without disease. 1/2 dead with disease.	

Plasmacytoma (Bone & Extramedullary) (Continued)

Author, Year	Total # Patients	Treatment	Results	Notes
Davis and Drachman, 1972	2	Radiotherapy: 3750–4000r.	Remission of the neuropathy and myeloma for 10 and 1.5 years.	Solitary plasmacytoma associated with peripheral neuropathy. Location of lesions: Right acrominon process (1) Left humerus (1). Authors also include a review of the literature of plasmacytoma associated with neuropathy.
Panovich and Griem, 1972	1	Series of radiation treatment over a period of 24 years. Each treatment consisted of 1980–5091r. Second lesion (humerus) irradiated with three courses (1980–2600r each).	Initial lesion of the right ischium. Relief of pain after irradiation but lesion is still active after 30 years. Second lesion, of humerus, responded to irradiation and there is no evidence of recurrence.	Original lesion was of the right ilium. Patient also had a lesion of the left 7th rib which was not treated and remains unchanged. Other treated lesion was in the right humerus.
Remigio and Klaum, 1971	13	1. Surgical resection alone (7). 2. Surgical resection plus radiotherapy (3). 3. Radiotherapy only (1). 4. Biopsy only (1). Radiation doses: 1700–2500r.	1. 3/7 died of gastric plasmacytoma within 2.5 years. 3/7 died of post-op complications. 1/7 well at 8 years. 2. 1/3 died of disseminated disease at 16 months. 2/3 well at 7 months and 6 years (after recurrence at 5th year). 3. Died of disseminated disease at 5.5 years. 4. Died of post-op complications.	All were cases of extramedullary plasmacytoma of the stomach. One case report and review of twelve cases in the literature are given.
Toland and Phelps, 1971	1	Radiotherapy, 2500r to the tumor plus oral cyclophosphamide.	Condition remains unchanged two years later. No evidence of systemic disease.	Plasmacytoma of the skull base.
Touma, 1971	1	Primary treatment: Preoperative radiotherapy with radon seeds then surgery followed by radiotherapy, 2400r. Secondary treatment: Excision followed by radiotherapy, 5000r.	Free of symptoms for ten years. Then presented with second lesion which was treated by surgery and radiotherapy. Patient died of other causes nine years later with no evidence of disease.	Extramedullary plasmacytoma of the head and neck.
	1	Radiotherapy, 6000r, Co^{60}. Subtotal maxillectomy when lesion started to spread again.	Initial regression but lesion started to spread again. Uneventful post-op course. No long term follow up as yet.	
	1	Partial laryngectomy and right radical neck dissection followed by total laryngectomy three years later (to correct difficulty with aspiration).	No residual tumor was found at second operation.	
Someren et al, 1971	1	Surgical excision plus post-op radiotherapy, 3500r/4 weeks to the posterior fossa.	No recurrence or dissemination of disease at sixteen month follow up.	Solitary intracranial plasmacytoma involving the inner surface of the dura of the posterior fossa and the tentorium cerebelli.

Plasmacytoma (Bone & Extramedullary) (Continued)

Author, Year	Total # Patients	Treatment	Results	Notes
Rainer, 1970	2	Radiotherapy (6950r/51 days in one patient), no details on the other.	Case #1: Patient free of disease at 2.5 years. Case #2: Patient developed lesions at several other sites each treated by radiotherapy. Patient eventually died seven years after initial treatment.	Extramedullary plasmacytoma of the upper respiratory tract.
Rosenbaum et al, 1970	1	Surgery followed by radiotherapy 4000r/34 days.	Some diminution in proptosis, but the patient was blind in the involved eye. No evidence of dissemination at 2.5 years.	All three patients had plasmacytoma causing exophthalmos.
	1	Surgery followed by radiotherapy 3600r/5 weeks.	Symptoms recurred six months later. Patient lost to follow up.	
	1	Radiotherapy 2000r/12 days.	Proptosis resolved but patient died of systemic disease ten weeks later.	Patient had systemic disease and multiple bone lesions.
Chang and Jin, 1969	1	Surgical excision.	Patient well at three year follow up.	Solitary intracranial plasmacytoma extradural lesion of the right parietal lobe not involving the skull.
Maruyama and Thomson, 1970	1	Radiotherapy: First course, 2000r/11 days 250 Kv. Excision Second course, 4000r/4 weeks 250 Kv and Co^{60}.	Mass decreased in size and serum electrophoretic pattern returned to normal. Recurrence (different site) four years later treated by excision. Recurrence of original site four years later. Full regression of mass and return of serum following radiotherapy. Patient died suddenly four years later. Cause of death was not determined, but could have been due to myelomatosis.	Original lesion-sternal region. Recurrences: sternum and right clavicle sternal region.
	1	Excision plus post-op radiotherapy, 3000r/11 days, 250 Kv. Treatment of recurrences: Pre-op radiotherapy (1800r/8 days) followed by excision in one instance. All other recurrences treated by radiotherapy alone (4000r/18-29 days).	Recurrence eight years later. New lesions occurring eight years, seventeen years, nineteen years and twenty years following treatment of original lesions. Some response of gamma globulin level after each treatment. M peak disappeared completely following last treatment. No evidence of disseminated myelomatosis after twenty-one years.	Original lesion - right mandible and maxilla. Recurrences: Left upper alveolus and maxilla Manubrium sterni Right mandible Right proximal humerus
Chan and Tam, 1969	1	Radiotherapy: 4800r/42 days to nasal lesion. 3000r (central dose) 24 days to lower and left humerus.	Nasal region: Rapid relief of symptoms and subsidence of swelling. Humerus: Pain relieved and range of motion increased. Paper electrophoresis returned to normal.	Extramedullary plasmacytoma followed by skeletal lesions.

Plasmacytoma (Bone & Extramedullary) (Continued)

Author, Year	Total # Patients	Treatment	Results	Notes
Wey, 1969	1	Surgery followed by radiotherapy: 5000r, Co^{60}.	No recurrence at three years.	Plasmacytoma of the tonsils.
Poole and Marchetta, 1968	8	1. Excision plus radiotherapy (3). 2. Curettage plus radiotherapy (1). 3. Biopsy plus radiotherapy (4). Radiotherapy: Doses ranged from 2887r/44 days to 5400r/43 days. 200-250 Kv was used in four cases, 2 Mev used in three cases. Radium pack was used in one.	1. 1/3 alive with no evidence of disease at 2.5 years. 1/3 died with no evidence of disease at four years. 1/3 died of disease at 3.5 years. 2. Died of disease at 1.5 years. 3. 4/4 alive with no evidence of disease at 3.5-12 years.	All were cases of extramedullary plasmacytomas of the head and neck.
Valderrama and Bullough, 1968	6	Partial excision plus radiotherapy or radiotherapy alone. Radiotherapy: 2200-3400r.	5/6 alive and well without signs of dissemination 4-14 years after diagnosis. 1/6 scattered osteolytic lesions after 10 years.	Solitary myeloma of the spine.
Moossey and Wilson, 1967	1	Surgical excision. A series of complications necessitated four operations. Surgery was followed by radiotherapy 2260r/3 weeks.	Patient was asymptomatic at 4.5 years follow up.	Solitary intracranial plasmacytoma.
Graffman et al, 1967	1	High energy protons: 2000r/2F and x-rays, 3500r, 220 Kv.	Good tumor response.	Nasopharyngeal tumor.
Lindberg, 1966	5	1. Radiotherapy, 4000-5400r/38-51 days, 250-400 Kv (3 patients). 2. Surgical excision only (2 patients).	1. 3/3 no evidence of disease at 6, 10 and 16 year follow up. 2. One patient has no evidence of disease at 15 months. One patient died of intercurrent disease at 3 months.	Plasmacytoma of the head and neck.
Todd, 1965	30	Radiotherapy (x-rays, radium or both).	Five year survival: 18/30(60%) Dosage comparison: 2500r: 6/11(54%) residual or recurrent disease. 2500-3000r 1/6(17%) residual or recurrent disease. 3000r: 0/8(0%) residual or recurrent disesase.	Includes plasmacytoma of bone (9) Upper air passages (16) Other extramedullary sites (5)
Weiner et al, 1966	1	Surgery plus radiotherapy, 3400r, Co^{60}.	Post-op the patient had left hemiparesis, right ophthalmoplegia and left facial and sixth nerve palsies. In the year following radiotherapy, the patient had gradual improvement in neurologic status and there has been no evidence of extracranial myeloma or recurrence of the intracranial lesion.	Intracranial plasmacytoma of the base of the right middle fossa with nodules on both medial and lateral temporal lobe surfaces.

Plasmacytoma (Bone & Extramedullary) (Continued)

Author, Year	Total # Patients	Treatment	Results	Notes
Helmus, 1964	37	1. Surgery 2. Irradiation 3. Surgery plus irradiation.	Recurrences: 1. 9/13(69%) 2. 4/11(36%) 3. 9/13(69%)	Extramedullary plasmacytoma of the head and neck.
Batsakis et al, 1964	13	1. Radiation only (6) 2. Excision plus radiation (2). 3. Excision only (4). 4. Excisional biopsy (1).	1. 5/6 recurrences. 2. 2/2 recurrences. 3. 3/4 alive 3-5 years. 4. 1/1 recurrences.	Upper respiratory tract plasmacytoma.

References

1. Dobson TA (1975) Solitary extramedullary plasmacytoma of the head and neck. *Am Acad Opth & Otol* **80**: 472-274.
2. Jacobson RJ, Levy JI, Shulman G and deMoor NG (1975) Solitary myeloma: A study of black patients during an 8 year period. *S Africa Med J* **49**: 1347-1351.
3. Noorani MA (1975) Plasmacytoma of middle ear and upper respiratory tract. *J Laryng & Otol* **89**: 105-113.
4. Catalona WJ and Biles JD (1974) Therapeutic considerations in renal plasmacytoma. *J Urol* **111**: 582-583.
5. Griffiths C and Brown G (1974) Extramedullary plasmacytoma. *Canada J Otol* **3**: 81-85.
6. Kutcher R, Ghatak NR, and Leeds NE (1974) Plasmacytoma of the calvaria. *Radiology* **113**: 111-115.
7. Meyer JE and Shulz MD (1974) Solitary myeloma of bone. A review of 12 cases. *Cancer* **34**: 438-440.
8. Castro EB, Lewis JS and Strong EW (1973) Plasmacytoma of paranasal sinuses and nasal cavity. *Arch Otol* **97**: 326-329.
9. Gromer RC and Duvall AJ III (1973) Plasmacytoma of the head and neck. *J Laryng & Otol* **87**: 861-872.
10. Moazzenyadeh A, Potter RT, Castellaneta C, Westring D, Son YH and Perfetto JA (1973) Solitary plasmacytoma of sternum. *NY St J Med* **73**: 275-278.
11. Van Wart CA, Dedo HH and McCoy EG (1973) Carcinoma of the sphenoid sinus. *Ann Otol* **82**: 318.
12. Davis LE and Drachman DB (1972) Myeloma neuropathy. *Arch Neurol* **27**: 507-511.
13. Kotner LM and Wang CC (1972) Plasmacytoma of the upper air and food passages. *Cancer* **30**: 414-418.
14. Panovich AM and Griem ML (1972) Plasma cell myeloma. A thirty-year follow up. *Radiology* **104**: 521-522.
15. Remigio PA and Klaum A (1971) Extramedullary plasmacytoma of stomach. *Cancer* **27**: 562-568.
16. Someren A, Osgood CP and Brylski J (1971) Solitary posterior fossa plasmacytoma. *J Neurosurg* **35**: 223-228.
17. Toland J and Phelps PD (1971) Plasmacytoma of the skull base. *Clin Rad* **22**: 93-96.
18. Touma BYB (1971) Extramedullary plasmacytoma of the head and neck. *J Laryng & Otol* **85**: 125-130.
19. Chang SC and Jin BS (1970) Solitary plasmacytoma in the cranial cavity. *J Neurosurg* **33**: 471-474.
20. Maruyama Y and Thomson J Jr (1970) Radiotherapeutic response of plasma cell tumors associated with monoclonal gammopathy. *Cancer* **26**: 110-113.
21. Rainer EH (1970) Extramedullary plasmacytoma of upper respiratory tract. *J Larng & Otol* **84**: 909-919.
22. Rosenbaum AE, Zingesser LH, Reiss JH, Schechter MD and Sanders CD (1970) Myeloma: Unusual cause of exophthalmos. *Radiology* **94**: 379-386.
23. Chan KP and Tam CS (1969) Plasmacytoma. Report of a case. *Cancer* **23**: 694-698.
24. Wey WA (1969) Rare tumors of the tonsils. *EENT Monthly* **48**: 406-409.
25. Poole AG and Marchetta FC (1968) Extramedullary plasmacytoma of the head and neck. *Ca* **22**: 14-21.
26. Valderrama JAF and Bullough PG (1968) Solitary myeloma of the spine. *J Bone & Joint Surg Br* **50**: 82-90.
27. Graffman S, Nohrman BA and Juna BH (1967) Supplementary treatment of nasopharyngeal tumors with high energy protons. *Acta Rad* **6**: 361-368.
28. Moossy J and Wilson CB (1967) Solitary intracranial plasmacytoma. *Arch Neurol* **16**: 212-216.
29. Griffiths DL (1966) Orthopedic aspects of myelomatosis. *J Bone & Joint Surg Br* **48**: 703-728.
30. Lindberg R (1966) Unusual malignant tumors of the head and neck. *Radiology* **86**: 1090-1095.
31. Weiner LP, Anderson PN and Allen JC (1966) Cerebral plasmacytoma with myeloma protein in the cerebrospinal fluid. *Neurol* **16**: 615-618.
32. Todd IDH (1971) Treatment of solitary plasmacytoma. *Clin Rad* **16**: 395-399.
33. Batsakis JG, Fries GT Goldman RT and Karlsberg RC (1964) Upper respiratory tract plasmacytoma. *Arch Otol* **79**: 613-618.
34. Helmus C (1964) Extramedullary plasmacytoma of the head and neck. *Laryngoscope* **74**: 553-559.

Pterygium

Carefully administered radiation using a ^{90}strontium applicator can decrease recurrence of pterygium. A "wipe test" prior to application must assure the therapist of no ^{90}strontium shedding from the applicator. Treatment should be administered shortly after excision. Calibrate the ^{90}strontium source and calculate radiation doses to the conjunctiva and critical normal structures prior to treatment. Fractionated doses in the range not exceeding 1800 rad seem optimal. Radiation has been shown to decrease vascularization at the operative site, and thus decrease recurrence. Ninety-five percent of radiation oncologists in the national survey would treat pterygium of the eye.

Pterygium of the Eye Radiotherapy

Author, Year	Treatment	Results	Side Effects or Complications	Notes
Tong, Zaret and Rubenfelds, 1969	Excision followed by Sr^{90} treatment beginning 3-4 days post-op. 3000 reps in 3 fractions at weekly intervals to the surface of the conjunctiva.	8/78(10%) recurrences	21(27%) telangiectasis of the conjunctiva. 1 showed keratitis (had received 5000 reps to two adjacent fields)	
Cameron, 1965 and 1968	Excision immediately followed by 2,200r in one application (Sr^{90}) using 9 x 5mm applicator.	Primary cases: 75/83(96%) satisfactory Recurrent cases: 10/13(77%) satisfactory		Results were just as good with the 9 x 5mm applicator which irradiates only one fourth the area that the 10mm applicator does. Therefore, the 9 x 5mm applicator is preferred.
	Excision immediately followed by 2,200r in one application (Sr^{90}) using 16mm circular applicator	Primary cases: 48/57(84%) satisfactory Recurrent cases: 35/47(74%) satisfactory		
	Excision only.	8/81(10%) satisfactory		
	Excision followed by irradiation restricted to cut edge of conjunctiva only.	17/28(61%) satisfactory		Restriction of irradiation to cut edge of conjunctiva does not fully inhibit the regrowth. Therefore the bare area should be included.
Herbstein and Donovan, 1968	Excision immediately followed by 2,000r with Sr^{90} in a single application.	No recurrence		
Rowen, 1968	Excision followed within 24 hrs by 1,380r with Sr^{90} applicator. Treatment repeated in two weeks.	2/27(7.4%) recurrences		A third radiation treatment may be given if pterygium is especially vascular.
	Excision only.	17/46(37%) recurrences		

Historical Data: Pterygium of the Eye Radiotherapy

Author, Year	Treatment	Results	Side Effects or Complications	Notes
Von den Brenk, 1968	Excision followed by irradiation with Sr^{90} applicator according to one of the following techniques: 1. 1000r or 1750r single treatment given within 12 hrs post-op. 2. 1800r, 2000r or 3000r given in 2 fractions on post-op days 0 and 7. 3. 2400r, 3000r or 3600r given in 3 fractions on post-op days 0, 7 and 14. 4. 3200r given in 4 fractions on post-op days 0, 7, 14 and 21.	1. 3/7(43%) recurrences 2. 5/39(13%) recurrences 3. 14/1053(1.3%) recurrences 4. 0/1 recurrences	4/1000(0.4%) cases of scleral or corneal damage (scleral ulcer, scleral necrosis or corneal ulcer). All occurred with technique 3.	Best cosmetic results were obtained with 2400r in 3 fractions at weekly intervals. 5/349 or 1.4% recurrence rate.
Duggan, 1966	Excision followed by 1000-1200 rep Sr^{90}.	24/25 good results	Telangiectasis(1)	
	Radiation only (3 cases): 1. 1,000 rep. 2. 4,800 rep. 3. 10,104 rep.	3/3 good results		Possible that a very thin pterygium could be treated primarily by irradiation.
Haik, 1962 and 1966	Excision followed immediately by 900r (Sr^{90})	2/314(0.6%) recurrences		
	Excision followed immediately by 900r (Sr^{90})	0/249 recurrences		
	Excision followed immediately by 900r (50mg radium applicator)	2/131(1.5%) recurrences		
	Excision only	6/44(14%) recurrences		
Hilgers, 1966	Excision followed in most cases within 3 days by irradiation (Sr^{90}): 1. 1,000-3,000 rep. 2. 3,000-4,000 rep. 3. 5,000 rep. Irradiation dose at 1,700 rep in one treatment was never exceeded.	1. 7/33(21%) recurrences 2. 3/18(17%) recurrences 3. 1/32(3%) recurrences	1. Telangiectasis(1) 2. Telangiectasis(1) Irradiation vacuoles(3) Opacities(1) 3. Telangiectasis(3) Irradiation vacuoles(4) Opacities(2)	Surgical parotitis
Bernstein and Unger, 1960	Excision followed by irradiation of 3000-4000 rep. in 3-5 fractions at weekly intervals.	2/46(6.5%) recurrences		
	Excision only	16/27(59%) recurrences		

Historical Data: Pterygium of the Eye Radiotherapy (Continued)

Author, Year	Treatment	Results	Side Effects or Complications	Notes
Lentino et al, 1959	Excision followed within one week by 2500 reps, Sr^{90}. the majority of patients received two irradiation treatments at an interval of two weeks for a total of 5000 reps.	6/166(3.6%) recurrences	Telangiectasia of the conjunctiva in 50%. Keratinization of the conjunctival epithelium (1)	

Historical Data: Pterygium of the Eye Alternate Modes of Treatment

Author, Year	Treatment	Results	Side Effects or Complications	Notes
Kleis, 1973	Excision plus thiotepa solution (1: 2000) applied 6 wks after operation.	4/48(8.3%) recurrences		
	Excision only	15/48(31.3%) recurrences		
Asregadoo, 1973	Excision followed by thiotepa (1: 2000) for 6 wks post-op.	Primary cases: 6/89(6.7%) recurrences Recurrent cases: 1/13(7.7%) recurrences.	Depigmentation of skin of eyelids and cilia(2), black deposits in the cul de sac(1) in patients who had exposed themselves to sunlight for long periods while on medication.	
Cassady, 1966	Excision followed by thiotepa (1: 2000) within one day to one week post-op continued for 6-8 weeks.	0/17 recurrences		
Liddy and Morgan, 1966	Excision followed by thiotepa therapy beginning on 2nd post-op day and continuing for 6 wks.	1/23 recurrences		
Joelson and Muller, 1966	Excision followed by Thio-tepa (1: 2000) beginning on 2nd post-op day and continuing for 6 wks.	Primary cases: 1/32 recurrences Recurrent cases: 1/14 recurrences	Severe conjunctival hypertrophy(3) - disappeared after discontinuation of medication. Granuloma formation(1)	
	Excision only	3/11(27%) recurrences		
Trivedi, Massey and Rohatgi, 1969	Excision followed by graft with mucous membrane from the mouth.	0/140 recurrences		

Historical Data: Pterygium

Author, Year	Total Cases	Site and Age	Treatment	Results	Notes
Nowell, 1986	205	Conjunctiva and corneal surface of eye.	Excision with immediate pure beta irradiation 500–1000r before suturing conjunctiva. Strontium ^{90} application was used. Single application.	205 treated eyes, 2 pterygia have recurred (1.46% recurrence rate). Duration of follow-up 20 years.	Early surgical intervention. Irradiation used as part of the primary procedure and not reserved for recurrences only. No complications observed.
Monselise et al, 1984	169 (213 eyes)	Conjunctiva invading cornea of eye	Excision followed by corticosteriod and thiotepa, and later beta irradiation 600–2400r (most–1800r) administered in consecutive doses of 600r. First dose given within 3 days of excision.	Bilateral cases Recurrence rate: 2/60 eyes treated with beta rays 4/18 non-treated ($p<0.10$) Unilateral cases Recurrence rate: 8/73 eyes treated with beta rays 18/41 non-treated ($p<0.025$) TOTAL EYES Recurrence rate: 10/135 eyes treated with beta rays 22/61 non-treated ($p<0.05$)	The difference in the recurrence rate between the eyes submitted to beta rays (strontium ^{90} applicator), and those not, is statistically significant. No complications. Strontium applicator put on the limbus and sclera at excision site and did not cover cornea by more than 1–2mm of its surface. Beta irradiation, thiotepa, and corticosteriods all work by preventing vascularization at operative site, and thus prevent recurrence of pterygium.
Bahrassa and Datta 1983	69 (83 eyes)	Edge of cornea and surgical bed of the pterygium in the conjunctiva	Excision followed in 2–48 hours by beta irradiation. 1800–2200r is equivalent to the surgical site	Thirty-nine percent of non-irradiated eyes recurred; 5% of the irradiated eyes recurred.	Cataract occurred in 5% of irradiated eyes and 10% of non-irradiated eyes. Lens dose = 70–90r Retinal dose = 4–8r
Alaniz-Camino, 1982	483	Conjunctiva Ages: 14–76 years	Surgical excision followed by 2800r in 4–5 days using strontium applicator	Recurrence rate – 4.32%	Radiation within the initial 24 hours of surgical excision is most effective in decreasing recurrence rate. Ninety-nine percent of the cases involved the nasal (medial) part of the eye.
Tarr and Constable 1980	57 (63 eyes)	Conjunctiva Ages: 27–69 years (mean-48)	Excision followed by beta irradiation, 720–5200r (mean-3475)	Complications: Scleral ulceration – 51 eyes, lens opacities – 19 eyes, cataract with reduced vision – 3 eyes Endophthalmitis – 4 pts. Also: ptosis, symblepharon and iris atrophy.	Significant cause of iatrogenic ocular disease in this series demands a need to modify radiation technique, dose and dosimetry.

Historical Data: Pterygium (Continued)

Author, Year	Total Cases	Site and Age	Treatment	Results	Notes
Cooper and Lerch, 1980	403 (526 eyes)	Conjunctiva Age: 16–80 years	Excision followed by beta irradiation, 1860–3720r (most-2790r) in 3 equal fractions over 3 weeks.	Recurrences ranged from 7%–27%. Patient beginning radiation > 4 days after surgery had fewer recurrences than those irradiated within 3 days of surgery.	Results regarding timing of irradiation in this study are at variance with other series.
Pinkerton, 1979	(975 eyes)	Conjunctiva	Excision and immediate strontium ^{90} application <3000r	Recurrence rate 6%	20 year follow-up. A survey and individual author's opinion.
Rahman et al, 1979	25 (28 eyes)	Conjunctiva Age: 30–75 years Average: 55 years	Excision and beta radiation beginning immediately after surgery. Dose – 3750r given over 4 weeks in 5 weekly 750r fractions.	Recurrence rate 3.5%	
Cooper, 1978	403 (526 eyes)	Conjunctiva Age: 16–80 years	"Bare sclera" excision followed by Sr^{90} beta irradiation	Recurrence 32/272(12%) 80% of the failures were salvaged by a second course of treatment.	50% of the recurrences occurred > 1 year after treatment, 25% of these were after 2 years of treatment. Long term follow up is essential.
Ozarda, 1977	211	Conjunctiva	Surgical excision followed by Sr^{90} beta ray therapy. Started within 24 hours post-operatively.	Recurrence rate: 1 in 211(<0.5%)	No apparent complications, follow-up in at least 6 months.

References

1. Nowell JF (1986) Management of pterygia 20 years later. *South Med J* **79**: 1382–1384.
2. Monselise M, Schwartz M, Politi F and Barishak YR (1984) Pterygium and beta irradiation. *Acta Ophthalmol* **62**: 315–319.
3. Bahrassa F and Datta R (1983) Postoperative beta radiation treatment of pterygium. *Int J Radiat Oncol Biol Phys* **9**: 679–684.
4. Alaniz-Camino F (1982) The use of postoperative beta radiation in the treatment of pterygia. *Ophthalmic Surg* **13**: 1022–1025.
5. Tarr KH and Constable J (1980) Late complications of pterygium treatment. *Br J Ophthalmol* **64**: 496–505.
6. Cooper JS and Lerch IA (1980) Post-operative irradiation of pterygium: an unexpected effect of the time/dose relationship. *Radiology* **135**: 743–745.
7. Pinkerton OD (1979) Surgical and strontium treatment of pterygium: recurrence and lens changes. Age statistics. *Ophthalmic Surg* **10**: 45–47.
8. Rahman SM, Chung CK and Constable WC (1979) Post-operative beta irradiation in the treatment of pterygium. *South Med J* **72**: 823–826.
9. Cooper JS (1978) Postoperative irradiation of pterygia: Ten more years of experience. *Radiology* **128**: 753–756.
10. Ozarda AT (1977) Evaluation of post excisional strontium^{90} beta ray therapy for pterygium. *South Med J* **70**: 1304.
11. Kleis W and Pico G (1973) Thio-tepa therapy to prevent postoperative pterygium occurrence and neovascularization. *Am J Ophth* **76**: 371–372.
12. Asregadoo ER (1973) Thio-tepa, and corticosteriod in the treatment of pterygium. *Am J Ophth* **74**: 960–963.
13. Cameron ME (1973) Preventable complications of pterygium excision with beta-irradiation. *Brit J Ophth* **56**: 52–56.
14. Tong EKC, Zaret MM and Rubenfelds S (1969) Cellular changes in the conjunctiva after strontium 90 treatment for pterygium. *Am J Roent Rad Ther & Nuc Med* **106**: 848–853.
15. Trivedi LK, Massey DB and Rohatgi R (1969) Management of pterygium and its recurrence. *Am J Ophth* **68**: 353–354.
16. Cameron ME (1968) Beta-irradiation of pterygia. *Brit J Ophth* **52**: 562–563.
17. Herbstein AV and Donovan JK (1968) Pterygium removal. *Br J Ophth* **52**: 162–165.
18. Rowen GE (1968) Pterygium - surgical excision followed by beta irradiation. *Rocky Mt Med J* **65**: 47–49.
19. Von den Brenk HAA (1968) Results of prophylactic post-

operative irradiation in 1,300 cases of pterygium. *Am J Roent Rad Ther & Nuc Med* **103**: 723-733.
20. Cassady JR (1966) The inhibition of pterygium by thio-tepa. *Am J Ophth* **61**: 886-888.
21. Duggan HE (1966) Results using the strontium [90] beta-ray applicator on eye lesions. *J Canad Ass Radiol* **17**: 132-137.
22. Haik GM (1966) The management of pterygia. *Am J Ophth* **61**: 1128-1134.
23. Hilgers JH (1966) Strontium[90], b-irradiation, cataractogencity and pterygium recurrence. *Arc Ophth* **76**: 329-333.
24. Joelson GA and Muller P (1966) Incidence of pterygium recurrence. *Am J Ophth* **61**: 891-892.
25. Liddy BSL and Morgan JF (1966) Triethylene thiophosphoramide (thio-tepa) and pterygium. *Am J Ophth* **61**: 888-890.
26. Cameron ME (1965) Pterygium throughout the world. Springfield, IL: Thomas Press
27. Haik GM, Ellis GS and Nowell JF (1962) The management of pterygia with special reference to surgery combined with beta irradiation. *Tr Am Acad Ophth Otolaryng* **66**: 776-784.
28. Bernstein M and Unger SM (1960) Experiences with surgery and strontium[90] in the treatment of pterygium. *Am J Ophth* **49**: 1024-1029.
29. Lentino W, Zaret MM, Rossignol B and Rubenfeld S (1959) Treatment of pterygium by surgery followed by beta radiation. *Am J Roent Rad Ther & Nuc Med* **81**: 93-98.
30. Lederman M (1957) Radiotherapy of non-malignant diseases of the eye. *Brit J Ophth* **41**: 1-19.

Pyogenic Granuloma

Pyogenic granuloma often of the middle ear is a benign proliferation of newly formed capillaries associated with inflammatory infiltrate. It should be managed by local surgical excision and/or electrocautery. There is no scientific evidence of the value of radiation therapy in this disorder. Ninety-six percent of radiation oncologists in the national survey would not treat pyogenic granuloma.

Pyogenic Granuloma of the Middle Ear

Author, Year	Total # Pts.	Site and Age	Treatment	Results	Notes
Aristizabal SA and Runyon TD, 1981	1	Middle ear, 64 years	2000r/10 fractions, 23 days	No evidence of disease, normal hearing @ 4 years, 4 months.	

Reference

1. Aristizabal SA and Runyon TD (1981) Radiotherapy of unusual benign disease. *Int J Radiat Oncol Biol Phys* **7**: 1437-1440.

Salivary Gland Adenoma

There is very limited published experience using radiotherapy in addition to surgical excision for benign tumor of the salivary glands. Conclusions drawn in regard to local control and/or malignant transformation remain speculative. In the national survey, 73% of the radiation oncologists would not treat salivary gland adenomas.

Salivary Gland (Pleomorphic Adenoma)

Author, Year	Total # Pts	Site, Age	Treatment	Results	Notes
Watkin and Hobsley, 1986	65; 17 given radiotherapy	parotid gland 14–62 years (mean age 33.5 years)	Radiotherapy either first local excision (primary XRT), or following later recurrence (secondary XRT) 4500–6000cGy (2 pts brachytherapy)	44% of irradiated patients developed local recurrence within first 5 years, not different from the 50% recurrence rate among those who did not undergo post-operative radiotherapy	All recurrent pleomorphic adenomas of the parotid gland 2/17 irradiated patients developed malignant transformation of their tumors Non-randomized study
Dawson and Orr, 1985	311	parotid gland 11–78 years	Surgery (local excision) and irradiation 5500–6000cGy via radium needle implant or 4meV linear accelerator	1–1.5% recurrence rate at 0–5, 5–10 years (benign recurrence) 8% cumulative risk of recurrence at 20 years (mostly malignant tumors)	All primary pleomorphic adenomas of the salivary gland Malignant transformation occurs as a late event
Armitstead et al, 1979	76	parotid gland 12–83 years	Extracapsular enucleation and irradiation Co-60, linear accelerator 4800r/3wks	1/76 recurred with a malignant tumor	All primary pleomorphic adenomas of the parotid gland Median follow up is not provided

References

1. Watkin GT and Hobsley M (1986) Influence of local surgery and radiotherapy on the natural history of pleomorphic adenomas. *Br J Surg* **73**: 74–76.
2. Dawson AK and Orr JA (1985) Long-term results of local excision and radiotherapy in pleomorphic adenoma of the parotid. *Int J Radiat Onc Biol Phys* **11**: 451–455.
3. Armitstead PR, Smiddy FG and Frank HG (1979) Simple enucleation and radiotherapy in the treatment of the pleomorphic salivary adenoma of the parotid gland. *Br J Surg* **66**: 716–717.

Sarcoidosis

Sarcoidosis is predominantly managed by medical means if it causes significant symptoms. Steroids, when used in the management, are not without serious sequelae. A series of lesions in atypical sites such as the brain, larynx and penis can lead to significant medical morbidity and may be life threatening. The limited available literature indicates objective responses both by physician report and radiologic evaluation with the use of 3000 rad. Thus, we conclude that should primary medical treatment fail to induce a remission in critical sites, the use of radiation would remain appropriate. In the national survey, ninety-two percent of radiation oncologists would not treat sarcoidosis.

Sarcoidosis

Author, Year	Total # Pts.	Sex/Age	Treatment	Results	Notes
Bejar et al, 1985	1 (CNS)	Male Age 44 years.	3000r in 300r fractions.	Complete resolution of radiographic findings with signs and symptoms. Author recommends XRT when steroids fail.	Neurosarcoidois. One year follow-up.

Sarcoidosis (Continued)

Author, Year	Total # Pts.	Sex/Age	Treatment	Results	Notes
Fogel et al, 1984	1 (Larynx)	Male Age 36 years.	3000r in 30r fractions.	Complete resolution sixteen months after treatment. Confirmed by tomograms.	Larynx involvement refractory to steroids.
Grizzanti et al, 1982	1 (CNS)	Male Age 26 years.	Whole brain radiation, 1000r in 200r fractions.	Responded dramatically. Died one year later of other causes. Had fibrotic granuloma in brain.	Sarcoid meningitis. Refractory to steroids.
Whittaker et al, 1975	1 (Penis)	Male Age 59 years.	Partial amputation and steroids with recurrence in one month. Given 3200r to penile stump.	Dramatic improvement.	One year follow-up.

References

1. Bejar JM, Kerby GR, Ziegler DK and Festoff BW (1985) Treatment of central nervous system sarcoidosis with radiotherapy. *Annals of Neurology* **18**: 258–260.
2. Fogel TD, Weissberg JB and Dobular KA (1984) Radiotherapy in sarcoidosis of the larynx: Case report and review of the literature. *Laryngoscope* **94**: 1223–1225.
3. Grizzanti JN, Knapp AB, Schecter AJ and Williams MH (1982) Treatment of sarcoid meningitis with radiotherapy. *Am J Med* **73**: 605–608.
4. Whittaker M, Anderson CK and Clark PB (1975) Sarcoidosis of the penis treated by radiotherapy. *Br J Urol* **47**: 325–330.

Skin Disorders

Superficial x-rays and grenz rays were commonly used in the past to treat a multitude of benign and inflammatory skin conditions including lichen simplex chronicus, lichen planus, pruritis ani, pruritus vulvae, seborrheic dermatitis, hidradenitis suppurativa, chronic eczema and psoriasis. Data regarding the effectiveness of this dermatologic treatment in the modern era are very sparse to nearly non-existent, and often accompanied by statements which are empirical. Alternative effective therapies are now available for many of these conditions with few exceptions. Grenz-ray therapy (5–20Kv) has limited penetration and thus is not associated with systemic risk if proper radiation safety measures and dose limits are used. Low energy orthovoltage has been utilized in the treatment of some of these disorders as well, although the use of such irradiation in these patients has not been associated with results warranting its general use.

In the national survey 96% of radiation oncologists would not treat eczema with radiation; 98% would not treat contact dermatitis, pruritis ani et vulvae or lichen planus; 98% would not treat granuloma annulare, pityriasis rosea or seborrheic keratosis; 78% would not treat hidradenitis suppurativa; 94% would not treat psoriasis; and 95% would not treat folliculitis barbae.

Skin Disorders

Historical Data: Lichen Simplex Chronicus

Author, Year	Total # Pts.	Site and Age	Treatment	Results	Notes
Jansen, 1978			Using grenz rays (depth 0.2–0.8mm) 150–300r weekly or twice monthly for 3–4 exposures. The schedule may be repeated after 6 months. Doses below 5000r.	No data. Author's opinion that it is effective.	Jansen recommends this therapy for: Pruritus ani et vulrae Seborrheic dermatitis Nummular eczema Dyshidrosis Persistent eczema Psoriasis Lichen planus

Historical Data: Paronychia

Author, Year	Total # Pts.	Site and Age	Treatment	Results	Notes
Jansen, 1978				No data	Jansen does not consider grenz ray treatment appropriate.

Historical Data: Pruritus Ani et Vulvae

Author, Year	Total # Pts.	Site and Age	Treatment	Results	Notes
Jansen, 1978			Grenz rays 150–300r weekly or twice monthly for 3–4 exposures. May be repeated after 6 months. Keep total dose < 5000r	No data. Author's opinion is that it is effective.	Author recommends some therapy for: Lichen simplex chronicus Seborrheic dermatitis Nummular eczema Dyshidrosis Persistent eczema Psoriasis Lichen planus

Historical Data: Lichen Planus

Author, Year	Total # Pts.	Site and Age	Treatment	Results	Notes
Jansen, 1978			Grenz rays 150–300r weekly or twice monthly for 3–4 exposures. Total dose < 5000r, depth 0.2–0.8mm tissue.	No data. Author's opinion is that it is effective.	Jansen recommends some therapy for: Lichen simplex chronicus Pruritus ani et vulvae Seborrheic dermatitis Nummular eczema Dyshidrosis Persistent eczema
Lukacs et al, 1978			Grenz rays 200–300r given in 3–4 fractions of 75–150r at weekly intervals.	No data. Author recommends for severely pruritic refractory cases, particularly verrucous forms of lichen planus.	

Historical Data: Seborrheic Dermatitis

Author, Year	Total # Pts.	Site and Age	Treatment	Results	Notes
Jansen, 1978			Grenz rays 150–300r weekly or twice monthly for 3–4 exposures. Total dose < 5000r.	No data. Author's believes treatment is effective.	Author recommends same therapy for: Lichen simplex chronicus Pruritus ani et vulvae Nummular eczema Dyshidrosis Persistent eczema Lichen planus

Historical Data: Eczema

Author, Year	Total # Pts.	Site and Age	Treatment	Results	Notes
Fairris et al, 1985	25	(lesions on hands)	300r superficial x-ray vs 900r grenz rays.	300r superficial x-ray superior to 900r grenz rays by both patient and physician evaluation at 12 weeks.	Patients resistant to topical treatment; double-blind trial
Fairris et al, 1984	14	(lesions on feet)	100r on 50Kv x-ray vs placebo with continual topical therapy to both feet	No statistical improvement in irradiated group as compared to controls.	Double-blind trial
Lukacs et al, 1978	46		75–100r at weekly intervals over 3–4 weeks. Total dose < 1000r superficial x-rays or < 5000r grenz rays.	34 of 46(74%) improved 9 recurred 7 no improvement	
Jansen, 1978			150–300r weekly or twice monthly; scheme may be repeated; total dose < 5000r grenz rays (depth 0.2–0.8mm)	No data. Author feels it is effective therapy. Particularly nummular eczema	

Historical Data: Psoriasis

Author, Year	Total # Pts.	Site and Age	Treatment	Results	Notes
Dabski and Stoll, 1986	1	Psoriatic plaques, 30 years	Grenz rays 8–10Kv and 10mA 200r given at 2–4 week intervals. Total dose – approximately 3000r to a single skin area over 20 years.	Developed 5 squamous cell carcinomas within 7 years following a 16 year period of grenz irradiation for psoriasis.	
Johannesson and Lindelof, 1985	16	Skin-symmetrical lesions (scalp) 27–71 years	4 Gy Grenz rays applied on 6 occasions at 1 week intervals vs placebo. X-ray: 11Kv, 10mA, 0.03mmA1 HVL, 20SSD, beryllium window	14/16(87%) healed completely. Significant improvement over placebo (p < 0.0001) 9 of 14 pts free from relapse 3 mos no prescription. 3 pts healed @ 6 mos.	A double-blind bilateral trial.

Historical Data: Psoriasis (Continued)

Author, Year	Total # Pts.	Site and Age	Treatment	Results	Notes
Schothorst et al, 1984	68	Skin, mean ages: 34-44 yrs.	High output UV-B radiation generated with Sylvania UV-6 or UV-21 tubes, maximal exposure time of 5 minutes per session.	80% of patients cleared of lesions. No difference in time to clearing, percentage of lesions improved, etc.	A controlled trial.
Brodersen and Reymann, 1981	20	Skin with symmetrical lesions. 20-60 years	Systemic steroids and either grenz ray, 12Kv, treatment of 1/2 lesions, or sham radiation. Radiation was 150r three times 1 week at weekly intervals.	Treatment with local steroids plus grenz rays was significantly better than steroids alone ($p < 0.005$).	Double-blind study.
Jansen, 1978			Grenz rays 150-300r weekly or twice monthly for 3-4 exposures. Total dose < 5000r.	No data	Author recommends same therapy for: Lichen simplex chronicus Lichen planus Pruritus ani et vulvae Seborrheic dermatitis Eczema Dyshidrosis
Lukacs et al, 1978	75		Grenz rays 200-300r in 3-4 fractions of soft x-rays 75-100r in weekly intervals. Total dose < 1000r.	42 of 75 improved 22 improved but recurred 18 no improvement	Main indication is involvement of nails

Historical Data: Hidradenitis Suppurativa

Author, Year	Total # Pts.	Site and Age	Treatment	Results	Notes
Lukacs et al, 1978			Superficial x-rays 40-80r at 1-2 day intervals.	No data	Use in combination with antibiotics.
Jansen, 1978			Grenz rays 150-300r weekly or twice monthly for 3-4 exposures	No data, but author considers it effective therapy.	For dyshidrosis

References

1. Dabski K and Stoll HL (1986) Skin cancer caused by grenz rays. *J Surg Oncol* **31:** 87-93.
2. Goldschmidt H (1986) Dermatologic radiotherapy. The risk-benefit ratio (editorial). *Arch Dermatol* **122:** 1385-1388.
3. Fairris GM, Jones DH, Mack DP and Rowell NR (1985) Conventional superficial x-ray versus grenz ray therapy in the treatment of constitutional eczema of the hands. *Br J Dermatol* **112:** 339-341.
4. Johannesson A and Lindelof B (1985) The effect of grenz rays on psoriasis lesions of the scalp: A double blind bilateral trial. *Photodermatol* **2:** 388-391.
5. Eells LD, Wolff JM, Garloff J and Eaglstein WH (1984) Comparison of suberythemogenic and maximally aggressive ultraviolet B therapy for psoriasis. *J Am Acad Derm* **11:** 105-110.
6. Fairris GM, Jones DH, Mack DP and Rowell NR (1984) Superficial x-ray therapy in the treatment of constitutional eczema of the feet (letter). *Br J Dermatol* **111:** 500-502
7. Schothorst AA, Boer J, Suurmond D and Kenter CA (1984) Application of controlled high dose rates in UV-B phototherapy for psoriasis. *Br J Dermatol* **110:** 81-87.
8. Boer J, Schothorst AA and Suurmond D (1981) Influence of UVA on the erythematogenic and therapeutic effects of UVB irradiation in psoriasis; photoaugmentation effects. *J Invest Dermatol* **76:** 56-58.

9. Brodersen I and Reymann F (1981) Effect of grenz rays on psoriasis treated with local corticosteroids. *Dermatologica* **162**: 327–329.
10. Goldschmidt H (1980) FDA recommendations on ionizing radiation therapy of benign diseases [editorial]. *J Am Acad Dermatol* **3**: 307.
11. Lavery HA and Burrows D (1980) PUVA therapy for psoriasis and other skin diseases. An initial report. *Ulster Med J* **49**: 48–53.
12. Goldschmidt H (1978) FDA recommendations on ionizing radiation therapy of benign diseases. *J Dermatol Surg Oncol* **4**: 619.
13. Jansen GT (1978) Grenz rays: Adequate or antiquated? *J Dermatol Surg Oncol* **4**: 627–629.
14. Lukacs S, Braun-Falco O and Goldschmidt H (1978) Radiotherapy of benign dermatoses: Indications, practice and results. *J Dermatol Surg Oncol* **4**: 620–625.
15. A review of the use of ionizing radiation in the treatment of benign diseases. US Dept of Health, Education, and Welfare [publication]. Public health Service, 78-8043.

Therapeutic Castration

The use of therapeutic castration by radiation has diminished in the last decade due to effects such as irregular and slower hormonal decrease compared to surgery. However, it may be used if appropriate in special circumstances in the advanced breast cancer patient. Seventy-five percent of radiation oncologists would treat for therapeutic purposes in the national survey.

Castration

Author, Year	Total # Patients	Treatment	Results	Notes
Nissen-Meyer, 1967	112	Prophylactic Castration: Premenopausal poor risk patients: 1. Ovarian irradiation 2. Oophorectomy	Premenopausal poor risk patients: 1. Ovarian irradiation. 62% free of disease at 5 years*. 71% crude survival*. 2. Oophorectomy 54% free of disease at 5 years*. 68% crude survival*. *These values were taken from the author's graphs. The differences are not significant.	Randomized prospective study showed no difference either in irradiation or surgical castration in poor risk premenopausal patients. Prophylactic versus therapeutic castration showed benefit in post-menopausal stage two patients.
Kennedy and Fortuny, 1964	177	Therapeutic Castration: 1. Ovarian irradiation (123 patients). 2. Bilateral ovariectomy (54 patients). Of the total number of patients, 177 were premenopausal, seven with vaginal smear estrogen activity within five years of menopause.	Responders (objective remission): 1. Irradiation: 56/123(45.5%). 2. Ovariectomy 28/54(51.8%) Mean duration 18 months, median 12 months.	Previous study by the same author showed no advantage to prophylatic versus therapeutic castration.
Block et al, 1960	60	Therapeutic Castration: 1. Irradiation (14 patients). High voltage irradiation. 625–1100r/10 days or less. 2. Oophorectomy (46 patients).	Objective remission: 7/14(50%) irradiation group 12/46(28.4%) oophorectomy group. Subjective remission: 8/14(57.1%) irradiation group 16/46(34.7%) oophorectomy group	Non-randomized series with small numbers of patients which seems to favor irradiation castration.

Historical Data: Castration

Author, Year	Total # Patients	Treatment	Results	Notes
Treves, 1957	152	Prophylactic Castration: 1. Ovarian irradiation (84 patients). Dose range of 300–1899r, majority in the range 1000–1499r. 2. Oophorectomy (68 patients).	Five year survival: 54.4% controls 58.1% irradiation castration 79.4% oophorectomy Ten year survival: 33.8% controls 42.3% irradiation castration 58.3% oophorectomy Interval between castration and recurrence: 19.6 months in irradiated series 25.3 months in oophorectomy series Interval between mastectomy and recurrence: 23.3 months in irradiated series 32.7 months in oophorectomy series	There is a statistical difference between the controls and the surgically castrated at five years, becoming more marked at ten years. Irradiation castrated patients benefited most at ten years but not as much as those who were surgically castrated.
Smith and Smith, 1953		Prophylactic Castration: 1. Ovarian irradiation (41 patients). Twenty patients with positive nodes. 2. Surgical castration (60 patients). Twenty-three patients with positive nodes.	Five year survival (Overall results): 75% surgically castrated* 46% not castrated* Five year survival (Patients with axillary metastases): 75% surgically castrated* 40% irradiation castrated 31% not castrated* Five year survival (Patients without axillary metastases): 82% surgically castrated* 76% not castrated* *These values were taken from the authors' graphs.	Authors give no figures but state that the 10 and 15 year survival rates for the irradiation castrated group are the same as for the surgical group.
Douglas, 1952	184	1. Ovarian irradiation (175 patients) 700–800r/1 week. 2. Surgical castration plus testosterone (9 patients).	1. Ovarian irradiation. 36/175(21%) favorable response. 2. Surgical castration. 1/9 slight response.	
Adair et al, 1945	335	1. Irradiation (high voltage x-rays or intrauterine radium) (304 patients). 2. Surgical castration (31 patients).	1. Irradiation Castration. 47/304(15%) improved. 57/304(19%) uncertain. 200/304(66%) no improvement. 2. Surgical Castration. 4/31(13%) improved. 7/31 uncertain. 20/31(64%) no improvement.	

References

1. Fisher B (1973) Cooperative clinical trails in primary breast cancer: A critical appraisal. *Cancer* **31**: 1271–1286.
2. Stein JJ (1969) Surgical or irradiation castration for patients with advanced breast cancer. *Cancer* **24**: 1350–1354.
3. Nissen-Meyer R (1967) The role of prophylactic castration in the therapy of human mammary cancer. *Europ J Cancer* **3**: 395–403.
4. Kennedy BJ, Mielke PW Jr and Fortuny IE (1964) Therapeutic castration versus prophylactic castration in breast cancer. *Surg Gynec & Obst* **118**: 524–540.

5. Kennedy BJ and Fortuny IE (1964) Therapeutic castration in the treatment of advanced breast cancer. *Cancer* **17**: 1197-1202.
6. Lewison EF (1962) Prophylactic versus therapeutic castration in the total treatment of breast cancer. *Obst & Gynec Survey* **17**: 769-801.
7. Block GE, Lampe I, Vial AB and Coller FA (1960) Therapeutic castration for advanced mammary cancer. *Surgery* **47**: 877-884.
8. Treves N and Finkheiner JA (1958) An evaluation of therapeutic surgical castration in the treatment of metastatic recurrent and primary inoperable mammary carcinoma in women. *Cancer* **11**: 421-438.
9. Treves N (1957) An evaluation of prophylactic castration in the treatment of mammary carcinoma. *Cancer* **10**: 393-407.
10. Smith GV and Smith OW (1953) Carcinoma of the breast. Results evaluation of x-radiation and relation of age and surgical castration to the length of survival. *Surg Gynec & Obst* **97**: 508-516.
11. Douglas M (1952) The treatment of advanced breast cancer by hormone therapy. *Br J Cancer* **6**: 32-45.
12. Adair FE, Treves N, Farrow JH and Scharnagel IM (1945) Clinical effects of surgical and x-ray castration in mammary cancer. *JAMA* **128**: 161-167.

Thymus

The treatment of status thymicus lymphaticus was an intellectual error in interpretation of the so-called disorder as well as a therapeutic venture which was inappropriate.

Tinea

Between 1950 and 1960 approximately 20,000 Israeli children were treated for tinea capitis by x-ray therapy as part of a large public health campaign to eradicate the disease. Approximately 20 years later it became clear that this treatment was associated with a multitude of undesirable late effects including cancers of the face, scalp, thyroid, brain, and parotid. In addition these unfortunate children appear to have sustained central nervous system injury resulting in poor scholastic aptitude, IQ and psychologic tests, poor school performance, and an increased number of psychiatric disorders. Many authors have confirmed these observations. This treatment has been abandoned. Although inhibition of fungal growth may be achieved by altering the skin and subcutaneous tissue, the risk-benefit ratio and alternate therapies available make radiation treatment unacceptable. In the national survey 98.6% of radiation oncologists would not treat tinea with radiation.

Tinea: Radiotherapy

Investigator, Year	Cases	Site, Age	Treatment	Results	Notes
Rubinstein et al, 1984	201	Scalp; 25-63 yrs, with mean of 45 yrs (at time of meningioma)	X-ray doses <850r with brain doses ranging from 70-175r Some patients received more than a single treatment	43/201(21.4%) with intracranial meningioma had previously received x-ray for tinea capitis	Patients were all Jewish Latent period 38 yrs Data compared with patients with meningioma without prior x-ray exposure
Shore et al, 1984	2226	Scalp; median age 7.9 yrs	300-380r to 5 overlapping fields on the scalp to cause depilation. This delivered doses of 300-600r to various portions of scalp, lower doses to face and neck	80 basal cell carcinomas of the scalp or face have occurred among 41 irradiated children The cumulative incidence of skin cancer 35 yrs post-irradiation was 4.9 per hundred persons The risk increases with time	Minimum latent period was 20 yrs Skin cancers were most prevalent in Caucasians and on the face where there was additional UVR exposure Data obtained via questionnaire and compared with non-irradiated controls

Tinea: Radiotherapy (Continued)

Investigator, Year	Cases	Site, Age	Treatment	Results	Notes
Soffer et al, 1983	42	Scalp; 45 yrs (at time of meningioma)	Patients previously had scalp irradiation for tinea capitis	Patients had statistically significant higher number of calvarial tumors ($p < 0.001$) Multiple meningioma, with high recurrence ($p < 0.02$) Histologically malignant ($p < 0.01$)	Data were compared to patients with meningiomas, without prior history of x-ray
Ron et al, 1982	10,842	Scalp; mean age 7.1 yrs	Mean brain dose of 130r from x-ray treatment for tinea capitis 75Kv x-ray machine	Irradiated children had poorer scholastic aptitude, IQ, psychologic tests; completed fewer school grades; had an increased risk for mental hospital admissions; slightly higher frequency of mental retardation	Data compared to ethnic, sex and age matched people from the general population, and to siblings
Yaar et al, 1982	44	Scalp	Cortex doses of 121–139r 2.5cm deeper – 95–121r when scalp treatment given	Increased abnormalities in EEG power values compared to controls, suggesting permanent change in EEG activity	Treatment administered 20 years previously
Ron and Modan, 1980	10,842	Scalp	Thyroid dose 9r when scalp x-ray given	An excess risk of 8.3 cases/yr/r/million population of benign and malignant thyroid neoplasms among persons given x-ray for tinea capitis	Data compared to matched controls Children irradiated under age 6 had the highest risk for developing carcinoma
Yaar et al, 1979	10,842	Scalp; ages 3–13 yrs, average age 7 yrs	Cortical doses 121–139r when scalp treatment given	Significant radiation effects were seen in visual evoked responses in adults irradiated as children	Data compared to non tinea, non irradiated matched controls
Pousti, 1979	7	Scalp; childhood	Scalp x-ray for tinea capitis to achieve epilation	All developed malignant tumors of the scalp 5 basal cell carcinoma 2 squamous cell carcinoma	Intervals 18 yrs – 50 yrs
Spallone et al, 1979	2	Scalp; infancy and 5 yrs	Scalp x-ray for tinea capitis	Both developed meningioma	Latency period 25–45 yrs
Omran et al, 1978	177	Scalp; average age 7.8 yrs	Scalp x-ray for tinea capitis	Irradiated group had more psychiatric symptoms and abnormal MMPI (Minnesota Multiphasic Personality Inventory) scores, and more psychiatric disorders	X-ray treatment 10–29 yrs earlier

Tinea: Radiotherapy (Continued)

Investigator, Year	Cases	Site, Age	Treatment	Results	Notes
Modan et al, 1977	10,902	Scalp; ages 2–10 yrs	Scalp x-ray delivered at thyroid dose of <9r	Increased rate of malignant thyroid tumors of $6.3/10^6/\text{yr}$ among irradiated children compared to controls	Data compared to non irradiated sex, age, ethnic matched controls, and non irradiated matched sibling controls
Harley et al, 1976			Scalp x-ray delivered: Thyroid dose – 6r Pituitary dose – 49r Parotid dose – 39r Skin dose 20–40r	Linear dose-response relationship within the first 30–40yrs after exposure, with a risk of 0.04%/r	
Shore et al, 1976	2215	Scalp; childhood	Scalp x-ray, 100 Kv unfiltered x-ray; 450–850r to scalp 400r to cranium 70–175r to brain 6r to thyroid	Excess incidence in the irradiated group of tumors of the head and neck, including skin, brain, thyroid, and parotid. No excess mortality. In white patients, a 40% excess of treated psychiatric disorders, but not in blacks	Data compared to non irradiated age, sex, race controls

References

1. Rubinstein Ab, Shalit MN, Cohen ML, Zandbank U and Reichenthal E (1984) Radiation-induced cerebral meningioma: a recognizable entity. *J Neurosurg* **61**: 966–971.
2. Shore Re, Albert RE, Reed M, Harley N and Pasternack BS (1984) Skin cancer incidence among children irradiated for ringworm of the scalp. *Radiat Res* **100**: 192–204.
3. Soffer D, Pittaluga S, Feiner M and Beller AJ (1983) Intracranial meningiomas following low-dose irradiation to the head. *J Neurosurg* **59**: 1048–1053.
4. Ron E, Modan B, Floro S, Harkedar I and Gurewitz R (1982) Mental function following scalp irradiation during childhood. *Am J Epidemiol* **116**: 149–160.
5. Yaar I, Ron E, Modan B, Rinott Y, Yaar M and Modan M (1982) Long-lasting cerebral functional changes following moderate dose x-radiation treatment to the scalp in childhood: an electroencephalographic power spectral study. *J Neurol Neurosurg Psychiatry* **45**: 166–169.
6. Ron E and Modan B (1980) Benign and malignant thyroid neoplasms after childhood irradiation for tinea capitis. *JCNI* **65**: 7–11.
7. Yaar I, Ron E, Modan B, Modan M and Perentz H (1979) Long-term effects of small doses of x-radiation applied in childhood, as manifested in adult visually evoked responses. *Trans Am Neurol Assoc* **104**: 264–268.
8. Pousti A (1979) Malignant tumors of the scalp resulting from x-ray treatment of tinea capitis. *Br J Plast Surg* **32**: 52–54.
9. Spallone A, Gagliardi FM and Vagnozzi R (1979) Intracranial meningiomas related to external cranial irradiation. *Surg Neurol* **12**: 153–159.
10. Omran AR, Shore RE, Markoff RA, Friedhoff A, Albert RE, Barr H, Dahlstrom WG and Pasternack BS (1978) Follow up study of patients treated by x-ray epilation for tinea capitis: psychiatric and psychometric evaluation. *Am J Public Health* **68**: 561–567.
11. Modan B, Ron E and Werner A (1977) Thyroid cancer following scalp irradiation. *Radiology* **123**: 741–744.
12. Harley NH, Albert RE, Shore RE and Pasternack BS (1976) Follow up study of patients treated by x-ray epilation for tinea capitis. Estimation of the dose to the thyroid and pituitary glands. *Phys Med Biol* **21**: 631–642.
13. Shore RE, Albert RE and Pasternack BS (1976) Follow up study of patients treated by x-ray epilation for tinea capitis. *Arch Environ Health* **31**: 21–28.

Tonsillitis

Radiation can reduce chronic inflamed tonsils. There are clear long-term sequelae to radiation treatment, however, that include thyroid tumors, salivary gland tumors, parathyroid tumors and neural tumors. In the follow up of 2,311 patients who received childhood irradiation of inflamed tonsil and adenoids, there were 31 neural tumors and 54 salivary gland tumors, all related to the treatment region and evidencing occurrence as late as 30 years after initial treatment. Particularly striking was the occurrence of 10 acoustic neuromas clearly related to treatment portals. Further, it should not be concluded that the 1983 reported incidence of these tumors is the final incidence since there is reason to believe tumor incidence will continue to increase with time. Although, as recently as 1975, Russian physicians reported ^{32}P plaque applications for tonsillitis, a 1976 survey of 49 academic and private practice centers revealed complete consensus for non-treatment of tonsillitis with irradiation. Thus, we conclude that treatment of tonsillitis should be restricted to antibiotics and/or surgery in chronic circumstances, and we cannot justify the use of radiation. Ninety-nine percent of radiation oncologists in the national survey would not treat tonsillitis.

References

1. Shore-Friedman E, Abrahams C, Recant W and Schneider AB (1983) Neurolemmomas and salivary gland tumors of the head and neck following childhood irradiation. *Cancer* **51**: 2159-2163.
2. Rao SD, Frame B, Miller MJ, Kleerekoper M, Block MA, Parfitt AM (1980) Hyperparathyroidism following head and neck irradiation. *Arch Int Med* **140**: 205-207.
3. Christenson T (1978) Hyperparathyroidism and radiation therapy. *Am Int Med* **89**: 216-217.
4. Schneider AB, Favus, MJ, Stachura, ME, Arnold J, Arnold MJ, and Frohman LA (1978) Incidence, relevance and characteristics of radiation induced thyroid tumors. *Am J Med* **64**: 243-252.
5. Kopicky J and Order SE (1977) Survey and Analysis of the Radiation Treatment of Benign Diseases: A Review of the Use of Ionizing Radiation for the Treatment of Benign Diseases. U.S. Dept of HEW FDS Vol II Append B, pp 15-25.
6. Filatov VF (1975) Use of beta applications in the treatment of inflammatory diseases of the palatine tonsils. *Vestn-Otorinoloringol* **6**: 29-34.
7. Modan B, Badatz D, Mait H, Sternitz R, Levin S (1974) Radiation induced head and neck tumors. *Lancet* **11**: 277-279.
8. Ju DMG (1968) Salivary gland tumors occurring after radiation of the head and neck. *Am J Surg* **116**: 518-523.
9. Hazen RW, Pifer JW, Tozooka E, Lurngood J, and Empelmann L. (1966) Neoplasm following irradiation of the head. *Ca Res* **26**: 305-311.

Tuberculosis

As with other inflammatory conditions, tuberculosis lymphadenitis responded to relatively superficial x-ray. The availability of modern antibiotics obviates the need for x-ray treatment of tuberculosis.

References

1. Autre JN, Kasuga K and Sanderson SE (1953) X-ray therapy of peripheral tuberculosis lymphadenitis. *Am Rev Tubercul* **68**: 157.
2. Lampe I, Chrest CP and Koch DA (1949) Concentrated roentgen therapy of cervical tuberculosis lymphadenitis. *Am J Med Sci* **217**: 632-636.

Xanthoma

Corneal xanthomas appear in association with generalized juvenile xanthogranuloma, with disseminated xanthoma, and with generalized histiocystosis. In the patient with normal cholesterol levels, the process consists of histiocytic proliferation and lipid accumulation. The role of radiotherapy as an integral part of therapy has been described, but its benefit has not been established. Risks are related to dose and dose-distribution. Gain is ill-defined. The review by Liebman et al., 1966, will prove helpful prior to any consideration of therapy. We find no evidence for the basis of orthovoltage radiation, but strontium^{90} application may be of value in preventing progression.

Corneal Xanthomas

Author, Year	# Cases	Age	Treatment	Results	Notes
Liebman et al, 1966	2	4 1/2 years	400-2000r external beam with up to 6000 rep strontium.	Inconclusive with regard to response.	Occurs in association with generalized xanthomas and histiocytosis.

Reference

1. Liebman SD, Crocker AC and Geiser CF (1966) Corneal xanthomas in childhood. *Arch Ophthalmol* **76**: 221-229.

Subject Index

abortion 9
acne 9
acromegaly 10
acyclovir 100
adamantinoma (ameloblastoma) 10-14
aggressive fibromatosis 71-74
aneurysmal bone cysts 14-18
angiofibroma, nasopharynx 18-20
ankylosing spondylitis 20-26
anovulation 26
arachnoiditis 142-144
arteriovenous malformations 26-28
arthritis 28-31
astrocytoma 31, 32
autoimmune disease 132-138

Bowen's disease 32-34, 77-79
bromocriptidine 10
bronchial adenomas 35-43
bronchial carcinoids 55
bursitis 43-47

carcinoid 52-55
carotid body tumor 55-62
chemodectoma (non-chromaffin paraganglioma) 55-62
chordoma 63-65
choroid plexus papilloma 65, 66
cimetidine 175-179
complications pituitary tumor 55
condyloma acuminata 140, 141
contact dermatitis 202-206
craniopharyngioma 66
Cushing's disease 67
cutaneous leishmaniasis 139
cylindromas (adenocystic carcin.) 35-43
cystic hygroma (lymphangioma) 67-71

desmoid 71-74
Dupuytren's contracture 74, 75

eczema 202-206
epithelial hemangioendothelioma 76, 77
erythroplasia of Queyrat 77-79
exophthalmos 125-132
extramammary Paget's disease 79-82
extramedullary hematopoiesis 113

federal tort claims 4
fibrosclerosis 83
follicultis barbae 202-206
fungal infections 83, 84

Gardner's syndrome 71
giant cell tumor 84-88
glomus jugulare 55-62
granuloma annulare 202-206
Grave's disease 116-132
guidelines 7
gynecomastia 88

heart transplantation 132, 136-138
hemangioma
  bone 89, 91, 92, 98-100
  cutaneous 95, 96, 98-100
  G. I. Trace 89, 96-100
  joint 89
  liver 89, 94, 98-100
  subglottic 94, 98-100
  urinary tract 89, 98-100
hemolytic anemia 112
herpes zoster 100-103
heterotopic bone formation 103, 104
hidradenitis suppurativa 202-206
histiocytosis 104-112
homograft rejection 132-134, 136-138
hypersalivation, ALS 112
hypersplenism 112-115
hyperthyroidism 116-125
hyperthyroid ophthalmopathy 125-132

immunosuppression 132-138
infections disorders 139-141
informed consent 5, 6
intracranial angiofibromas 18-20
intracranial angiomas 97-100
inverted papilloma 147

keloid 147-153

lethal midline granuloma 153-156
leukemia 112-115
lichen planus 202, 203, 205
lichen simplex chronicus 202, 203, 205
lupus erythematosus (nephritis) 132, 135
lymphangioma 67-71
lymphoid hyperplasia 156, 157
lymphoma 112-115

malpractice 3-7
meningioma 157, 158
MIGB (I-131) 52
Mikulicz syndrome 158-161
mucoepidermoid carcinomas 35-43
multiple sclerosis 132, 135, 136, 138
myasthenia gravis 161-164
myelosclerosis 112-115

neurofibroma 165

ocular histoplasmosis 141
ophthalmopathy 125-132
optic nerve glioma 165-168
organ transplantation 132, 136-138
osteoblastoma 168, 169
osteoid osteoma 168, 169
otitis media 169, 170

pancreatic fistulae 170
pancreatitis 170
paraganglioma (chromaffin positive) 170-172
praquat poisoning 1
paronychia 203, 205
parotitis 172-175
perifolliculitis capitis 179, 180
Peyronie's disease 180-185
pinealoma 185, 186
pituitary adenomas 55, 67, 186-188
pituitary tumors 55, 67
plantar fibromatous 188
plantar warts 140, 141
plasmacytoma 189-194
platelet consumption 112-115
polymorphic reticulosis 153-156
prostate cancer (DES) 88
pruritis ani 203, 205, 206
pseudotumor 156, 157
pseudotumor orbit 156, 157
psoriasis 202-206
pterygium 195-200
pyogenic granuloma 200

radioactive colloids 30, 31
radioactive isotopes 116-125
ranitidine 175
Rathke's pouch 66
renal transplantation 132-134, 137, 138
rheumatoid arthritis 29-31, 132

salivary gland adenoma 200, 201
sarcoidosis 201, 202
seborrheic keratosis 202, 204, 205
sinusitis 142
skin disorders 202-206
standard of care 3-6
status thymicus lymphaticus 208
^{90}Strontium 195-200
subglottic hemangiomas 89, 90, 98-100
synovitis 43, 47-52

tendonitis 43, 142
therapeutic castration 206-208
thymoma 161-164
thyroid cancer 9
thyroiditis 142, 144-146
tinea 83, 84, 208-210
tonsillitis 210, 211
total lymphoid irradiation 132-138
tuberculosis 211

von Recklinghausen disease 165

Wegener's granulomatosis 153-156
wipe test 195

xanthogranuloma, iris 211, 212
xanthoma 211, 212

Medical Radiology

Diagnostic Imaging and Radiation Oncology

Edited by **L. W. Brady**, Philadelphia; **M. W. Donner**, Baltimore; **H.-P. Heilmann**, Hamburg; **F. Heuck**, Stuttgart

The series recognizes the demand for an international state-of-the-art account of the developments reflecting the progress in the radiological sciences. Each volume conveys an overall picture of a topical theme so that it can be used as a reference work without taking recourse to other volumes. The contents of the volumes concentrate on new and accepted developments in a manner appropriate for review by physicians engaged in the practice of radiology.

G. E. Laramore, University of Washington (Ed.)

Radiation Therapy of Head and Neck Cancer

Foreword by L. W. Brady and H.-P. Heilmann

1988. 123 figures. XII, 237 pages. Hard cover. ISBN 3-540-19360-X

This volume considers the treatment of head and neck cancer from the point of view of the radiation oncologist. The epidemiology of head and neck cancer, evaluation of the patient, and basic treatment issues are discussed and the separate chapters are devoted to specific head and neck sites.
The book provides a valuable summary of treatment approaches and results representing the best standard of care in the United States, Canada, and Europe. It offers a consensus approach and does not set forth the particular attitudes of any single institution. A comprehensive survey of the relevant literature is presented at the end of each chapter. Material is treated in such a way as to be relevant both to the practicing clincian and the resident in training.

R. R. Dobelbower, Jr., Medical College of Ohio, Toledo (Ed.)

Gastrointestinal Cancer

Radiation Therapy

1989. 82 illustrations. Approx. 450 pages. Hard cover. ISBN 3-540-50505-9

The intricate role of radiation therapy in the management of GI cancer is comprehensively reviewed in this timely volume. It offers unique coverage of the entire gastrointestinal tract, from the esophagus to the anus. Although the work focuses clearly on the radiotherapeutic management of tumors of the GI tract, reviews of anatomy, epidemiology, and other pertinent topics are given. The volume is generally organized by disease site, but extensive special sections amplify important aspects related to GI cancer. These include the radiographic evaluation of GI malignancy and tumor markers, an up-to-date review of chemotherapeutic treatment of gut cancers, and patient follow-up. Edited by an internationally known leader in the field of radiotherapy, this volume represents a compilation of years of research and experience utilizing today's technology and state-of-the-art techniques.

Springer-Verlag Berlin
Heidelberg New York London
Paris Tokyo Hong Kong

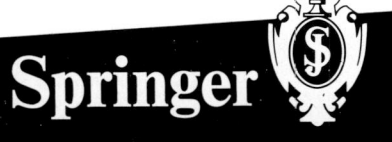

Medical Radiology

Diagnostic Imaging and Radiation Oncology

Edited by **L. W. Brady,** Philadelphia; **M. W. Donner,** Baltimore; **H.-P. Heilmann,** Hamburg; **F. Heuck,** Stuttgart

The series recognizes the demand for an international state-of-the-art account of the developments reflecting the progress in the radiological sciences. Each volume conveys an overall picture of a topical theme so that it can be used as a reference work without taking recourse to other volumes. The contents of the volumes concentrate on new and accepted developments in a manner appropriate for review by physicians engaged in the practice of radiology.

C. W. Scarantino, Wake Forest University, Winston-Salem (Ed.)

Lung Cancer

Diagnostic Procedures and Therapeutic Management With Special Reference to Radiotherapy

1985. 42 figures. XI, 173 pages. Hard cover. ISBN 3-540-13176-0

This up-to-date reference book covers a broad range of topics regarding lung cancer.
There is an extensive review of recent epidemiological and early detection studies, as well as of current histological observations of the tumor heterogeneity of lung cancer. It presents an up-to-date examination of the latest clinical developments in diagnosis and treatment as well as results of clinical trials employing irradiation chemotherapy and surgery.

H. R. Withers, University of California at Los Angeles; L. J. Peters, University of Texas (Eds.)

Innovations in Radiation Oncology

Foreword by L. W. Brady and H.-P. Heilmann

1987. 111 figures. XVII, 329 pages. Hard cover. ISBN 3-540-17818-X

Contents: General Aspects. – Conservation Therapy. – Extended Field Therapy. – Restricted Field Therapy. – New Imaging Technologies and Radiotherapy. – Modified Fractionation. – Drugs and Radiation. – Neutrons. – Adjunctive Therapies. – Subject Index.

This book contains up-to-date reports of areas of growth in radiation oncology written for the practicing radiation oncologist.

Springer-Verlag Berlin
Heidelberg New York London
Paris Tokyo Hong Kong

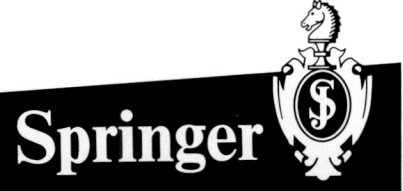

DATE DUE

GAYLORD   PRINTED IN U.S.A.

WITHDRAWN